HANDBOOK
OF
MAMMOGRAPHY

by

Shirley M. Long, RTR, CBI

Co-authors:

Louise C. Miller, RT (R)(M)
Margaret A. Botsco, RT (R)(M)
Linda L. Martin, BSc, OT, MEDes

Fourth Edition
(January, 2000)

Mammography Consulting Services Ltd., Edmonton, Alberta, Canada

This handbook was designed to accompany the **C.A.M.R.T. (Canadian Association of Medical Radiation Technologists)** Mammography Correspondence Courses.

It is also, in its own right, a valuable reference for mammographers.

First Edition 1990   Second Edition 1991
Third Edition 1994   Fourth Edition 2000

The authors and publisher of this handbook have checked with sources believed to be reliable in a conscientious effort to provide information that is complete and congruent with acceptable standards at the time of this publication. However, the dynamic nature of mammography leads us to anticipate frequent changes and updates. Therefore, readers are encouraged to confirm with other reliable sources to ensure that they will receive complete, accurate, and current information.

Mammography Consulting Services Ltd.
1024-82nd Street, N.W.
Edmonton, Alberta, Canada T6K 1X6
Telephone or Fax 780-462-2615
http://www.mammography.com
e-mail: info@mammography.com

Canadian Cataloguing in Publication Data

Main entry under title:

Handbook of Mammography

Includes bibliographical references and index.
ISBN 0-9694867-2-3

1. Breast—Radiography. I. Long, Shirley M., 1951 II. Mammography Consulting Services (Edmonton, Alta.).
RG493.5.R33H36 2000   618.1'907572   C99-910591-4

Cover design and artwork by Dennis R. Long. Illustrations by Dennis R. Long.
Typesetting and layout by Satoo Design & Graphics Inc., Edmonton Alberta, Canada.
Printed by Art Design Printing Inc., Edmonton Alberta, Canada.

Dedicated to
Claire Trenchie

A dear friend and colleague
whose vivacious spirit and fresh, unassuming
nature continue to inspire me every day.
A spirit such as yours is very rare indeed.

*"The greatest use of life
is to spend it on something
that outlasts it."*
A very wise but unknown author

PREFACE

A *handbook* can be defined as a concise reference book.

The *Handbook of Mammography*, 4th edition was conceived on this basis. It is not large or bulky. It was designed to ensure durability — an important feature for a handbook that is frequently referenced. In many areas, it is indeed concise. There are many excellent references that provide detailed information on equipment, image quality, radiographic technique, and quality control; their use and study is recommended.

Chapter four falls short of the definition of *handbook*. Ironically, it also is the very essence of this handbook, as is evident by its comprehensive nature. The authors have endeavored to describe mammographic positioning as completely as possible and to include an abundance of complementary information gained through their combined extensive practical experience; they feel this will assist the mammography technologist to perform her job with a greater degree of professionalism. A number of topics have been included (body mechanics and patient relations) that are not frequently encountered in mammography literature. Also, a new way of understanding breast positioning, Breast Mapping, has been described in detail. Many technologists have found the visual component of this technique to be a refreshing and informative teaching tool.

We openly acknowledge that a variety of opinions will always exist in a dynamic field of study. This, we believe, is beneficial and to be welcomed. Our technology has developed through the thought process and stimulation of controversy; further growth and development will only be accomplished in the same manner. Such must be our approach as we evaluate new ideas that will enrich our current knowledge base.

This handbook concludes with a list of common abbreviations and a glossary of medical terms that will facilitate comprehension with technical readings and clinical situations that the mammographer may encounter.

There are many excellent mammography references available to the technical community. However, we believe a void exists for a reference with the complete, well-rounded approach that you will find in the *Handbook of Mammography*, 4th edition. It is our sincere hope and desire that this handbook will serve as a valuable and enjoyable reference and guide for technologists, residents, radiologists, and other related professionals.

FOREWORD

Professionals in the field of breast care are indeed a fortunate lot. We are grateful for and respectfully acknowledge the contributions of the pioneers of mammography. Despite unbelievable skepticism and opposition, they persevered to establish mammography as a viable, indeed invaluable, diagnostic specialty. They are responsible for establishing the foundation of state-of-the-art mammography as we enjoy it today.

Therefore, today we find ourselves in a most auspicious position. We have the technology. We have the knowledge. We have trained and dedicated professionals. We stand on the brink of major advancements in the field of breast disease. Pre-clinical, minimal, in-situ carcinomas can be diagnosed. For the first time in decades, we are in a position to truly make an impact on breast disease.

Women, who comprise a significant segment of the population, would certainly welcome this prospect. Men also hold a vested interest through their mothers, sisters, sweethearts, wives, and daughters. Therefore, it is apparent that every single human being will benefit from and sincerely appreciate progress of this nature.

Throughout this century, no disease has received as much publicity as breast disease. The previous skepticism toward and disapproval of mammography occurred as a result of a void in information and an unfounded fear of radiation. Although we occasionally still encounter opposition, we have progressed to the stage where mammography is now widely recognized and utilized. Women themselves, out of concern for their personal health and well being, are now embracing regular breast health care. The contribution of mammography to the early detection of breast disease is now universally acknowledged.

The authors of this publication would like to take this opportunity to propose a toast to the art and science of mammography and to the state of refinement that we currently enjoy. The ongoing commitment to the early detection of breast disease will continue to be of the highest caliber as we enter the new millennium. Our goal is, through increased awareness, to bring quality mammography to all women in the hands of competent professionals.

ACKNOWLEDGMENTS

When a task such as this handbook is completed, it is important to reflect upon the sources of assistance and encouragement that have made this work a reality. It is a great pleasure to take this opportunity to acknowledge and to express my sincere appreciation to a number of people.

To Rod and Bob, the talented photographers who are responsible for the extensive visual element of this material. Thank you for your patience and for your professional suggestions that have helped us to convey our message in pictures. To all the models: we are truly grateful for your patience in enduring the lengthy sessions and the hot lights; you have been so valuable in allowing us to clearly demonstrate so many ideas that are difficult with only words.

To Dennis, the graphic artist whose creative talents you will enjoy through the abundance of illustrations and drawings that adorn these pages. With only rough ideas scratched out in primitive form, you have brought to life ideas in ways that still amaze us. Your dedication to the artistic component of this material has been invaluable: you kept us all focused on the *big picture* and the importance of consistency and harmony in the material. Your contribution has brought an impressive professional finish to this project. Thank you, Dennis. Through your patience, your hard work, and your professional talent, this book is truly a work of art.

The assistance and guidance of Herb Ratsch of Art Design Printing Inc. of Edmonton, Alberta have been invaluable in coordinating the preparation and printing of this material. Thank you, Herb, for your patience, guidance, and for the critical eye that has brought a truly professional presentation to this book. To Adolph, and all the others who assisted Art Design with the folding, collating, and binding of the *Handbook of Mammography*, 4th Edition, thank you all; your labor has added a beautiful finishing touch to this work.

The mammography examinations throughout this text have been photo-graphed with the permission and blessing of Dr. N. Horeczko, of the Lendrum

Breast Centre in Edmonton, Alberta. Thank you so much for your generosity in opening your files to us and offering us the opportunity to represent such a variety of interesting and informative examinations; your dedication to education is always close at hand. Your wonderful staff — Judy, Arlene, Lori, Ellamay, Marjorie, Judy, Madeline, Tammy, and Amanda: it is a privilege to know and work with each and every one of you. Thank you for your help with the cases for this book, and of course, for the great work that you all do every day — the evidence is here on these pages. Your patients are so fortunate to experience the work and dedication of such a fine team.

The growth and development of this handbook is the cumulative result of years of experience and opportunities in the field of mammography. We have had the good fortune of working with many extraordinary people; they have enriched our experience. My personal list includes Jake Enns, for introducing me to mammography; Dr. W.R. Castor, of the Cross Cancer Institute in Edmonton, Alberta, for the experience of supervising the mammography department, teaching radiology students and residents and working with other related modalities such as thermography, transillumination, and research projects; Dr. N. Horeczko of the Lendrum Breast Centre, for support and growth that has enriched my experience in this field. Many other wonderful people — Dr. A.E. Nett, Dr. P. Burns, Dr. M. Jones, Cheryl, Claire, Debra, Carol, Denise, Olga, Jeanette, Paula, Louise, Margaret, Nancy, and finally, the many technologists that I have met and worked with — I thank you all.

With this edition of the *Handbook of Mammography*, I have had the wonderful opportunity to enjoy the company and the professional association of three talented and competent women. Louise C. Miller, who has developed and authored the technique of *Breast Mapping* that is represented in Section I of the chapter on *Mammography Positioning*. This fresh, new approach to understanding mammography positioning has helped many technologists make sense of patient postioning. As well, Louise co-authored the chapter on *Patient Relations* with Sandy L. Thoma and me; her dedication to creating a positive experience for the mammography patient is evident throughout this material. Thank you, Louise, for all the hard work and the hours you dedicated to present this interesting and useful material to the mammography community. Your contribution to education (on an international level) has had a significant impact on our field of practice. Margaret A. Botsco, another colleague whose focus and attention on the technical components of quality control, film processing, artifacts, and mammography accreditation, has brought the most current information and distinct credibility to the chapters on *Quality Control*, *Artifacts* and *Image Problem Solving*. Thank you Margaret for sharing your expertise with us and for your work in preparing this material for the book. Your contribution has been most valuable. Finally, thanks to Linda Martin, a consultant in ergonomics, who was instrumental in preparing and presenting the material in the chapter on *Preventing Musculoskeletal Discomfort and Injury in Mammography*. Your expertise in preparing the information in this seldom-discussed area of concern for all mammographers has been very enlightening. Your expertise provided a sound basis for your task in preparing material specific to mammographers as you followed us around, observing our true work environment and questioning us on our work habits and concerns. Thank you for your dedication to this project.

It seems that the best individuals to pursue for this type of collaborative effort are always those who have the least amount of *spare time*. Ironically, this is, in fact, what makes them the best choice — each of my co-authors are masters in their own right, an observation supported by their obvious dedication and the busy schedule that commands their expertise. Therefore, it has been an interesting experience connecting and working with these three very busy professionals. We have communicated from around the world to complete the task of preparing this material for mammographers. I am sincerely grateful for the professional affiliation of these women. Thank you all for your time, your dedication, and your invaluable expertise.

A special acknowledgment goes out to our many friends who have so generously allowed us *time out* to compile and complete this publication. Thank you for permitting us to *sign off* for a significant period of time, for understanding, for checking with us periodically, but not pressuring us for time we could not afford.

One of the *we's* that I refer to is my support, my strength, my source of inspiration and encouragement, and my manager, Bob. This would never have been completed without his unwavering focus, drive, and foresight. Many times when I felt overwhelmed, he sat me down and said, *Shirley — this is you — now finish it!* Thank you so much Bob; you have made an outstanding contribution to this book and to my career. Thank you for making this project a reality.

Last, and by far the most important of all, is the special recognition that goes out to my family. Only those who have undertaken a task such as this can appreciate how it completely absorbs your time, your energy and, in fact, your whole being. I am sincerely grateful for the sacrifices you have made in allowing me the freedom and the space to complete this fourth edition. Only you know the personal satisfaction and meaning this holds for me; I am eternally indebted to you for everything you have endured as a result of this project. You are the most important people behind this endeavor; your contribution will never be forgotten. You have shared my dreams and desires and brought them to fruition. I thank you from the bottom of my heart.

Shirley M. Long, R.T.R., C.B.I.

I would also like to express my gratitude to my family for their support through all my endeavors. I would like to thank Auntie Gertie, friend and support, June Leong, graphics artist, and Faye McCoole, chapter support, for their contributions. Thank you all.

Linda Martin

ABOUT THE AUTHORS

Shirley M. Long, RTR, CBI
Mammography Consultant and Educator

Shirley has been involved in the field of mammography since 1971. She supervised the Mammography Department at the Cross Cancer Institute in Edmonton, Alberta for 10 years where she developed a teaching module for student technologists and for radiology residents. She was also directly involved with the introduction of new modalities — thermography and diaphanography (breast light scanning) — as well as with research projects relating to breast cancer. She has set up the radiology department at two private breast imaging facilities in Edmonton, Alberta, and the Quality Control component of the provincial breast screening program where she worked as a consultant for three years. Shirley has served on the Clinical Practice Guideline Committee of Alberta. She authored previous editions of the *Handbook of Mammography* and two C.A.M.R.T. mammography correspondence courses, of which she is also the instructor. Shirley lectures in both the USA and Canada and is directly involved with instruction in mammography basics, patient positioning, quality control, and interventional procedures. Shirley is indeed a pioneer in mammography education. Currently, she manages her own consulting business (Mammography Consulting Services Ltd.), which assists sites with mammography accreditation, imaging film trials, educational seminars, and on-site mammography education and training.

Louise Miller, RT (R)(M)
Mammography Consultant and Educator

Louise is the Director of the Mammography Practicum at the School of Medicine at the University of California, San Diego, and the instructor of mammography at San Diego Mesa College. She is also a coordinator and faculty for the QCC (Quality, Care and Commitment) National Mammography Viewbox Seminars which has trained over 10,000 technologists since 1991. Louise has served on numerous national committees which determine educational standards for mammography technologists, including the American College of Radiology,

Technologist Education Committee, and the American Society of Radiology Technologists National Committee on Mammography, which she has chaired for two years. Louise has lectured for such internationally recognized radiologists as Daniel Kopans, MD, Lásló Tabár, MD, and Edward Sickles, MD. She devotes most of her time to technologist education and works as an independent mammography consultant and volunteer to various national and international endeavors. She devotes most of her time to technologist education and mammography consultation. In recent years she has volunteered her time to help develop screening programs and increase the level of competency in mammography in the countries of Cuba, Ukraine, and China. Most importantly, Louise continues to work as a mammography technologist in San Diego, on a per diem basis.

Margaret A. Botsco, RT (R)(M)
Mammography Consultant and Educator

Margaret has been a registered radiologic technologist since 1973. She was the Associate Technical Director of the Mammography Technologist Training Program for the University of Southern California. She is a coordinator for the QCC (Quality, Care and Commitment) National Mammography Viewbox Seminars, now in their ninth year of providing mammography education. Margaret co-authored the Quality Determinantes of Mammography guidelines for the Agency for Healthcare Policy and Research. She has served as a member of the Committee for Mammography Quality Assurance for the American College of Radiology since 1990. She was appointed to the National Mammography Quality Assurance Advisory Committee, advising the Food and Drug Administration on the implementation of the Mammography Quality Standards Act in the United States. She was a member of the American College of Radiology/Centers for Disease Control Cooperative Agreement Committee on Technologist Education. She is a member of the Breast and Cervical Cancer Detection Quality Assurance Taskforce for the state of California.

Linda Martin, BSc, OT, MEDes
Ergonomics Consultant

Linda has a Bachelor's degree in Rehabilitation and a Master's degree in Environmental Design. She is currently working on her PhD at the University of Calgary. Linda has extensive presentation experience at conferences and association meetings and is a sessional instructor at the University of Alberta, teaching ergonomics to occupational therapy students. Linda is a member of the Alberta Association of Registered Occupational Therapists and the Canadian Association of Occupational Therapists, and she is a full member of the Human Factors Association of Canada (HFAC). She is also a student affiliate of the Human Factors and Ergonomics Society.

TABLE OF CONTENTS

CHAPTER 1: SENSITOMETRY

CHAPTER 2: FILM PROCESSING

CHAPTER 3: QUALITY CONTROL

CHAPTER 4: POSITIONING FOR MAMMOGRAPHY

Section I: The Breast MAP*
*Mammography Aid for Positioning

Section II: A Technologist's Approach to Mammography

Section III: Mammography Projections / Views

CHAPTER 5: FILM CRITIQUE

CHAPTER 6: IMAGE QUALITY

CHAPTER 7: ARTIFACTS

CHAPTER 8: VIEWING CONDITIONS

CHAPTER 9: IMAGE PROBLEM SOLVING IN MAMMOGRAPHY

CHAPTER 10: RADIATION EXPOSURE AND DOSE

CHAPTER 11: PREVENTING MUSCULOSKELETAL DISCOMFORT AND INJURY IN MAMMOGRAPHY

CHAPTER 12: PATIENT RELATIONS

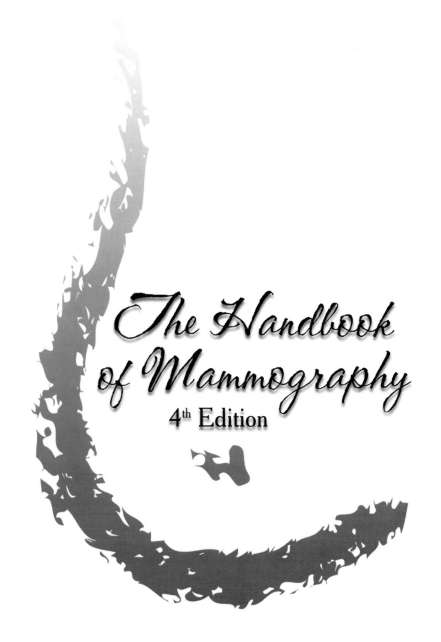

The Handbook
of Mammography
4th Edition

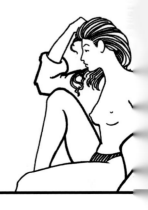

CHAPTER 1:
SENSITOMETRY

SENSITOMETRY

A. INTRODUCTION

Sensitometry is a method of quantitatively estimating the relationship between exposure and density. More specifically, sensitometry is the study of how photographic emulsions respond to specific conditions of exposure and the corresponding densities produced by unique development conditions. These principles are the foundation of daily processor monitoring. A sensitometric strip is exposed and developed; a densitometer is used to measure film densities and the appropriate information is then plotted on a trend or control chart. The technologist must understand the information presented by the processing control chart in order that she may appropriately manage the variants that are inherent in this dynamic environment.

B. EQUIPMENT REQUIRED FOR SENSITOMETRY

1. Sensitometer

A sensitometer is a special instrument that contains a constant light source of known luminous intensity and spectral quality, and an optical step wedge. It is designed to produce an image containing a series of incremental, step-like densities representing a wide range of film exposure levels. The densities of these steps are measured and used to predict and evaluate the critical parameters of an imaging system. Most step wedges consist of 21 steps; they are designed to produce a 0.15 optical density difference between adjacent steps. The complete range of steps and corresponding film densities should simulate the full spectrum of optical densities that a clinical image may display. The densities on a typical mammography film would range between 0.16 (B+F)

---

optical density to 4.00 (D-Max) optical density. Many sensitometers are exposure adjustable; a series of dipswitch selections will *customize* the output, allowing the user to produce the most appropriate density range for an individual film product. The spectral quality of the sensitometer must match the sensitivity of the film being exposed; for green sensitive film, a green emitting sensitometer should be used. The vast majority of mammography film falls into this category. Many sensitometers provide selectable spectral emission (green or blue); always ensure that the correct setting for the film type in use has been selected before performing sensitometry every morning. Dual emulsion film should be exposed with a sensitometer that is able to expose both sides of the film simultaneously. Most sensitometers are designed for single emulsion film. It is important to orient the emulsion side of the film down (adjacent the light source) when inserting it into the sensitometer for exposure.

Whenever the sensitometer is changed for any reason, a crossover should be performed using both instruments for several days. New operating parameters may need to be established when a new sensitometer is introduced to the QC program; even sensitometers from the same manufacturer may exhibit minimal performance variations that need to be incorporated into the QC program.

It is important to note that the response of a film to exposure from the simulated light source in a sensitometer and the light from an intensifying screen (during an actual exposure to radiation) is markedly different. For this reason, *sensitometry images should never be used to compare film imaging characteristics when evaluating a variety of film products.*

The consistency of a sensitometer's light output is very difficult to verify; cross-referencing with another similar unit on a regular basis is recommended. This comparison must be made with the same control film developed in the same processor; the optical density values from both films can then be compared. Sensitometers may require recalibration when light output diminishes as the tungsten light source and the electroluminescent panel age. The manufacturer should be contacted for information regarding recalibration recommendations.

 The spectral quality of the sensitometer must match the sensitivity of the film being exposed; for green sensitive film, a green emitting sensitometer should be used.

It is important to orient the emulsion side of the film down (adjacent the light source) when inserting it into the sensitometer for exposure.

Most sensitometers can operate with standard batteries or with an electrical adaptor. Batteries should be replaced periodically; this should be the first troubleshooting measure to perform whenever problems arise.

2. Densitometer

A densitometer is an instrument used to measure optical densities by means of transmitted light. Film can be oriented emulsion up or down in a densitometer; consistency is the only recommendation. Densitometers should contain a white light source. They must be able to read optical densities up to 4.00 with an accuracy of close to 2.0%. Changes in illumination and collection technology make it difficult to compare readings between older and newer generations of densitometers.

Two varieties of densitometers are commercially available: spot reading densitometers and automatic scanning densitometers. With a spot reading densitometer, the operator must manually position the area to be measured over the densitometer light source. These densitometers often come with a variety of light aperture sizes, frequently 1.0, 2.0, and 3.0 millimeters in diameter. The operator may choose which size to use routinely, keeping in mind that a larger diameter will provide more reliable density averaging, but will require more precision in positioning over the individual density steps.

Whenever a change in densitometer is made, a crossover procedure, similar to that described above for sensitometers, should be performed and the new operating parameters must then be introduced into the site's QC program.

A calibrated step wedge image with sample density readings accompanies new densitometers to provide a means of verifying the calibration of the meter. Densitometer readings should be checked with this reference strip at least annually. Physical damage or fingerprints on the test strip may invalidate the density readings; therefore, care must be exercised with these images. Also, because film quality may degrade with age, these test strips may also have an expiry date. Automatic scanning densitometers are frequently self-calibrating and come accompanied with a calibration strip.

Densitometers can operate on battery or electrical adaptor.

3. Thermometer

Every morning, after the processor has reached its operating temperature; a thermometer should be used to verify the correct developer temperature *before sensitometry is performed* and *before patient films are processed.*

A reliable thermometer that is able to differentiate 0.5°F (0.3°C) should be used; its accuracy should be periodically compared to another thermometer of known accuracy. It should be inserted in a consistent location in the tank, usually beside the main rack on the non-gear side of the processor. Rinse the stem well between readings and before storing to prevent corrosion. A digital thermometer is recommended for the purpose of obtaining exact and reproducible readings. Dial-type thermometers require a subjective interpretation of the temperature reading; this can easily introduce variability due to differences in operator readings. Glass thermometers break easily and are not recommended. *Never use a mercury thermometer.* Mercury is a sensitizing agent and, in the event of breakage, even a minute amount of free mercury will result in serious processor contamination. Clinical fever thermometers available in drug stores and pharmacies are both accurate and reasonably priced. Unfortunately, they are frequently only suitable for developer temperature measurement; their working range may not extend below 90°F (32°C) and therefore they cannot verify the fixer and water temperatures.

 A digital thermometer is recommended for the purpose of obtaining exact and reproducible readings.

4. Control Film

The same type of film used in the clinical setting for patient examinations must be used for sensitometry in order to provide meaningful and appropriate data. Reserve an entire box in the film bin for quality control testing; this will limit the need to perform frequent crossover procedures since the same emulsion number will be available for an extended period of time. When a new emulsion batch is introduced into the system, a crossover procedure must be performed in order to determine whether the film response of the two emulsions is similar. This procedure is outlined in Chapter 3, Quality Control. Some sources now recommend that the crossover procedure be performed with every new box of film used for quality control, even if it has the same emulsion number as the previous box. This will allow the site to incorporate any aging effects that may

The same type of film used in the clinical setting for patient examinations must be used for sensitometry in order to provide meaningful and appropriate data.

have influenced the response of the film when a number of boxes have been reserved for the QC program.

5. Control Charts

A variety of control (trend) charts are available from the various film manufacturers; they are all acceptable for monitoring quality control and plotting sensitometric information. Control charts are extremely valuable because they provide a quick, easy reference of the parameters that the quality control program is monitoring. All pertinent data should be plotted *as soon as new (testing) information is obtained* in order that an accurate and current indication of operating conditions is always available. Any action with the potential to influence operating conditions must be documented (change in developer temperature or replenishment rates, new chemistry, processor cleaning, etc.). The trend chart should be posted near the film processor for easy and immediate reference throughout the workday. The information in these charts is important to facilitate the immediate management of processing problems as well as to appreciate the development of trends in processing conditions.

Refer to Chapter 3, Quality Control for additional information regarding establishing operating levels for control charts and their acceptable performance variations.

C. CHARACTERISTIC CURVE

The sensitometric curve is a graphic representation of the relationship between the exposure given to a photographic material and the resulting optical density. Other common names for a sensitometric curve are characteristic curve, D log E curve, and H & D (Hurter & Driffield) curve. The curve represents the film density changes that occur as exposure increases. While density increases along the vertical axis, the relative exposure increases logarithmically along the horizontal axis (film responds in a logarithmic, rather than a linear manner). This is reflected on the sensitometric strip by a doubled exposure value with every second step.

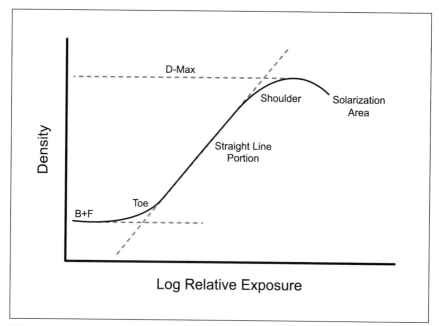

Figure 1.1 The individual parts of a typical Characteristic Curve.

The characteristic curve is typically S-shaped with the exact configuration reflecting the individual characteristics of the film type and the developing conditions. It can be divided into five distinct areas, each representing specific density parameters.

- The Base Plus Fog (B+F) area represents a minimal density due to the tint of the film base as well as any fog that the film has been unintentionally exposed to. This measurement can be made on step 1 of the sensitometry strip or on any clear area of the film.
- In the Toe or Threshold area, the graph slowly begins to climb upward as light gray tones appear. The first measurable density above base plus fog is known as D-min. Contrast is at a minimum in the toe area; minimal density differences limit the perception of image detail.
- The Straight-Line Portion represents usable film densities. In this area, density builds rapidly and the graph rises sharply. This area provides information that is important to evaluate the imaging characteristics of a film product.
- The Shoulder area represents an ongoing increase in density, beyond the straight-line region. Here density builds rapidly to a maximum level.
- The D-Max area represents the maximum film density when *all the silver crystals have been exposed and developed*; density cannot in-

crease beyond this point. The human eye cannot differentiate density differences approaching D-max, making the perception of image detail impossible. This region generally represents areas of overexposure on an image.

- The Solarization Region lies beyond the D-max area of the characteristic curve and represents large exposures beyond the useful range for medical radiography. In this region, increased exposure results in decreased film density. Some emulsions contain restrainers that prevent the image reversal that would occur in this area. Duplicating film has been solarized. This area of the sensitometric curve is seldom charted.

 The sensitometric curve is a graphic representation of the relationship between the exposure given to a photographic material and the resulting optical density.

D. SENSITOMETRIC PARAMETERS

The characteristic curve demonstrates the following sensitometric paramaters:

- Speed (Sensitivity)
      Latent Image Fading
- Contrast
      Average Gradient
- Latitude
- Fog
- D-Max

1. Speed or Sensitivity

Film speed is designated on a sensitometric strip as the step whose density most closely matches a value of 1.0 plus base + fog. For a film with a base + fog of 0.20, the ideal speed step would be 1.20. In reality, your closest step may have an optical density of 1.30 or perhaps even higher. Rarely will you achieve the precise, numerical value of 1.0 plus base + fog. This should not be a concern; simply choose the nearest density value over 1.20 and use this step on a regular basis to plot and monitor speed.

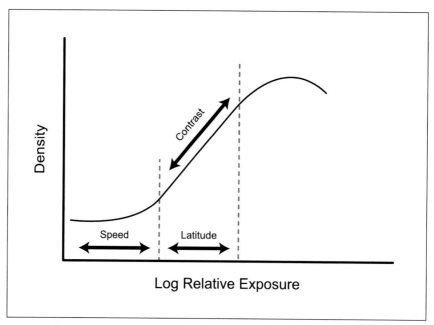

Figure 1.2 Graphic representation of sensitometric parameters

A relative indication of speed can be obtained by observing the proximity of the characteristic curve to the vertical axis of the graph (Figure 1.2). The further to the left that the curve is located, the faster the film speed will be. Speed is affected by film type, screen type, processing conditions, ambient environmental conditions, and latent image fading. Ambient conditions such as age, high temperatures or humidity, chemical fumes, or other poor storage conditions will influence the film speed.

a. Latent Image Fading

When excessive time passes between the exposure and the development of an image, a lower optical density than expected may be noted due to a phenomenon know as *latent image fading*. The degree of film speed loss varies with individual film products. An average estimation of the expected loss of speed with delayed processing is outlined in Figure 1.3.

 When excessive time passes between the exposure and the development of an image, a lower optical density than expected may be noted due to a phenomenon known as latent image fading.

Delay (Hours)	% Speed Loss
4	10
8	12
24	18
48	23

Figure 1.3 Approximate loss of speed when image processing is delayed.

Latent image fading should *rarely* be encountered in clinical practice. In an unusual situation, exposure factors can be adjusted to accommodate delayed processing and the loss of speed that will be apparent. Mobile mammography units that do not have access to immediate film processing must factor latent image fading into their exposure techniques. To minimize latent image changes, films are frequently sent to a home base every evening for processing the following morning.

The image change that is known to occur with delayed processing is the reason why pre-exposed sensitometric strips must *never* be used for quality control purposes.

2. Contrast

Contrast can be defined as the density difference between any two areas on an image. These areas may be directly adjacent to one another; they may be two specifically selected areas on an image; or they may even be the lowest and the highest measurable density of a specific film. Images will only *become* visible through a difference in density, or through varying tones of black and white on a radiograph.

The straight-line portion of the characteristic curve is the graphic representation of contrast. Contrast must be maximized in order to enhance subtle architectural changes. Information about contrast can be determined by the rate of change of density in this area. A rapid, sharp rise in density in the straight-line portion indicates a film of high contrast whereas a slow, gradual density rise depicts a low contrast film, also frequently referred to as *latitude film*. High contrast film, also referred to as *contrast film*, will be represented by large density differences between the steps of the sensitometric strip. Smaller density differences spread over a longer range is characteristic of low contrast and latitude film.

a. Average Gradient

Average gradient is another term that is used to describe the slope of the straight-line portion of the curve. Contrast and average gradient are related: the steeper the slope, the higher the contrast; and the flatter the slope, the lower the contrast. Average gradient, however, includes only the useful densities on our mammography images between 0.25 and 2.0 plus B+F (0.45 and 2.20). This represents the useful range of densities for medical radiography. Therefore, average gradient gives us an indication of contrast relative only to the useful densities we frequently encounter on our images. Average gradient provides the most accurate and reliable indication of film contrast in a given chemical environment.

Film manufacturers frequently quote average gradient values; the value can, however, be mathematically calculated from a characteristic curve. Refer to the diagram below for an example of this calculation.

Determining the average gradient from the characteristic curve: Average gradient for medical x-ray films incorporates the density range of 0.25 to 2.0 above base plus fog. The formula for average gradient is:

$$\text{Average gradient} = \frac{E_2 - E_1}{\text{Log } E_2 - \text{Log } E_1}$$

Where E_1 is the exposure corresponding to the density of 0.25 above base + fog and E_2 is the exposure corresponding to the density of 2.0 above base + fog.

For a film with a base + fog of 0.20:

$$\text{Average Gradient} = \frac{2.21 - 0.45}{1.15 - 0.60} = \frac{1.76}{0.55} = 3.2$$

Should the calculated average gradient for the specific film and chemistry that you are using vary significantly from the manufacturer's suggested performance criteria, the reasons for diminished performance should be investigated and corrected. Your film representative may be very helpful in troubleshooting possible areas of concern in order to restore image contrast to its achievable value.

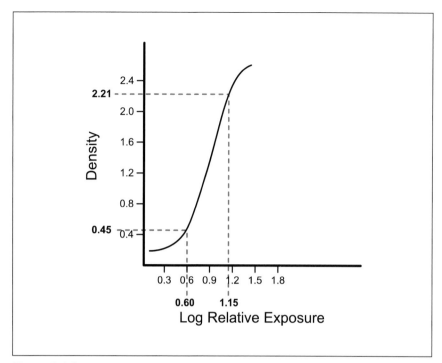

Figure 1.4 Average gradient can be calculated from a characteristic curve.

The following parameters should be checked when attempting to improve average gradient: developer temperature, developer replenishment rates, blocked replenishment lines, correct developer type, possible developer contamination, processor ventilation, and film emulsion variation.

When the correct average gradient has been achieved sensitometrically but the user is still unhappy with clinical image quality, the film processor can be eliminated from the troubleshooting process. Other imaging parameters such as breast compression, equipment features (tube, focal spot, kVp and mAs accuracy, exposure technique), viewing conditions, and safelight and darkroom integrity must then be investigated.

3. Latitude

The characteristic curve can also provide useful information regarding the latitude of a film product. Latitude can be defined as the range of exposure values that will produce image densities between 0.25 and 2.00 above the base plus fog density. As described above in the discussion on film contrast, a sharp, rapid rise in the average gradient portion of the characteristic curve is noted

Average gradient gives us an indication of contrast relative only to the useful densities we frequently encounter on our images.

with a contrast film; the exposure range (along the horizontal axis) is relatively small between the low and the high end of the average gradient for this particular film product. This indicates that the exposure range that will produce an acceptable image is relatively limited. On the other hand, consider the exposure range (along the horizontal axis) for a latitude film, where the average gradient portions of the characteristic curve rises much more gradually, producing a much flatter slope. The exposure range in this situation is much greater from the low to the high end of the straight-line portion of the curve; this means that a greater range of exposure techniques will produce acceptable images, within the operating contrast limits of the system.

4. Base plus Fog

Fog, base plus fog, and gross fog are all terms used to describe the optical density reading of a film on step 1 of the sensitometric strip or on any area that has not received intentional exposure. The base plus fog density of an x-ray film will vary with the individual manufacturer's product thickness, transparency, tint density, and base hue. The base plus fog density also reflects any fog that the film may have unintentionally been exposed to as a result of poor storage conditions, darkroom conditions, light leaks, and chemical fog. This density is usually very low and, in general, should be negligible. However, should the base plus fog density increase by more than 0.03 of your standard operating level, image contrast will suffer, and clinical images must not be processed until the factors responsible for this occurrence have been investigated and corrected.

5. Maximum Density or D-Max

The maximum density of an image will vary with the type of film used and with the conditions of exposure and development. The new generation of high contrast mammography films introduced in the mid 1990s has increased the maximum density levels on mammography films. Contrast is significantly enhanced with *blacker* blacks; this is particularly apparent when fatty tissue is imaged directly adjacent to glandular tissue in the breast. With the previous generation of mammography film in general, high intensity mammography illuminators could easily create a gray, washed out appearance to the exposed background area of mammography images. In addition to the significant improvement in image contrast, the blacker D-max density of our current products is much more esthetically pleasing when images are brightly illuminated during interpretation.

E. CONCLUSION

Sensitometry is the cornerstone of quality mammography imaging. Managing the variables inherent in the processing environment requires an in-depth knowledge of the individual systems and components as well as experience with the interactions that are frequently encountered. Mastering these skills is a complex but essential process for the mammography technologist.

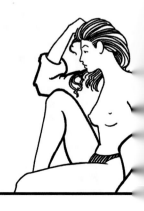

CHAPTER 2:
FILM PROCESSING

CHAPTER 2:
FILM PROCESSING

A. INTRODUCTION

Through a number of recent technological advancements we have access to exceptional quality and variety in dedicated mammography equipment and film-screen combinations. An abundance of literature and educational opportunities allows us to enrich our knowledge base and improve our technical skills. There remains one element which persists as a perpetual challenge for us. That element is film processing. Its dynamic environment preserves its reputation as the most variable element of the entire mammography system. Its very nature precludes the aspiration of control; our goal is to diligently monitor and to skillfully manage its fluctuations.

B. THE PROCESSING CYCLE

After exposure, the latent image must be chemically treated or processed in order to produce a permanent visible image. The goal of film processing is to produce a hard copy of the x-ray image which can be conveniently handled, illuminated, interpreted, and then stored for an extended time without significant deterioration. To accomplish this end, the film must be developed, fixed, washed, and dried.

1. Development

The most critical segment of film processing is image development; hence the intense focus on this component of the cycle. During development, the latent image becomes visible, the appropriate optical density level is achieved, and contrast in the final image is accomplished through a well-organized pattern of metallic silver deposits in the emulsion layer of the film.

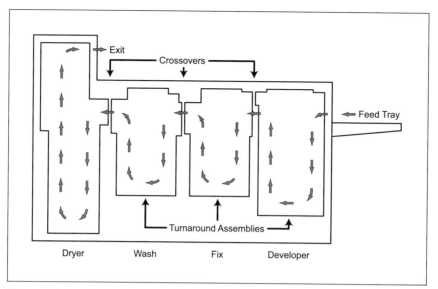

Figure 2.1 The automatic film processor

Typical developer tank volumes range from 1 to 3 gallons (3.8 to 11.4 liters) in size. Continuous motion of the developer solution is accomplished by the recirculation system. This is important to maintain even temperature and chemical activity throughout the tank; it also provides a continuous supply of fresh, active chemicals to the emulsion surface as the film passes through the developer rack.

The squeegee action of the rollers removes as much developer solution as possible from the emulsion as the film leaves the developer tank. However, the swollen, softened emulsion layer still contains a considerable amount of developer when it enters the crossover rack on its way to the fixer tank. Also, the process of reducing the latent image to black, metallic silver consumes some of the chemical components and alters the chemical activity of the developer solution. Therefore, the replenishment system is needed to add fresh chemicals to the tank on a regular basis in order to maintain both the volume and the chemical activity of the developer solution.

Starter solution must be added to the developer when fresh chemicals are used to refill the tank after a thorough cleaning. Starter solution begins the process of *seasoning* the chemicals, mainly through the addition of bromide ions. Consult the individual film manufacturer's literature for detailed information regarding the recommended volume of starter to use.

With flooded replenishment, starter is added to the replenishment tank instead of the processor tank at a rate of 3.0 fl oz (89 ml) per US gallon (3.8 liters) or 25.0 ml per liter.

In most cases, fresh developer is usually very active; this is reflected by higher-than-average readings on the sensitometry strip and by a higher optical density on clinical images. As films are developed, chemical agents are consumed and bromide ions and other by products are released into the working solution. At some point, the chemical activity of the developer will stabilize and settle into its *average* sensitometric operating range. These chemicals are now considered *seasoned*. In general, the developer is considered to be seasoned after three times the volume of the tank has been added to the chemicals through replenishment.

Finally, the temperature control system must maintain the very rigid parameters required for optimum film development. The developer solution must be maintained within 0.5°F (0.3°C) of its ideal temperature range.

2. Fixing

In an ideal setting, when a film emerges from the developer tank, every exposed silver halide crystal has been converted to black metallic silver. The remaining unexposed crystals have not been affected by development and remain intact in the emulsion layer. The process of fixing removes these unexposed, undeveloped silver halide crystals from the emulsion, making the image permanent; the next task is to begin to shrink and harden the emulsion layer. Therefore, fixing is accomplished in two distinct stages: clearing and hardening. Fixer chemistry is also composed of an intricate mixture of ingredients; however, the operating parameters of this segment of film processing are far less critical than those required of the development process.

The goal of film processing is to produce a hard copy of the x-ray image which can be conveniently handled, illuminated, interpreted, and then stored for an extended time without significant deterioration.

The average fixer tank size is 1 to 3 gallons (3.8 to 11.4 liters). As with the developer, a recirculating system maintains uniform temperature and chemical activity throughout the tank.

In general, fixer operating tolerances are much less stringent. Ideally, sufficient fixer activity is required to clear the emulsion of all undeveloped silver halide crystals; the archival quality of the film depends on this premise. Higher chemical activity will not harm the film in any way; it will simply result in wasted chemicals. The replenishment system adds fresh chemicals to the tank to replace the chemical components that have been consumed by the fixing process and to maintain the required volume of working solution in the tank.

The fixer temperature is not as strictly controlled as that of the developer; it also has a wider acceptable operating range.

3. Washing

In the wash section, all traces of chemicals are removed from the emulsion layer to ensure long-term stability of the image for archival purposes. This is the last of the wet sections of the processing cycle.

As with the other tanks, agitation is important to adequately wash the film and remove residual chemicals from the emulsion. In some geographical locations, filtration may be needed to remove particulate matter and minerals from the water supply.

The temperature of the wash water is not strictly controlled in the processor. However, the wash water is often used to cool the developer solution; therefore, the upper temperature limit of the water tank should be between 5°F to 10°F (2.8°C to 5.6°C) below the desired developer temperature. Incoming water temperature should not be lower than 40°F (4.4°C).

 Starter solution begins the process of **seasoning** *the chemicals, mainly through the addition of* *bromide ions.*

4. Drying

The final stage, drying, removes excess water from the emulsion to set the image and to allow it to be safely handled and viewed. A heater rapidly heats the air and a blower delivers the warm air to the dryer section where it is uniformly distributed to the film surface through a series of hollow air tubes. An air exhaust is required to remove moisture-laden air from the processor and stabilize humidity. This exhaust must be properly vented to the outside, preferably through the building's exhaust system, to prevent a build up in the processor or in the darkroom. Alternately, drying is sometimes accomplished with infrared heat bulbs that are surrounded by a reflective shield which directs the heat toward the wet films.

A tendency to over-dry films is frequently noted in clinical practice. This results in surface artifacts and needlessly wastes energy. The dryer temperature should be kept just high enough to dry the films as they exit the processor.

C. PROCESSOR SYSTEMS

A number of individual systems work together to complete the complex and intricate process of developing film images. These systems are the:

- Transport System
- Replenishment System
- Recirculation System
- Temperature Control System
- Silver Recovery System

1. Transport System

A roller transport system moves the film through each of the processing sections. The time spent in each of the individual areas of the processor must be precisely controlled in order to achieve optimal film quality; this is accomplished with a constant speed motor. A rack driving system of either the gear or the chain drive type sets the rollers in motion and maintains smooth, uniform

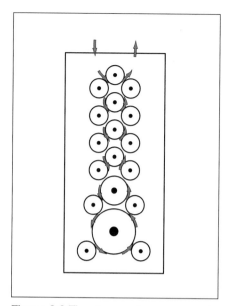

Figure 2.2 The staggered arrangement of rollers in a processing rack.

transport throughout the processor. A master rack in each individual tank transports the film throughout that particular section; the rollers are seated in either a staggered (Figure 2.2) or opposing (face-to-face) configuration (Figure 2.3) to move the film along. Rollers made from a variety of materials are found throughout the processor. Phenolic rollers provide uniform wetting and good contact with the film surface; plastic rollers are particularly suited to move the film throughout the tanks; silicon rollers minimize surface damage and abrasion; and stainless steel rollers provide pressure against the squeegee rollers to efficiently extract moisture from the emulsion. Some rollers have a textured surface designed to *hold* chemicals against the film surface as it travels through the processor. This roller style may be found in the fixer, where it is important to abruptly arrest film development. The film must accommodate numerous dramatic changes in direction as it travels throughout the system. A turnaround assembly consisting of a group of precisely aligned rollers is located at the bottom of each rack to turn the film 180 degrees when it reaches this point. Guide shoes are also used to turn the film when a relatively significant change of direction is required. Some manufacturers have developed a *smooth* guide shoe design for mammography processors to minimize surface damage to the films. Crossover racks are small groups of rollers that transport the film from one processor section to another; they are seated above and between the main processing tanks. An entrance roller assembly, located just beyond the feed tray, intercepts the film as it enters the processor to be devel-

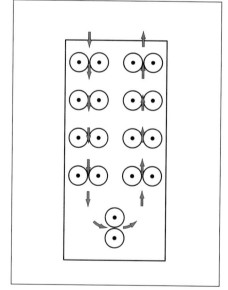

Figure 2.3 The face-to-face (opposing) arrangement of rollers in a processing rack.

oped. This assembly frequently contains sensors that measure film travel and initiate chemical replenishment based either on film length or film area.

Developer immersion time for both standard and extended cycles refers to the time from when the leading edge of film enters the developer to when this same edge enters the fixer. This time will vary among manufacturers and among individual film processors.

Total processing time for both standard and extended cycles refers to the time from when the leading edge of a film enters the processor until the trailing edge of the film exits the processor. A 24 cm film size is routinely used when quoting mammography parameters such as this.

 Some manufacturers have developed a smooth *guide shoe design for mammography processors to minimize surface damage to the films.*

2. Replenishment System

As films are processed, the activity of the chemicals will gradually be depleted and the solution levels in the tanks will drop as the film emulsion absorbs chemicals. This progressive loss of activity and solution volume is compensated for by chemical replenishment. The amount of replenishment required is highly dependent on the individual processor, the processing cycle, the film type, and the volume of film processed. Consult your film representative for assistance in determining appropriate rates. The volume of replenishment added to the developer and fixer tanks can be individually adjusted; the quoted rate is usually based on 24 cm of film travel.

In general, a low film volume will require higher replenishment rates. Conversely, a high film volume requires less replenishment per film because the fresh chemicals entering the tank on a regular basis maintain high activity.

Low volume processing leads to the accumulation of chemical by-products that encourage oxidation. This will eventually seriously compromise film quality. Also, the accumulation of undesirable chemical by-products in the tanks would severely diminish chemical activity. *Flooded replenishment* is a process of using a timed-cycle circuit to automatically add a predetermined amount of developer and fixer replenisher to the processing tanks, usually every five minutes; this maintains chemical activity in a low volume situation. Replenisher solution is also added to the tanks each time a film is fed into the processor. When flooded replenishment is used, starter solution is added to the replenisher tank only; additional starter should not be added to the developer tank as well. Flooded replenishment systems maintain a fresh chemical environment; the effects of a seasoned chemical state are never achieved.

3. Recirculating System

Each section of the processor has an individual recirculation system. In the wet sections, agitation of the solutions is very important to maintain uniform chemical activity and temperature throughout the individual tank. Agitation also serves to continually provide fresh, active chemicals close to the emulsion surface as the film travels through each area of the processor. Agitation is accomplished by pumps that continuously circulate the chemistry and by means of roller contact and movement at the film surface. The recirculating pumps of both the developer and fixer operate at an average rate of 2 to 4 gallons (7.6 to 15.2 liters) per minute. In the wash tank, a flow rate of 0.25-1.5 gallons (0.95 to 5.7 liters) per minute is typical and acceptable to adequately remove chemicals from the film. In the dryer section, a blower assembly serves to circulate fresh dry air throughout the dryer section to facilitate the drying process. The blower circulates the air at a rate of 100 to 300 cubic feet (3 to 9 cubic meters) per minute. Infrared dryer systems do not require as great a volume of circulating air; this is accomplished with a small fan.

Filters are used in a number of locations throughout the processor. The developer chemicals circulate through a filter which removes debris and particulate matter from the working solution. A 75-micron filter is generally used, although the porosity required will vary with the local water conditions of each site. The developer filter should be replaced every time the chemicals are changed (approximately monthly) or after processing 5,000 films. For the wash tank, a 50-micron filter is usually adequate, although a finer filter may be required in areas where an abundance of minerals and particulate matter are evident. This filter should be replaced every 1 to 3 months, depending on how quickly it becomes saturated with debris. In areas where the water supply is particularly poor, a double, *piggy-back* filter system is very effective in control-

Low volume processing leads to the accumulation of chemical by-products that encourage oxidation.

With mammography film-screen processing, it is extremely important to follow the manufacturer's recommendations for processor selection, cycle time, chemistry selection, replenishment rate, temperature, and processor maintenance schedules in order to consistently produce optimal film quality.

ling the negative impact of these conditions on film processing. The fixer solution generally does not require a filter.

4. Temperature Control System

The critical impact of temperature on the activity of the developer solution requires that it be manually verified *on a daily basis* rather than relying on processor readouts. Refer to Chapter 1, Sensitometry, for detailed information on appropriate thermometers for manual verification of processor solution temperatures. Most dedicated mammography processors operate at a developer temperature of 95-96°F (35-35.6°C). A system of thermostats and heat exchangers maintain this temperature to within 0.5°F (0.3°C).

The operating fixer temperature is frequently within 5°F (3°C) of the set developer temperature. Its accuracy is not as critical as that of the developer and it is not necessary to verify on a daily basis. A higher fixer temperature will fix the films more quickly, but there will be no other adverse consequences.

Incoming water can be cold or tempered. Extremes in temperature can encourage the growth of algae; they will also promote poor washing, transport problems, and the frequency of film artifacts. Heaters, chillers, and mixing valves may be used to control incoming water temperature. Wash water is frequently used to cool the developer; should this be the case, its maximum temperature should be 9°F (5°C) below the desired developer temperature. Water temperature in the processor is maintained with heat exchangers from the developer and/or fix sections.

In the dryer section, temperature control is maintained with a thermostat and heater arrangement. Ideally, the lowest temperature that will adequately dry the emulsion should be used. Excessively high dryer temperatures have a tendency to promote surface drying artifacts; they also create a very brittle emulsion that is prone to physical damage and *pick-off*. An ideal dryer temperature ranges between 100°F and 160°F (37.8°C and 71.2°C). The infrared dryer system is also thermostatically controlled.

5. Silver Recovery System

Waste management for processor effluents must be conducted in accordance with regional environmental restrictions. An important by-product of film processing is silver; it is present in the fix solution and to a much lesser degree, in the wash water. Silver is considered an environmental pollutant by today's standards. Therefore it is both cost effective and environmentally sound to remove as much silver as possible from the used fixer solution before it is disposed of. Typically, 5.0 mg of silver per liter of solution is considered acceptable for solutions entering the sewage system. Individual local regulations should be verified, as they may be stricter. Silver recovery can be accomplished with a metallic replacement cartridge or by means of an electrolytic process.

Many variables are affected by the dynamic nature of the processing environment; they must be carefully monitored and skillfully managed on a regular basis.

D. OPTIMIZING FILM PROCESSING

The accuracy and consistency of film processing is critical to the imaging process; its value cannot be overemphasized. The manufacturer's specifications should be followed in order to achieve the expected performance for a particular film product. This is essential to achieve optimal processing conditions. Thereafter, an on-going quality control program is essential to maintain these conditions over an extended period of time. Many variables are affected by the dynamic nature of the processing environment; they must be carefully monitored and skillfully managed on a regular basis.

Trend charts with established levels of variability are essential to monitor the dynamics of film processing. Major changes, which result in sudden, abrupt performance variations, require immediate attention. Chronic, gradual changes should also be analyzed periodically by examining trend chart patterns over an extended period of time. Many processing variables can be accommodated by adjusting exposure parameters on the mammography unit. Unfortunately, this frequently results in increased patient dose. This is unacceptable; the correct approach is, instead, to restore processing parameters to an acceptable operating range.

With mammography film-screen processing, it is extremely important to follow the manufacturer's recommendations for processor selection, cycle time, chemistry selection, replenishment rate, temperature, and processor maintenance schedules in order to consistently produce optimal film quality.

Currently, sensitometric testing is the only reliable method of verifying the chemical activity of the processor with any degree of accuracy. Specific gravity is another test that can be performed; however, its value is limited to an indication of too little or too much water in the chemistry. The pH value is also not a good indicator of chemical activity; a relatively large change in activity would be required before it could be detected with pH testing.

1. Standard Cycle Processing

Film manufacturers are constantly striving to improve the quality of mammography images. Recently, a new generation of high contrast mammography screen-film systems has been introduced to the mammography community. Many of these new systems are optimally processed in standard cycle processing. In fact, their performance is diminished in the extended cycle systems that were considered state-of-the-art just a few years ago. New film types and emulsion variants are continually being developed; each product will require unique and individual operating parameters in order to achieve optimal imaging results. It is extremely important to follow the recommendations of the film manufacturer for the best possible environment for each individual film system.

Diligent monitoring is also essential in order to maintain the precise processing parameters required for mammography imaging.

The film processor is largely responsible for the majority of film artifacts that are evident on our finished radiographs. Proper processor maintenance will minimize their occurrence.

2. Extended Cycle Processing

Extended cycle processing has been popular for mammography images for a number of years. Again, the primary focus is development, which is extended to 47 seconds (compared to 23-32 seconds with standard processing) in order to achieve more complete development in the film processor. This usually translates to a 30-40% reduction in patient exposure. The benefit of extended processing and the resulting exposure reduction varies with individual film types. With extended cycle processing, the developer temperature and replenishment rate are carefully adjusted according to the developer tank size, the immersion time, and the film volume in order to accomplish the desired sensitometric values of speed, contrast, and base plus fog. The ideal conditions of a 44 to 47 second developer immersion at 95°F to 96°F (35.0°C to 35.6°C) with 600 ml of developer replenishment per square meter of film were pioneered and fine-tuned by Dr. László Tabár, MD of Sweden. He has demonstrated exceptional quality and consistency in his mammography images using the above operating parameters. Kits are available for most processors to accommodate these parameters. Individual film characteristics combined with specific chemistry features will have a direct effect on both contrast and sensitivity (speed).

E. PREVENTATIVE MAINTENANCE AND CLEANING

The importance of maintaining processor performance cannot be emphasized enough.

It is important to implement a preventative maintenance and cleaning schedule for the film processor that fulfills the requirements of the quality control program. This component of the mammography environment must be maintained within very strict tolerances. Refer to Chapter 3, Quality Control, for the protocol suggested by the ACR and the CAR mammography accreditation programs.

Automatic film processing involves a complex combination of chemical and mechanical variables that are intricately interconnected.

In order to maintain the high quality, trouble-free processing a dedicated mammography processor must consistently produce, a regular preventative maintenance program with a reputable service organization must be established. The integrity of the rollers, springs, sprockets, etc. should be checked regularly because of the wear and tear expected with extended use. Problems

New film types and emulsion variants are continually being developed; each product will require unique and individual operating parameters in order to achieve optimal imaging results. It is extremely important to follow the recommendations of the film manufacturer for the best possible environment for each individual film system.

can then be detected early and corrected before significant loss in film quality is apparent and before the inconvenience of excessive down time occurs. The film processor is largely responsible for the majority of film artifacts that are evident on our finished radiographs. Proper processor maintenance will minimize their occurrence.

F. CONCLUSION

It is essential that all mammographers possess a working knowledge of the components of film processing, acknowledge the potential danger areas, recognize when these factors are infringing on image quality, and understand the direction to proceed to remedy the situation.

Many facilities produce good mammography images; few produce exceptional examinations. The difference lies in their knowledge and understanding of all the working components of the mammographic chain and the meticulous attention they devote to the entire system.

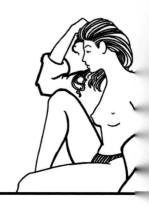

CHAPTER 3:
QUALITY CONTROL

QUALITY CONTROL

A. INTRODUCTION

Breast imaging requires strict quality control standards to consistently produce the highest quality films at the lowest dose to the patient and at the lowest possible cost to the facility. Mammography is technically demanding. All of the variables involved contribute in a positive or a negative manner to the quality of the images, depending on how closely the standards for quality are maintained. Each link in the chain — processing, film, equipment, viewing conditions, and technical competence on the part of the technologist with regard to positioning and technical factors — will contribute to the final product. If any part of the chain is weak or has been compromised, the resulting outcome will be negatively affected.

Quality Control (QC) refers to monitoring the technical variables that directly affect image quality. The Quality Assurance (QA) program is responsible for all aspects of mammography: from the time a woman makes an appointment with the facility, through the performance of the examination, the interpretation and reporting of results, and the monitoring of outcome data. Thus, Quality Assurance is a comprehensive program encompassing every aspect of patient care. Quality Control is the technical component of the QA program.

B. MAMMOGRAPHY ACCREDITATION

The American College of Radiology (ACR) established a comprehensive program for quality control in mammography in the early 1990s, and has continued to update procedures and standards as changes in the industry have warranted them. In 1994, the United States Congress implemented the Mammography

Quality Standards Act (MQSA) in the U.S. under the direction of the Food and Drug Administration (FDA). For the most part, MQSA follows the guidelines already set forth by the ACR with some minor revisions, which have been included in this material. A similar program has been implemented in Canada through the Canadian Association of Radiologists (CAR). Both the ACR and the CAR have established Mammography Accreditation Program(s) (MAP)(s) in order to improve the quality of mammography examinations on a national level. The CAR MAP has adopted the basic guidelines that have been established by the ACR MAP program.

The Mammography Accreditation Program (MAP) emphasizes the need for a *Team Approach* to quality mammography. Each member of the team is a vital component of the program. The goals of this program are:

1) To establish quality standards for mammography examinations

2) To provide the opportunity for mammography sites to compare their individual performance with nationally developed standards

3) To encourage quality assurance practices for mammography

4) To ensure that patients receive high quality examinations at low radiation doses

All members of the mammography team must have regular exposure to education and training programs. New information and improvements in basic procedures are released on a regular basis. Exposure to new data and ideas is important to maintain a current perspective of the specialty; it is also important to stimulate the interest and pride of the personnel involved in the program. Through a regular review of the QC data, shortcomings in the program and areas that require improvement may be identified and addressed; these measures are beneficial in stimulating growth in the program and in maintaining quality over an extended period of time.

The key roles of the individual team members are as follows:

1. The Radiologist

The radiologist is ultimately responsible for the quality of mammography performed at the facility. Any duties or responsibilities not assigned to other individuals are the responsibility of the interpreting physician (radiologist)

under MQSA requirements. It is therefore in the best interests of the facility and the radiologist to follow the eleven duties outlined by the ACR and the CAR accreditation programs.

The duties of the radiologist are to:

1) Ensure that technologists have adequate training and continuing education in mammography

2) Provide orientation for technologists and a written procedure manual prepared according to specific guidelines outlined in the program's quality control manual

3) Provide motivation, oversight, and direction to all aspects of the QC program

4) Select a single QC technologist to perform the prescribed QC tests and to oversee any tests that have been delegated to other individuals

5) Ensure the availability of appropriate QC test equipment and materials

6) Provide adequate time to perform, document, and interpret the QC tests

7) Provide frequent, consistent feedback (positive and negative) regarding clinical film quality and QC procedures

8) Select and collaborate with a medical physicist to oversee equipment-related QC issues and to perform the prescribed physicist's tests

9) Review the technologist's test results at least every three months and the physicist's test results annually or more frequently when required

10) Oversee or designate a qualified individual to oversee the radiation protection program for all employees and for patients

11) Ensure that all records are properly maintained and regularly updated in the QC manual

In addition to the technical components of the QC program, the radiologist is responsible for establishing an ongoing program to monitor the quality of mammography interpretation provided by the program.

2. The Medical Physicist

The role of the medical physicist has been expanded somewhat under MQSA legislation and subsequently by the ACR as well. While the medical physicist has always been considered a key member of the team, the new guidelines specify the medical physicist as the individual responsible for overseeing the entire quality control program. The physicist's role as an adviser and consultant in this regard is vital. The technologist responsible for QC is encouraged to meet with the physicist on an annual basis to review documentation and image quality and to provide recommendations for improvement.

The physicist's role relates to equipment performance; this should encompass image quality assessment, patient dose evaluation, and operator safety issues.

The parameters which must be evaluated annually by the medical physicist according to the ACR and CAR accreditation programs are as follows:

1) Mammogaphy unit assembly evaluation
   (Decompression assessment has been added under MQSA)

2) Collimation assessment

3) Evaluation of system resolution

4) AEC performance assessment

5) Uniformity of screen speed

6) Artifact evaluation

7) Image quality evaluation

8) kVp accuracy and reproducibility

9) Beam quality (HVL) assessment

10) Breast entrance exposure, AEC reproducibility, average glandular dose and radiation output rate

11) Viewbox luminance and room illuminance

As well, evaluation by the medical physicist is required following significant changes to the mammography equipment or film processor. A new baseline phantom image should be done after any of these changes, which include:

- New installation of x-ray unit (even if unit has been used previously)
- New installation of processor (even if used)
- Disassembled and reassembled x-ray unit or film processor
- X-ray tube replacement
- Collimator replacement
- Filter replacement
- AEC replacement

3. The QC Technologist

The QC technologist is responsible for the performance and documentation of the eleven tests outlined below. It is important that these tests be performed with as much consistency and meticulous methodology as possible. Therefore, it is ideal to have one individual assigned to specific tests so that variability in performance can be minimized. The more experience (through repetition) that a technologist has with these tests, the more competent she will become. She will also be able to readily determine where and why corrective action may be required.

Prompt and proper documentation of all results (whether within limits or not) and of any corrective measures taken is essential. It is important to note that perfection in the results obtained when performing these test procedures is neither expected nor reasonable; in fact, consistently perfect performance is likely to be suspect. The very nature of the imaging process predisposes the parameters involved to change and fluctuation. Documentation of problems that may be encountered followed by a corresponding corrective action that restores operating parameters to acceptable limits confirms with certainty that the QC program is being properly executed. It should also be apparent that it is extremely difficult, if not impossible, to solve problems in the imaging chain without an understanding of the QC testing procedures and their acceptance criteria.

The technologist's role focuses on patient care and image quality. This includes quality control, patient positioning, breast compression, image production, and infection control. In addition to performing a series of specific tests, the QC technologist should review the status of the quality control program with the responsible interpreting physician (radiologist) and with the medical physicist.

The eleven tests that the QC technologist is responsible for are:

1)	Daily	Darkroom cleanliness
2)	Daily	Processor QC
3)	Weekly	Screen cleanliness
4)	Weekly	Viewbox cleanliness and viewing conditions
5)	Weekly	Phantom imaging
6)	Monthly	Equipment evaluation (visual checklist)
7)	Quarterly	Repeat analysis
8)	Quarterly	Fixer retention testing
9)	Semiannually	Darkroom fog testing
10)	Semiannually	Screen contact testing
11)	Semiannually	Compression device testing

It should be emphasized that these are minimal test frequencies; when problems arise, they will need to be performed more often, at least until conditions stabilize. Testing must also be done when new equipment is installed and after service or preventative maintenance has been performed.

The procedures and acceptance criteria for each of these tests are clearly documented in the Quality Control Manuals that accompany the documenta-

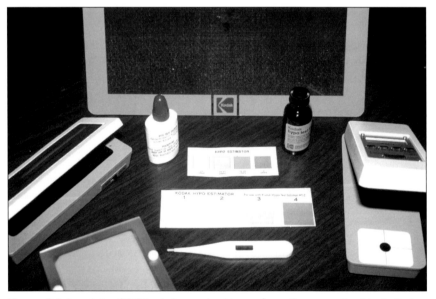

Figure 3.1 A variety of QC tools is required to perform the prescribed tests that are outlined in the QC technologist's component of the MAP.

tion for the ACR and CAR accreditation programs. It is important to refer to the appropriate accreditation manuals provided to your facility for detailed information pertaining to the performance of the QC tests, as it is not our intention to reiterate those specifics here. Key points and issues that are often overlooked are outlined briefly in this material.

It should be noted that many of the states (U.S.) and provinces (Canada) have individual quality assurance compliance programs. Each facility must investigate the regulatory requirements that apply to its individual location in addition to the standard guidelines described here for the ACR and CAR mammography accreditation programs.

C. IMAGE RECEPTOR

1. General Information

Increasing the speed of an imaging system will be accompanied with a corresponding increase in quantum mottle or noise in the image; this occurs because fewer x-rays are being used to produce the image. As well, high contrast systems will make noise even more visible; the sharpness of both anatomical structures and noise will be improved. Noise is particularly troublesome in mammography: it interferes with the ability to visualize fine detail, especially microcalcifications. System speed must always be balanced with acceptable levels of noise or mottle.

Each screen must be marked with a unique identifying number in an area that will not interfere with the image (to one side, along the edge away from the chest wall) using an opaque permanent number or letter. Also indicate this same number on the outside of the cassette to facilitate easy identification of problem screens during the workday. The manufacturer's recommendations should always be followed regarding what product is best to number or identify the screens. Always be very gentle with screens; they can easily be damaged. Unfortunately screen damage almost always means that the entire cassette must be replaced.

2. Screen Cleanliness

Clean screens as often as may be required. While the ACR and CAR guidelines recommend a weekly minimum frequency, many busy facilities will find it necessary to clean screens more often. If dust artifacts occur often, more frequent cleanings will be necessary. Excessive dust should always be investi-

---

gated, since poor darkroom design and/or maintenance may contribute to this occurrence. During the workday, any cassette that demonstrates dust artifacts should be removed from circulation until it can be cleaned and reloaded. Screen cleaners may build up on the surface of the intensifying screen; if this occurs, the manufacturer may recommend using alcohol to remove the buildup. Always verify the manufacturer's policy for using any substance other than screen cleaner. Also, be gentle when screen cleaner is applied. The solution should be lightly applied to a lint free cloth or gauze, then gently wiped across the screen surface. Vigorous *scrubbing* may result in premature wear to the protective surface of the screen. Without the protective layer, screen speed may be affected and substances may penetrate the phosphor, resulting in permanent image artifacts.

The manufacturer's recommendations for products that are appropriate for screen cleaning should always be followed; failure to do so may invalidate the manufacturer's warranty.

Canned, compressed air may be used periodically to eliminate dust in corners and difficult to reach areas (identification windows) of film cassettes. Only *pure*

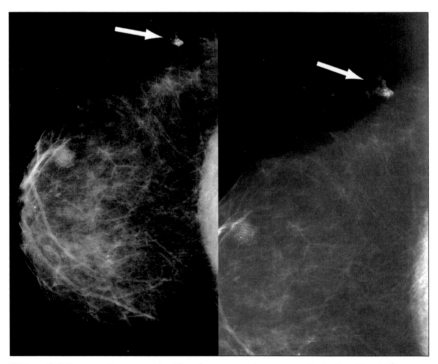

Figure 3.2 Screen damage resulting from spraying canned air directly at the screen surface from a very close range.

air should be used; many of these products contain oil or other contaminants that could damage screens. In particular, avoid compressed air that contains freon, such as that used for computers, as screen damage may result. Also, never spray the air directly at the screen surface; the high pressure can permanently embed debris in the surface of the screen (Figure 3.2).

a. Cassette Cleaning

In contrast to the fragile imaging screens that they house, the exterior surface of film cassettes are much more hardy and durable. Occasionally a site may choose to clean the outside of their cassettes; any general use cleaning compound can be used on the exterior cassette surface.

The interior surface of the cassette that lies adjacent to the screen should be wiped, whenever the screen itself is cleaned. A lint free cloth moistened with the manufacturer's recommended screen cleaner should be used.

3. Film Handling

Single emulsion film is very sensitive. It is also prone to handling artifacts. An extensive discussion of artifacts is included in Chapter 7. To avoid unnecessary artifacts, handle the film by the corners and ensure that hands are clean, dry, and free of lotions and creams. Double emulsion film has the advantage of two emulsion surfaces; damage on only one side will be effectively masked by the emulsion layer on the opposite side of the film. With single emulsion mammography film, any dirt on the screen surface or any scratches on the emulsion itself will result in a white/clear film artifact that will be very obvious, because there is no emulsion layer on the opposite side to mask its appearance.

4. Screen-Film Contact

Cassettes must be allowed to *rest* after film has been loaded in order to facilitate the expulsion (bleeding) of air that may be entrapped between the film and the screen. The ACR manual recommends that fifteen minutes be allowed following film loading to minimize this problem. While there is nothing magic about this number, the fact remains that pockets of trapped air may be present when cassettes are first loaded. Trapped air will result in an area of poor screen-film contact; this will be visualized as a localized area of blur on the clinical image. Unfortunately, it is often difficult to determine the source of image blur on a radiograph. In other words, what appears to be motion or blur on the image may in fact be the result of trapped air, poor screen-film contact, poor compression, patient motion, or equipment motion. In any case, the need to

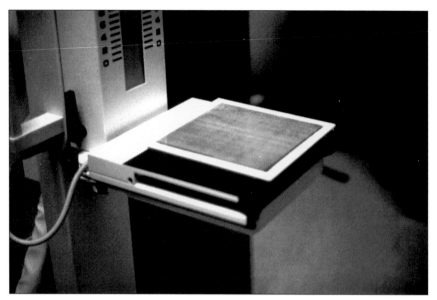

Figure 3.3 A 40-mesh screen contact test tool is used to evaluate the integrity of screen-film contact for every cassette in circulation in the mammography department.

repeat this image will always result in additional exposure for the patient. In a busy mammography department it may be difficult for the technologist to be certain that appropriate air bleed time has been allowed. Therefore, it is imperative that there be an adequate number of cassettes in both sizes for every mammography unit or room to allow for proper rotation as cassettes are reloaded during the workday.

Cassettes or screens in poor condition will impair diagnostic image quality. Cassettes should be checked regularly for wear; the closure mechanism must be very secure to prevent light leaks, yet easy to operate for the technologist. Fatigue or deterioration of the screen's foam backing material will result in screen contact problems that will consistently demonstrate localized areas of blur on radiographic images.

Cassettes with poor screen contact cannot be repaired by the user. Replacing screens in a cassette is a very delicate procedure requiring specialized equipment. Permanent screen damage frequently results when this task is attempted by an unqualified person.

A 40-mesh screen must be used for mammography screen contact testing. The larger mesh screens used for general radiography are not sensitive enough for mammography test purposes. Always store this mesh flat.

Freshly cleaned and loaded cassettes for screen contact testing should rest for fifteen minutes before exposure to allow any air that may be trapped in the cassette to *bleed* out. Air that remains within the cassette will result in large areas of poor contact; the test will need to be repeated. Likewise, entrapped air in the clinical setting will result in the need to repeat films (see above).

The sheet of acrylic, if used with screen contact testing, must cover the entire surface of the receptor. It should be placed on the compression paddle and raised up so that it is located distant from the film to prevent scatter from reaching the film. The basic purpose of the acrylic is to ensure an adequate exposure time to achieve an optical density of 0.70 to 0.80 for this test.

Screen contact test films are evaluated on viewboxes and at a distance (minimum one meter) rather than at close range and with a magnification glass. If areas of poor screen-film contact are noted, the screen should be cleaned and the test repeated. Screens that continue to demonstrate areas of poor screen-film contact (larger than one centimeter) despite repeated testing, should be taken out of circulation.

Although a minimum testing frequency of every six months has been legislated, this test should be performed any time that an increased occurrence of *patient motion* or *blurry areas* on clinical images is noted. It is helpful to record cassette identification numbers when these problems arise, in the event that a specific cassette (or cassettes) is consistently involved.

5. Archival Film Quality

The importance of preserving mammography films and maintaining image integrity over an extended period of time has become increasingly important. Regular mammography screening examinations have become part of many women's personal health programs. In order to facilitate adequate comparison with previous mammography examinations, it is imperative that the archival quality of mammography images is preserved. The processes of fixing the image and then washing the film are particularly critical in achieving good archival quality in processed radiographs.

An extensive and comprehensive quality assurance program will maintain the highest standard of image quality, even over an extended period of time. A mammogram is, in fact, an important legal document and should be regarded as such. MQSA requirements in the United States are very specific with regard to the retention of mammographic examinations for a period of ten years for future reference.

a. Fixer retention test

The fixer retention test should be performed in a room with average to subdued lighting. Either unexposed mammography film from the film bin or, alternately, the clear area on the daily processor sensitometric strip may be used to perform this test. A white piece of paper placed under the test film will assist with more accurate color perception; the estimator strip should remain in the protective sleeve when making the color comparison. A densitometer may be used to compare optical density values should you find this difficult to determine visually. The color of the stain will change with time, so documentation at the time of testing is critical.

High readings indicate problems in the wash section (flow rate, circulation problems, low temperature, blocked lines) or the fix section (depleted chemicals, loss of circulation, improper replenishment, low temperature).

This test is important for ensuring the archival properties of mammography images for future reference. The results must be documented in the QC manual.

The Mammography Quality Standards Reauthorization Act in the United States specifies the analysis of fixer retention in film for the reasons stated above. The ability of a mammography image to maintain its quality for an extended period of time is dependent upon the extraction of residual fixer from the emulsion during film processing.

This test must be performed at least semi-annually. To pass the stain test, no more than five micrograms of fixer per square cm. of film can be detected in a processed film.

D. EQUIPMENT

1. Mammography Unit

a. Visual Checklist

The visual checklist is performed monthly to ensure that mammography equipment system indicator lights, displays, mechanical locks, and detents are functioning properly. The mechanical rigidity and stability of the equipment is also checked for optimum performance. Although some of these items function primarily for operator convenience, others are essential for patient safety and for the production of quality images.

Additional items may be added to the visual checklist if they are appropriate for the equipment used at the facility.

b. Compression Device

The compression test is performed to ensure appropriate levels of compression in the manual and power modes for imaging. It is important also that the equipment does not provide too much compression, as patient injury may result.

The importance of proper compression in producing quality mammography images has been described in detail in Chapter 4 of this publication. Image quality is significantly improved with the use of appropriate compression.

The compression test is performed when equipment is initially installed, and every six months thereafter. It should also be done any time reduced compression is suspected. Digital bathroom scales should not be used, because they sample data and may not respond properly when additional compression is applied slowly. Analog bathroom scales are preferred for this test unless a digital scale that has been specifically designed to measure compression is available.

A compression force of at least twenty-five pounds must be achievable according to MQSA requirements; this value must not exceed forty-five pounds of force for the initial power drive. If these test results are outside of acceptable limits, the source of the problem must be identified and corrected before any further patient examinations are performed.

2. Viewboxes and Viewing Conditions

The importance of proper viewing conditions for mammography cannot be overstated. The standard optical film density that a site selects will be directly related to the viewing conditions at the facility. Often, facilities that fail accreditation or inspection due to clinical or phantom image underexposure are those with poor/inadequate viewing conditions, i.e., high levels of ambient lighting, low levels of viewbox output, and lack of appropriate masking. To make matters worse, technologists often do not have access to viewing conditions that match those of the interpreting physician. As a result, the clinical images the technologist reviews may appear quite different when the radiologist interprets them with optimum viewing conditions. It is important that the viewboxes used for QC meet the same quality requirements as those used by the interpreting radiologist.

For these reasons, it is important that the evaluation of viewing conditions be given the focus and attention it deserves. The medical physicist is responsible for measuring the actual light output of the viewboxes. However, the QC technologist should review the facility viewing conditions on a regular basis. Fluorescent tubes should all be replaced at the same time, rather than one at a time, as they burn out. Because the tubes slowly decrease in brightness over time, the tubes should be replaced every eighteen to twenty-four months. The color and luminance of the tubes should all be the same.

Viewboxes should be cleaned at least once a week according to ACR and CAR recommendations using window cleaner. Marks that cannot be easily removed with window cleaner should be removed with a safe and appropriate cleaner. It is also good practice to remove the front panels to wash behind them on occasion.

E. DARKROOM

1. Darkroom Cleanliness

The darkroom is a major source of potential problems for all mammography facilities. A clean darkroom will go a long way in controlling a multitude of predictable difficulties. A strict policy of no smoking, eating, or drinking in the darkroom must be established. A specific area, preferably near the film bin, should be designated for film loading and unloading; this area should not be used for any other purpose. There should be no shelves above this area; shelves are potential dust collectors and their presence in the darkroom should be minimized. Avoid positioning ceiling air ducts above the film loading area; they will be a constant source of dust and debris. In the unfortunate event that they currently are situated above the loading area, a filter should be installed to control dust. Note that this will only minimize dust; construction or remodeling in any part of the building will be reflected by an abundance of shadow artifacts on clinical images. The darkroom should have a solid ceiling. Sectioned tiles and panels introduce the potential for light leaks; they also collect dust that will inevitably sift down onto countertops.

Adequate darkroom ventilation is very important; ten air exchanges per hour inside the darkroom, and two per hour outside the darkroom is recommended for a healthy environment. All incoming air should be clean or filtered, especially for darkrooms used for mammography processing. In addition, darkroom air pressure should be greater than surrounding room air pressure to ensure that the air will be moving in the direction of film travel across the feed tray and not against it. This helps to minimize the opportunity for dust and other contaminates to be drawn into the processor along with the film.

Store film boxes on end to avoid pressure artifacts. Institute a system of stock rotation to ensure that the oldest film will always be used first. Check expiry dates; do not accept film that will not be used before this date.

The use of electrostatic air cleaners and humidifiers can be very helpful in controlling artifacts and minimizing static discharge in the darkroom.

2. Darkroom Fog

Darkroom fog is frequently encountered in clinical practice. It needs to be monitored regularly, at least semiannually, according to ACR and CAR guide-lines. Darkroom fog results in an overall plus density, and therefore has a negative effect on the contrast of films. Fog destroys contrast, and may be doing so clinically in a very subtle manner without being detected. Refer to the darkroom fog procedure in the ACR and CAR quality control manuals for a detailed description of the protocol for this test, utilizing the mammography accreditation phantom.

The phantom is used to evaluate levels of darkroom fog. The procedure is much the same as the procedure for phantom imaging, except that the cassette should be loaded in total darkness with the safelights turned off. Make the exposure as usual, then unload the cassette in total darkness. Place the film on the counter with the emulsion facing up. Cover half of the film with a piece of cardboard. Turn the safelights on and wait for two minutes. Remove the cardboard and process the film normally. The optical density of the background must be between 1.40 and 2.00. Unexposed or underexposed films are much less sensitive to the effects of darkroom fog.

Measure the density in the middle of the image on the unfogged side. Measure the density in the middle of the image on the fogged side. The measured optical density of the fogged side should not be greater than 0.05 OD more than that measured on the unfogged side of the image.

The darkroom fog test should be carried out using each of the films used for mammography at the facility; a minimum frequency of every six months is required.

Sources of darkroom fog can include such factors as damaged safelight filters, incorrect bulb wattage in safelights, locating safelights too close to working surfaces, and light leaks around doors, passboxes, processors, or ceiling tiles. Also, indicator lights on processors, clocks, timers, and other electronic devices may also result in fog on films.

F. FILM PROCESSING

1. General Information

It is important to establish a regular, comprehensive program for the cleaning and maintenance of the film processor. The importance of this component of the quality control program cannot be emphasized enough.

On a daily basis, the crossover racks should be removed and rinsed with warm water, rotating the rollers to expose and clean their entire surface using a synthetic sponge. They should be allowed to air dry, resting on their flat, upper surface. Pressure on the guide shoes will occur when crossover racks are placed on a countertop in their normal processor orientation. This must be avoided. Even minimal deviation or misalignment of the guide shoes will result in film artifacts. Occasionally (perhaps every two weeks) the entrance roller assembly should be wiped thoroughly; daily rinsing is not possible because this assembly requires forty-eight hours to dry. The main racks from the processor tanks should be removed and thoroughly cleaned every two weeks. Every day,

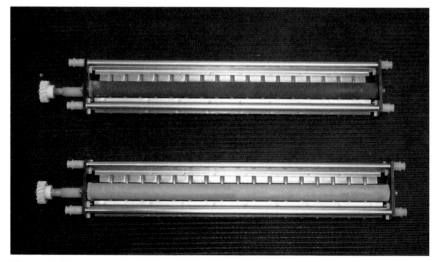

Figure 3.4 Crossover racks should be rinsed daily to remove chemical deposits and residue that could damage the softened emulsion during film processing.

before turning the processor on, wipe any chemical deposits that may have collected on the top rollers of the main processor racks, just above the level of the solutions in the tanks. Also, the feed tray in the darkroom must be cleaned daily before films are processed; occasionally it may need to be cleaned again throughout the workday if dust and debris collect on its surface.

Processor performance may be affected by factors such as film volume and chemical stability, resulting in the need to increase or decrease the frequency of changes to fresh chemicals. When in doubt, the film manufacturer should be consulted. The developer filter should be changed every time the developer chemicals are replaced.

Do not use chemicals that have been frozen or demonstrate any evidence of sediment in the bottles. Also, chemicals that have an unusual color, particularly if they are abnormally dark, may be oxidized and should be returned to the vendor.

Purchasing chemical concentrate and mixing the working solution as needed with an automatic mixer will provide the best possible chemical environment. Inconsistency and variability may occur when premixed chemicals are delivered by an outside source. If premixed chemicals are used, it is wise to monitor the specific gravity and acidity (pH) to verify proper mixing.

A floating lid that sits on top of the developer solution in the replenishment tank will help to minimize chemical oxidation. Not all mixing tanks are equipped with floating lids.

Never immerse an entire processor rack into systems cleaner. Removing all traces of the solution can be extremely difficult. Instead, working in small sections, spray the solution on the rack, then scrub and immediately rinse thoroughly.

Scotchbrite (tm) pads are very abrasive and should not be used on processor rollers, especially the *soft* rollers that dedicated mammography processors may have. Surface damage can occur and debris may be embedded in the roller surface. A lint free chamois or a synthetic sponge should be used instead. Rollers should be closely inspected during each cleaning to detect scratches or other surface flaws that may have developed. Defective rollers should be replaced before they cause film artifacts.

It is important to understand that each individual screen-film combination will exhibit a different film speed, contrast, and noise level that is dependent on a

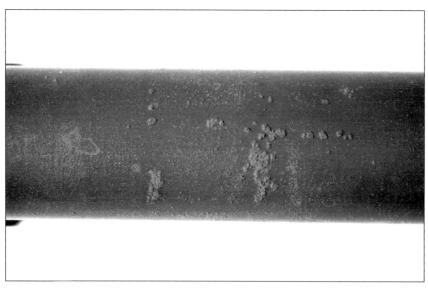

Figure 3.5 Careful inspection of processor rollers on a regular basis will facilitate the early replacement of defective rollers before they compromise the quality of clinical images. The pitted surface of this roller eventually created film artifacts.

variety of factors in the processing environment. Different products exhibit an individual and unique response to changes in these conditions. It is therefore critical that the recommendations of the film manufacturer be followed as closely as possible. It is impossible to expect optimum performance from any film when the processing conditions differ from what is recommended, or when processor maintenance is neglected.

A well-planned and executed approach for equipment maintenance and repair is essential to minimize equipment downtime and to address problems as they arise and before they become serious.

An effective quality control program requires that when problems are identified, they will be addressed and resolved in a timely manner. Consultation with other members of the mammography team should be readily available, particularly regarding problem issues, in order that appropriate remedial action can be taken to restore controlled conditions as quickly as possible.

Film manufacturers are constantly striving to improve the quality of mammography images. The goal continues to be high contrast (in order to enhance the visibility of detail) with the lowest possible dose to the patient. These efforts at improving mammography film have resulted in a trend, as of this writing,

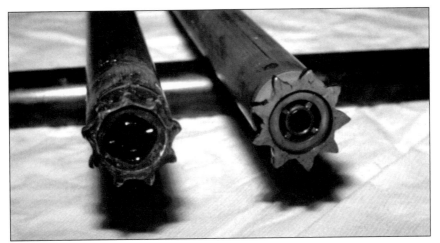

Figure 3.6 The regular inspection of processor racks, rollers, springs, guideshoes, etc. will help to ensure well-functioning, uninterrupted film processing. The worn gear on the left roller in this picture eventually created transportation problems and artifacts on the clinical images.

toward faster systems, with higher background density and lower image noise. Improvements in viewing conditions have encouraged increased overall image density, especially in the glandular tissue where the detection of microcalcifications is critical (suggested optical density of 1.0 in glandular tissue). Many of these systems are optimally processed in standard cycle processing conditions, as opposed to the extended cycle processing environment that was considered state-of-the-art only a few years ago. Since the development of new systems for mammography is likely to continue, it is critical to understand and implement the processing conditions that are optimal for the particular screen-film system that your facility uses.

2. Establishing Processor QC Operating Levels

Select a fresh box of film of the same type that is used for patient examinations. Reserve this box for QC purposes only. Set up the processor according to the specifications of the film manufacturer regarding chemistry, starter, temperature, replenishment rates, and cycle time. The processor control values should be established with seasoned chemicals; depending on film volume, this could take between one and two days. For five consecutive days, expose (emulsion side down in sensitometer) and process a sensitometric strip from the control box of film. Each day, before processing the strip, ensure that the processor has been running a minimum of thirty minutes. Manually verify that the correct developer temperature has been reached, and process several clean-up films to remove foreign material and chemical residue from the rollers. Feed the film into the processor on the same side of the feed tray that is routinely used (usually non-gear side), with the lightest density step being developed first to minimize the effects of bromine drag. The time frame between sensitizing and developing the strip should be the same each day; this will minimize latent image changes that could affect density readings. Do not use pre-exposed strips.

After the fifth day, read the densities of each step on all five films and determine the average for each step. Measure the density as close to the center of each step as possible to obtain the most accurate reading.

1. Mid-Density (Speed)
Determine the speed. Mid-density (MD) or speed is determined by selecting the step with the density closest to, but not less than 1.20. Designate this step as the (MD) step for your processor quality control chart. Other common names for the mid-density step are the speed step, speed index, speed point, or simply the speed.

2. Density Difference (Contrast)
Determine the contrast. Find the step with a density closest to 2.20 and also the step with a density closest to, but not less than 0.45. The difference in density between these steps will be the density difference (DD); this value is also called the contrast index or simply the contrast.

3. Base plus Fog
Determine the base plus fog (B+F). Read the density of step #1 or any unexposed area on the film to obtain the Base plus Fog measurement. This number represents the density of the base material that the emulsion is coated on as well as any film fog that may be present.

Record these readings on the processor quality control chart; this chart should be posted near the processor for easy and immediate reference.

4. Control Limits
Establish control limits according to the recommendations of the ACR and CAR mammography accreditation programs. The upper and lower control limits should be indicated for each of the control values on the processor chart. A range of +/- 0.10 for MD and DD, and a +0.03 change in the B+F is considered an acceptable operating range; +/- 0.15 values should also be indicated for both MD and DD to indicate the levels beyond which corrective measures must be initiated.

Over an extended period of time, should the operating control limits appear overly generous, an individual site may choose to restrict this range somewhat. This should only be initiated after consultation with the radiologist and the medical physicist. On the other hand, should the control limits be continually exceeded, never extend them to accommodate a greater degree of variability in your daily processor operation. The recommended control limits that have been established by the ACR and the CAR are reasonably achievable in all circumstances when a good quality control program is in place. Should the operating limits be frequently exceeded, the quality control program itself must be evaluated and improved. Again, perfection without variability is not expected; the goal is to maintain acceptable operating conditions despite normal fluctuations and variables. Finally, do not discontinue the quality control program if problems seldom occur. Acknowledge that you are doing a good job and are in control, but never lose sight of the potential for change that exists within your system. The dynamic nature of the processing environment promotes variability that must be monitored on a regular basis with strict parameters.

On a day-to-day basis, whenever the maximum control limits are exceeded, the test that indicated this occurrence should be repeated. If the control limits are still exceeded, corrective action must be taken prior to processing clinical images. Documentation must also verify that correct operating limits have been restored before patient examinations can be processed. Failure to do so is a violation of ACR, CAR, and MQSA guidelines and regulations.

3. Processing Control Charts

a. Daily Processor Quality Control

Processor quality control is the single most important task that the mammographer performs in order to ensure that consistently high quality images are produced every day.

Every morning the daily processor quality control must be completed before patient examinations can be processed. After the developer solution has reached its operating temperature and clean up film has been run, expose and process a sensitometric strip. The reserved box of QC film should be used and the procedural steps described above regarding the exposure and processing of the strip should be followed.

Measure the density of the previously established steps for MD, DD, and B+F. Enter this data on the processor control chart. Ideally, we want our MD and DD readings to be situated between +/- 0.10 of their ideal operating levels

---

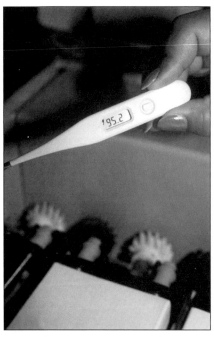

Figure 3.7 The temperature of the developer solution must be verified before the sensitometric strip is processed every morning.

and the B+F measurement to be within + 0.03 of its standard value. Should the MD or DD readings fall between +/- 0.10 and 0.15 of their established level, proceed with patient examinations, noting this discrepancy on the control chart. Should the MD or DD exceed the +/- 0.15 limits, patient examinations must not be processed until the source of the problem has been discovered and corrected. If necessary, continue to perform the patient examinations, but do not process the images until controlled processing conditions have been restored. Should the B+F level rise above the 0.03 control limit, repeat the strip to verify this finding. If the out-of-control conditions are confirmed by the second strip, you must discontinue processing patient examinations until the source of the problem has been determined and corrected.

On a day-to-day basis, small changes may appear insignificant and very acceptable. It is important to maintain a broad perspective of the *big picture* to appreciate subtle, steady changes in performance.

Note any trend that may be developing on your control chart. Any directional change that persists for three consecutive days is considered a trend and must be investigated and addressed. This indicates a slow, steady deterioration of control limits.

Record all data that pertain to processing conditions: changes in chemistry, temperature or replenishment rates, new control film emulsion number, new operating parameters (and reason for change), processor maintenance or service, cleaning schedule, etc.

Control charts indicate consistency of day-to-day processing conditions; they do not indicate that processing conditions have been optimized. Control charts provide an easy and convenient means to review relevant processing data in order to detect subtle trends that could indicate an unstable process. Processor

QC control charts must be retained in the QC records for a period of one year; the actual sensitometry films themselves must remain on file for the previous full month.

QC tests must be performed regularly, using a consistent protocol. They may be performed with the minimum required frequency; however, when problems or trends become evident, they should be performed more often until conditions stabilize once again.

Test results should be reviewed on a quarterly basis with the medical physicist and/or the radiologist.

The date must be included in the identification of every film exposed as part of a quality assurance program. Documentation is of the utmost importance. Equipment service that may affect film density, image quality, or radiation output requires that appropriate tests be conducted to verify the operation of the unit before patient examinations are performed. New techniques or exposure parameters may need to be established and posted for the mammography technologists.

Testing frequency may need to be increased if the mammography equipment exhibits significant change between scheduled inspections or if it is consistently subjected to an exceptionally high workload.

The purpose of processor sensitometry is to ensure appropriate processor activity before processing clinical exams. Therefore, it is essential that the strip be exposed, processed, read, and charted before processing patient exams. Do not delay this test until later in the day or week. This only monitors past performance (good and bad) and will result in inconsistent image quality.

Do not visually compare density steps on your sensitometric strips. Use a densitometer for accurate readings. Also, measure the density of any given step as close to the center as possible; this will provide the most accurate and consistent density reading.

Do not use pre-exposed sensitometric strips. They will exhibit the effects of latent image fading and will not be as sensitive to processing variations.

Circle any out of control data points on your processor quality control charts and indicate the corrective action that was taken on each occasion. Dramatic, sudden changes are usually a result of a mechanical breakdown such as the replenisher pump or the thermostat. Whenever out of control data is discovered, immediately repeat the test that indicated this occurrence, in case an error was made in the testing protocol. The resulting return-to-normal data must also be confirmed with a sensitometric strip and recorded on the chart as well.

4. Crossover Procedure

A crossover procedure is performed when a new emulsion of film is to be used for processor QC. The purpose of this procedure is to adjust operating levels for the subtle differences that can occur in manufacturing with individual emulsion batches. It is not advisable to set aside more film from one emulsion than can be used in a timely fashion, as film performance deteriorates with time and may be prone to fog and sensitometric changes under these circumstances. Often it is easier to perform the crossover procedure at the end of the month (for documentation purposes) rather than when the box of film runs out. In any event, placing a cardboard sheet in front of the last five sheets of film will help avoid inadvertently using them. Seasoned chemicals should be used for the crossover procedure.

Expose and process five strips from both the old and the new film emulsions at the same time, on the same day. Using the previously established quality control steps read and record the optical densities (OD) on each of the films. Average the density values for mid-density (MD), density difference (DD), and base plus fog (B+F) for the five old emulsion films. Do the same for the five new emulsion films. Determine the difference between the old and the new values for MD, DD, and B+F. It is important to note whether these numbers have increased or decreased for the new emulsion. If the number has increased, the number difference must be added to the current operating level average (used on current processor QC chart); this number represents your new operating level average for your daily processor quality control chart. If the number has decreased, the number difference must be subtracted from the current operating level average (used on current processor QC chart). Again, this number will be your new operating level average for your daily processor quality control chart. At this point, a new chart is started, using the adjusted operating levels and noting the new emulsion number. Five-day averages should only be performed when a major change is made; examples would be the type of chemicals, film, or processing cycle time for the facility.

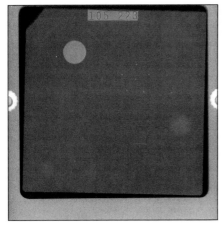

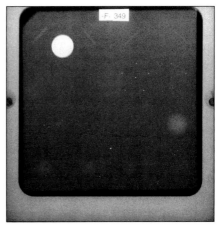

Figure 3.8 The RMI mammography accreditation phantom.

Figure 3.9 The Nuclear Associates mammography accreditation phantom.

G. IMAGING THE MAMMOGRAPHY PHANTOM

1. General Information

The phantom is an important tool in a mammography quality control program. It provides a measurable and more objective indication of image quality. The phantom is used to determine whether imaging conditions and parameters are adequate based upon the standards imposed by government or accrediting body regulations. In addition, the phantom is very useful for analyzing imaging problems, including artifacts. The more familiar and comfortable the QC technologist becomes with phantom imaging and interpretation, the easier it will be to evaluate differences in films, screens, processing conditions, and equipment. Both phantom images and clinical images demonstrate the cumulative effects of all imaging parameters in a system.

The mammography phantom can be used for a number of purposes because it represents an *average* breast (50% glandular tissue and 50% fatty tissue) in thickness and x-ray absorption and also because it contains objects that simulate anatomic breast structures. Therefore, it can simply be used to evaluate the optical film density of an imaging system to determine, on a regular basis, that the correct optical density will be achieved on clinical images. Second, it is most often used to evaluate image quality, based on the number of objects visualized (fibers, speck groups, and masses). Finally, it is also frequently used to analyze image artifacts.

Currently, two phantoms are acceptable for mammography accreditation and inspection purposes in the United States and Canada. One phantom is manufactured by RMI (Radiation Measurements Incorporated), model RMI-156; the other phantom is manufactured by Nuclear Associates, model 18-220. These phantoms are designed to simulate a 4.2 cm compressed, 50-50 glandular-fatty breast. Each is made of acrylic, with a wax insert that has embedded fibers, specks, and masses of decreasing diameters. Other models of breast phantoms are also commercially available, including one that simulates natural breast tissue; these phantom models can be very helpful in evaluating the performance of mammography systems in the clinical setting. It is also possible that new phantoms will be developed and accepted by governing bodies in the future.

It is essential that proper procedures be followed for imaging the phantom. In the United States, the Mammography Quality Standards Act (MQSA) requires weekly phantom imaging for all certified facilities. Canada's accreditation program also requires regular phantom imaging, scoring, and documentation. As well, the phantom must be imaged and a new baseline established whenever major changes that involve mammography equipment, processing, or image receptors have occurred. Refer to the Medical Physicists duties, outlined near the beginning of this chapter, for additional information on this subject.

Since the phantom is designed to simulate breast imaging, it is important to utilize the same exposure technique that is routinely used for clinical mammography imaging. One cassette should be selected for phantom imaging, and clearly designated as such. Although this cassette may also remain in circulation for everyday clinical imaging, it is imperative that the same cassette is used each time the phantom is imaged. This will eliminate inconsistencies that may occur as a result of individual screen or cassette variability.

To perform the phantom image test, load a sheet of the mammography film that is used for patient imaging into the cassette. Allow time for the cassette to rest in order to obtain good screen-film contact. Place the cassette in the cassette holder so that the chest-wall edge of the phantom is aligned with the chest-wall side of the image receptor. Center the phantom from left to right. The acrylic disc should be positioned consistently, just below the two largest fibers and just above the two smallest fibers.

Lower the compression device to rest lightly on the phantom (do not compress vigorously because the compression paddle can be damaged).

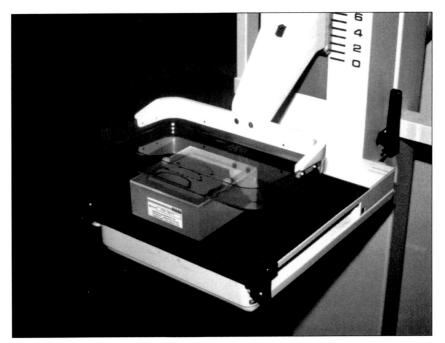

Figure 3.10 The RMI 156 phantom. The mammography phantom must be imaged at least weekly.

The AEC detector should be positioned under the pink wax insert (close to the center of the insert is ideal).

As always, consistency is important. Make an exposure using the technical factors that are currently used for clinical images (i.e. kVp, density control setting, target, filter, and grid). Note and record the readout of mAs. Note the density setting, kVp, and any other pertinent variables. Mobile units without on-board processing capabilities may only have the mAs reading to evaluate whether problems have occurred as a result of moving the unit. If mammograms are batch-processed at the end of the day due to distance from the processing facility, the phantom image should be run first after processor QC has been verified. The mAs noted on the generator readout should not change by more than +/- 15% with the same technical factors selected. MQSA regulations state that density settings should not be adjusted to compensate for quality control fluctuations.

If density-setting selection is changed deliberately to adjust the background optical density, or to accommodate differences in film speed between batches, the operating level for mAs should be adjusted and documented appropriately.

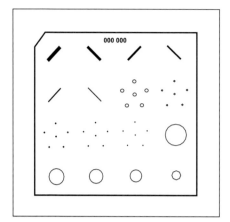

Figure 3.11 The fibers, speck groups, and masses in the RMI 156 phantom are used to evaluate image quality.

Process the film in the processor used for mammography film processing, using the same orientation each time. Film optical densities should be measured at three locations. The background optical density is measured at the geometric center of the phantom. The background density of the phantom must never be below 1.20 OD. This means that the operating level must be at least 1.40 OD; the control limits, once the background density has been established, are +/- 0.20 OD. To determine density difference (DD), the measured optical density in the center of the acrylic disc is subtracted from the optical density measured immediately adjacent to and to the right of the disc. These measurements must be made consistently in the same locations every time. In general, the operating level for DD with the 4.0-mm acrylic disc should be at least 0.40 OD. The DD will vary depending on the type of film used, the processing conditions, and background density level. In addition, it is important to note that there may be variations in actual disk thickness. There may be an increase or decrease in density difference even when using the same film, as a result of different mAs and background optical density. Once the optimum operating level has been determined, the control limits for DD are +/-0.05 for subsequent phantom images. Note that the density difference measurement is for quality control purposes only, and may not be used as an absolute measurement of film or image contrast. If the background density operating level is changed for any reason, the density difference must also be adjusted accordingly. Plot the background density and the density difference results on the phantom control chart.

2. Phantom Scoring Protocol

- Scoring should be done using optimum viewing conditions. Room (ambient) lighting should be low and diffuse. Viewboxes should be of high intensity, and located away from other sources of bright light. Images should be masked to eliminate extraneous light. A magnifying lens should be used to score speck groups.
- First, evaluate the overall phantom image. Are there any obvious artifacts or inconsistencies? Artifacts should be investigated before scoring the image.

- To score the phantom, begin with the largest fiber in the upper left corner of the image. If the fiber is seen in its entire length and proper location and orientation, score one full point and go on to the next fiber. If a fiber is partially, but more than half visualized, the fiber is given 0.5 point. When a fiber is reached with a score of 0.5 or zero, do not count beyond this point. For example, if counting from the largest fiber down, you can clearly see the first, second, and third fibers; half of the fourth and half or all of the fifth, the fiber score is 3.5 fibers. The fifth fiber is not counted even if it is visualized, since the fourth fiber was only partially visible.
- The next step is to look for any fiber-like artifacts in the phantom image. If an artifact looks like a fiber but is not in the proper location or orientation, you deduct the *artifact* fiber from the last true fiber if the artifact fiber is equally or more apparent. The deduction is made only from the last real fiber visualized, not from additional fibers. Record the resulting score on the phantom image chart. The four largest fibers must be visualized for a passing score.
- Use a magnifying lens of at least 2X magnification to score the speck groups. There are six specks in each of five groups, in descending size from largest to smallest. If you can see four or more specks in the group, in the proper location and orientation, score one full point. If two or three specks are visualized, score 0.5. Again, if a point score of 0.5 or zero is reached, do not go on to the next group.
- Next, look for any speck-like artifacts in the image. The artifacts must be truly *speck-like*, and as apparent as the real specks. If such artifacts are visible, subtract them speck for speck from the last whole or half speck group counted. In other words, if the score is 3.5, with 2 specks visible in the last group, but there is one speck-like artifact, the score drops to 3.0 because there will be only one speck remaining in the last group. The minimum passing score for speck groups is three.
- The masses are three dimensional, and should be well circumscribed to count as a full point. If the mass is visible in the proper location and appears to be circular with more than 3/4 of the perimeter visible, count the mass as one full point. If a minus density object is visible, but the perimeter is not generally apparent, score the mass 0.5 point.
- Then evaluate the overall background for any mass-like artifacts in the wrong location. If such an artifact is seen, deduct the artifact from the last whole or half point scored for masses. It is often helpful to sit back from the viewbox to evaluate masses, as this improves depth perception. Three masses must be visible for a passing score.
- As a final step, closely evaluate the background of the image with the magnifying lens for any non-uniform areas. If any grid lines, dirt, dust,

or other artifacts are noted they should be circled and evaluated. If artifacts are difficult to identify and isolate, consult the medical physicist for assistance.

The phantom evaluation cumulatively includes all of the components in the imaging chain. Changes in image quality may result from any one or more of the components. Therefore, it will be necessary to evaluate each parameter individually in order to determine the factor (or factors) responsible for any loss of image quality. The processor is the foremost variable to eliminate in these circumstances. Once the processor has been determined to be in control, each of the other components can then be evaluated individually to detect areas of inconsistency.

The current criterion for the number of objects in the phantom, according to the American College of Radiology, is a minimum of the four largest fibers, the three largest speck groups, and the three largest masses. In addition, the number of test objects in each group may not decrease by more than one half from the current operating level. If a greater change is noted, the image should be compared with the original image used as a standard to determine whether or not the change is real and significant.

Summary of Performance Criteria:
- The four largest fibers, the three largest speck groups, and the three largest masses must be visualized and may not decrease by more than 1/2 from the operating standard.
- The background density of the phantom image must be at least 1.40 OD, and may not vary by more than +/- 0.20 OD from the operating standard.
- The density difference (DD) when measured with the 4 mm acrylic disc should be at least 0.40 OD, and should not vary more than +/- 0.05 from the operating standard.

If more than one type of film is used for mammography, the phantom image test must be done with each film that is used clinically. If the performance criteria established for this test are not met, a second phantom film should be imaged and evaluated. If criteria are still not met, the reason(s) for the discrepancies must be evaluated and corrected. Once corrective action is taken, a phantom image should be taken to confirm adequate performance. These results must be documented before clinical images are performed on patients. Failure to correct and document results before performing mammograms is unacceptable. This failure is generally accepted as a significant violation of good standards of practice, and may result in a Level 1 violation of MQSA in the

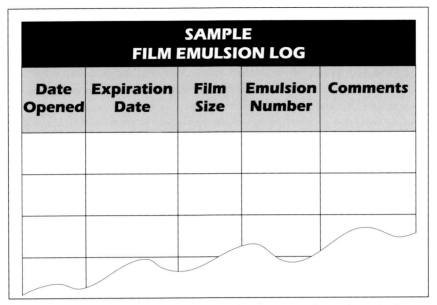

Figure 3.12 A film emulsion log can be used to document inconsistencies in film density that may be noted in the clinical setting.

United States, or failure during inspection in both the U.S. and Canada. In addition to phantom evaluation, other testing methods may be required to determine the source of the problem or change in system performance.

It is very difficult to maintain consistency whenever subjective measurements are involved. This difficulty can be minimized by making certain that the same individual views the images, under the same viewing conditions, using the same magnification glass, at the same time of day. It is also very helpful for the medical physicist and the radiologist to review the phantom images and scoring with the QC technologist on an annual basis to ensure agreement with results.

Any visual differences between the current phantom image and the original should be investigated. For this reason, it is often useful to maintain phantom images in the quality control records to use as a reference when imaging problems occur. (MQSA guidelines require retaining phantom images in the QC records for at least the last full year. Individual state requirements may vary. Many facilities keep the images for the full period of accreditation, or some-times even longer.)

When changes occur as a result of batch-to-batch differences with film, the film manufacturer should be consulted to determine whether the change is greater than what should be expected. If the change is significant, the non-compliant batch of film should be replaced. Recommended Specifications for New Mammography Equipment published in 1995 by the American College of Radiology, states that at an optical density of about 1.20 OD, a difference of 0.30 OD is the maximum variation that should be reasonably expected or accepted, given the same exposure parameters and equipment. A mammography film emulsion log (Figure 3.12) may be useful to aid in tracking the emulsions of film used clinically. These records help the film manufacturers compare differences in speed, contrast and maximum density (D-max) between film emulsions and from one period to another.

A *split-phantom test* may be performed to radiographically demonstrate relative speed differences between two different film emulsions when a significant change is suspected. This test requires that half of a film from each emulsion be loaded into a single cassette in total darkness. The mammography phantom is then exposed with the same parameters that are used clinically. The two film halves are then processed identically and the optical density for each is measured with a densitometer.

H. REPEAT-REJECT ANALYSIS

Rejected films should be distinguished from repeated films. Rejected films are all films that have been discarded for any reason. Repeated films are films that have been retaken in order to compensate for technical error, resulting in an additional exposure to the patient. Repeated films are not the same as additional views; a repeat is the same film taken again for a cause, such as improper positioning or exposure. Repeated films are often included in the patient film folder, rather than being discarded. It is important to record these films, however, because they must be included in a repeat/reject analysis. This can be accomplished with a list posted near the viewboxes; technologists can record the number, size of, and reason for repeated films each time this occurs.

When a repeat analysis is first introduced to a site, there may be a tendency for some technologists to alter their film acceptance criteria, feeling that their rejected films may have a negative impact on their performance evaluation. When this occurs, it is important to emphasize the objectives of a quality control program and to help them understand that the goal of the repeat analysis is to improve the overall quality of the facility's mammography examinations, rather than to conduct an individual audit. The repeat analysis provides valuable information with regard to a number of areas that may need improvement from patient positioning to equipment problems to film processing issues.

In the past, a great deal of emphasis was placed on specific numerical repeat rate percentages. Fortunately, it has now been recognized that the greatest value of this process lies in the analysis of an increase or a consistently high rating in any of the individual categories. Currently, if the repeat or reject rate changes by more than 2% from its previously reported rate, the contributing factors must be investigated and corrected. By determining the causes of such increases, the facility can implement appropriate corrective measures for improvement. Positioning and technical issues that are common to several individuals can be addressed by providing in-service education. There is an abundance of potential information that can be extracted from the repeat analysis; this is frequently overlooked. Productivity, film and chemical costs, and a reduction in radiation exposure can be documented by a more thorough analysis of the data provided. At a minimum, it is imperative that positioning, light and dark films, and motion repeats be counted and evaluated. Any increases in the rates of these categories should be investigated and documented. Individual states and provinces may have additional requirements with regard to the repeat analysis.

This test must be performed at least quarterly. To obtain meaningful results, a minimum of 250 patient examinations (or 1000 images) should be included in this evaluation; when this is not possible due to a low patient volume, a site must still comply with the minimum quarterly testing requirement. Whenever the number of images in the analysis is increased, more reliable data and more meaningful results will be extracted from the evaluation. High volume sites may choose to perform a repeat-reject analysis every month.

I. CONCLUSION

Mammography is an extremely technically demanding activity. Careful attention and monitoring of every component in the imaging chain is essential to the routine production of high quality examinations. Groups of test procedures have been established along with recommended test frequencies. The basic purpose of these tests is to ensure that minimum performance criteria are met and that the system parameters remain within acceptable operating levels. Although established regulations may not address every area relative to image quality, they should, nevertheless, not be overlooked. To do so is to risk compromising the quality of mammography performed at the facility.

Besides the tests that evaluate individual components, it is also important to include tests that evaluate the entire system as a whole.

The tools and instruments used for the QC testing must be appropriate for mammography. That is to say, the appropriate performance level must be evaluated with the required accuracy and precision that is relevant to mammographic imaging. The performance of these test tools and instruments should also be verified on a regular basis; recalibration or replacement should be pursued when required. The tests must be performed precisely each time to ensure that relevant and comparable data is collected with a minimum of variation. Precise documentation is also important to set the stage for meaningful interpretation of subsequent tests in order to detect changes and to expedite appropriate corrective measures. The QC test results should be reviewed regularly (ACR suggests quarterly) by the physicist and the radiologist.

The possibility of consistently producing high quality images at a low patient dose is within our control. It will only be achieved, however, with skill, dedication, and METICULOUS attention to quality control. Our rewards will be excellence in patient care and the satisfaction of generating, on a daily basis, exceptional image quality.

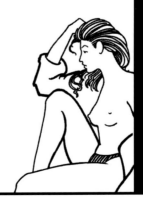

POSITIONING FOR MAMMOGRAPHY

SECTION I:
THE BREAST MAP*
*Mammography Aid for Positioning

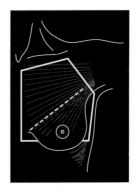

SECTION I:
THE BREAST MAP*
*Mammography Aid for Positioning

A NEW WAY OF UNDERSTANDING MAMMOGRAPHY POSITIONING

SECTION I:
THE BREAST MAP*
*Mammography Aid for Positioning

A NEW WAY OF UNDERSTANDING MAMMOGRAPHY POSITIONING

A. INTRODUCTION

The process of clinical image evaluation creates both an interactive and a dependent relationship between the mammography technologist and the radiologist. The radiologist must be confident that the technologist has included the maximum amount of breast tissue on the film; the technologist must trust that the radiologist knows that this is in fact the best she can do (often under less than optimal circumstances). Many times substandard films are evaluated by both parties and neither person has the knowledge or understanding required to identify and correct the positioning problem(s) that led to the exclusion of breast tissue on the standard CC and MLO mammographic images. Repeat views are often necessary.

Additional views may also be necessary for the evaluation of a specific area of breast anatomy and / or for the localization and clarification of abnormalities. Both the technologist and radiologist must have a clear understanding of breast anatomy and positioning and how each of these entities directly affects the mammographic evaluation process for standard and additional views.

Often technologists have received training in positioning techniques from many different sources. They may also have accumulated extensive clinical experience which supplements their expertise in patient positioning. As well, the vast majority of mammographers are well versed in the clinical analysis of the mammogram through the routine inspection of their images for both quality and content. Many times a technologist's knowledge is further advanced with practical clinical experience gained through the process of the diagnostic work-up, which frequently requires supplementary projections. The well-trained technologist should know what anatomic structures must be demonstrated radiographically and understand how to accomplish this.

An additional consideration is the radiologist's familiarity with mammography positioning. Although the radiologist is able to assess the mammogram to ensure compliance with clinical criteria and to confirm that the breast tissue has been adequately visualized, he or she is frequently unfamiliar with the intricacies of patient positioning techniques. In these situations, the well-trained mammographer can provide invaluable input regarding the direct relationship between the technique of patient positioning and the resulting clinical images.

A Mammography Aid for Positioning, or The Breast MAP has been developed to simplify the comprehension of this relationship. A breast map, or drawing, is used to visually *demonstrate* the effect of both proper and improper positioning techniques and their relationship to clinical film evaluation. It is important to clarify at this point that The Breast Map is a *teaching tool only*; it is *not* a new or alternate method of patient positioning.

There are many publications and other resources that describe the details of positioning techniques (see references). Instruction in these principles is essential; it is the cornerstone of quality mammography. Most technologists, however, when learning mammography positioning, are taught a *method* or given instructions on *steps* to perform. While this technique is practical and highly effective, it does not allow for the many variables that a mammography technologist will encounter. The variables are numerous:

- technologist size and shape
- patient size and shape
- equipment SID (source-to-image receptor-distance)
- tube head and face shield size and configuration
- bucky thickness and construction (corners)
- configuration of compression paddle
- accessibility of C-arm controls
- accessibility of collimator light control

Because of these variables, particularly height and weight differences, not all technologists can position all patients in the same manner. A tall technologist with long arms positions one way; her height and arm length work to her advantage. A short technologist with short arms will position in a manner that may be very different from that of her tall co-worker. The technologist who has large breasts herself will have difficulty standing close to her patient as many positioning protocols suggest. All of these variables affect *how* the technologist will actually go about *performing* a mammogram. Most technologists have learned to make *adjustments* in recommended positioning techniques in order to deal with their individual characteristics. This task will be much easier when she has developed a clear understanding of the relationship between the way the patient is positioned and the resulting clinical image. The Breast MAP can bridge this gap. It provides a strong foundation for understanding mammography positioning, based on anatomy. The positioning technique the technologist then uses will be a result of this understanding. The technique *variables* are less formidable and troubleshooting positioning problems becomes a simple, intuitive task. The mammographer who utilizes the concept of The Breast MAP will expand her positioning and technical expertise and become a more valuable member of the mammography team.

B. PATIENT AND BREAST ANATOMY

During any discussion on mammography and image evaluation, our attention must focus on the primary goal of mammography positioning: To visualize the maximum amount of breast tissue in the most effective and efficient manner. To be successful, the technologist must understand how anatomic structures will affect her ability to accomplish this goal.

In conventional radiography, anatomical structures are used routinely for positioning all body parts. For the pelvis, the ASIS and the symphysis pubis bone are used. When positioning the wrist, the radius and ulna are aligned so they are perfectly parallel for the lateral view. For the PA view we use the *heads* of these two bones as reference points to make sure the wrist is not rotated, and thus improperly positioned. Radiography of the skull is yet another example that demonstrates the use of anatomical structures to insure proper positioning. Here we often *connect* important landmarks with imaginary lines. The *Orbito Meatal Line* (OML) must be perpendicular to the table for some views; the *Acantho Meatal Line* (AML) is used for others.

The collimator light is also used in conjunction with the anatomical landmarks for all conventional radiographic positioning. The technologist checks to make sure that the *landmarks* are positioned accurately under the light ... and obviously that none of the body part is *coned* off (excluded from the image).

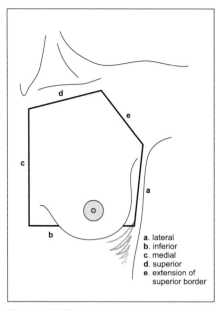

a. lateral
b. inferior
c. medial
d. superior
e. extension of
   superior border

Figure 4.1 The perimeter of the breast tissue.

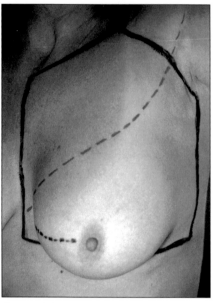

Figure 4.2 The perimeter of the breast, demonstrated on a patient.

The Breast MAP uses these same simple principles for mammography. By using anatomical landmarks of the breast and thorax, the mammography technologist can be assured that all the breast tissue will be included before making the exposure.

The Breast MAP can therefore help the technologist *see* mammography positioning in a *new light*.

ANATOMICAL STRUCTURES USED FOR POSITIONING AND IMAGE ANALYSIS

In order to relate the anatomical structures that are seen on the film to the patient, a number of relative structures must first be defined.

1. The Perimeter of the Breast

Perimeter of the Breast is defined by the following borders:
a. Lateral border .... Mobile   Axilla to IMF
b. Inferior border ... Mobile   IMF to sternum
c. Medial border..... Fixed   Sternum to sternoclavicular joint
d. Superior border . Fixed   Sternoclavicular joint to humeral head
e. Superior border . (extension)   Humeral head to axilla

The breast is physically defined by four borders. It is the goal of the technologist to include as much as possible of the breast tissue that lies within these borders on the combination of the two standard screening views. It is well documented that the MLO view demonstrates the maximum amount of breast tissue within this perimeter due to anatomical considerations and to the application of proven positioning techniques. The CC view is also necessary to provide additional information as well as a different imaging perspective that can be very helpful in sorting out superimposed structures on the MLO view. It is not that more breast tissue is seen by adding the CC projection, but the view does provide a valuable alternate image of the breast.

Two of the breast borders are mobile; two are fixed and immobile. The ability to move the two mobile borders is a critical component of optimum patient positioning. Both mobile borders are utilized for the positioning of both standard mammography views.

Lateral Border (Figure 4.1a)
This mobile breast border extends from the posterior aspect of the axilla, just anterior to the latissimus dorsi muscle down to the lateral border of the inframammary fold (IMF).

The lateral border is used to facilitate positioning of the MLO view. It is moved medially, to bring the nipple in line with the *free margin* of the pectoralis muscle which forms the *front* of the axilla. When the technologist performs this movement, she brings the breast tissue closer to the compression paddle and closer to the fixed medial breast margin, thereby including more medial breast tissue on the film. The bucky and compression paddle are angled to support and maintain the breast in this position for the MLO view.

For the CC view, the lateral, moveable border of the breast is again utilized to include more of the lateral glandular breast tissue on the film. The final positioning maneuver that the technologist performs, just as the compression is applied, is to pull the lateral breast tissue forward, onto the film. Proper compression will then maintain the breast in this position for the exposure.

Inferior Border (Figure 4.1b)
The inferior breast border is also mobile. It extends as a horizontal line from the inferior point of the lateral border to the inferior margin of the sternum.

The inferior border is elevated on both the CC and the MLO views so that the posterior nipple line (PNL) (page 92) is perpendicular to the chest wall. This will ensure the maximum visualization of breast tissue.

Medial Border (Figure 4.1c)

The medial border is a fixed border of the breast. It is essentially defined as a vertical line running along the mid-sternum. It extends from the inferior margin of the sternum up to the sternoclavicular joint.

Superior Border (Figure 4.1d)

The superior margin is also a fixed border of the breast. It extends from the sternoclavicular joint, under the clavicle, to meet the inferior medial margin of the humeral head.

An extension of the superior border (Figure 4.1e), continues from the inferior medial margin of the humeral head to the anterior margin of the latissimus dorsi muscle within the axilla.

This now completes the perimeter of the breast tissue that the technologist will focus on as she performs mammography examinations.

2. Pectoralis Muscle

The pectoralis major muscle plays a very important role in the mammography positioning process. Consideration for this anatomical structure is essential in understanding both patient positioning and the analysis of the clinical image. The pectoralis muscle has a major impact on the technologist's ability to demonstrate all of the breast tissue on the mammogram. It is interesting to note, however, that although the pectoralis muscle is NOT part of the breast, it does represent an important anatomical landmark during the positioning process and the subsequent evaluation of clinical images.

a. Anatomical Characteristics

Anatomically, the pectoralis muscle extends from the proximal humerus (just below the head of the humerus), where it is capped by the biceps muscle, across the thorax at varying degrees of angulation. It inserts along the lateral border of the sternum on the medial aspect of the thorax. The superior margin of the pectoralis muscle is horizontal. The lateral margin runs nearly vertical, along the lateral side of the thorax. Between these two margins, the muscle fibers fan out and are oriented at a variety of angles (Figure 4.3). These angulated muscle fibers are a primary focus when positioning the patient, particularly for the MLO view.

---

b. Mammography Angulation

Most technologists have been taught to *angle to the pectoralis muscle* when performing the MLO view. This is often confusing, given the variety of angles to choose from. The proper degree of angulation, chosen prior to patient positioning, does not relate to the variety of angles at which the muscle crosses the thorax. Instead, it is dictated by one particular segment of the muscle, specifically the free, mobile margin of the pectoralis muscle that forms the anterior margin of the axilla. The bucky should be angled so that it is parallel to this particular aspect of the pectoralis muscle (Figures 4.4 and 4.5).

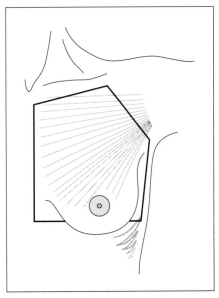

Figure 4.3 The orientation of the pectoralis muscle to the thorax.

In the process of positioning the MLO projection, the technologist's hand will elevate the lateral border of the breast, moving the tissue medially, toward the compression paddle. This position will be maintained by the angle of the bucky behind the breast laterally and the

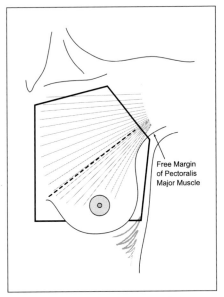

Figure 4.4 The "free margin" of the pectoalis muscle which determines the degree of angulation.

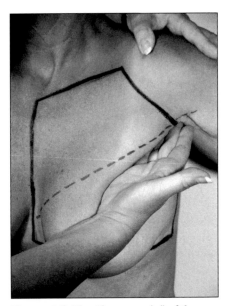

Figure 4.5 The "free margin" of the pectoralis muscle, demonstrated with a patient.

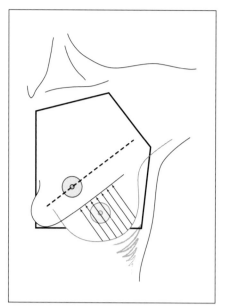

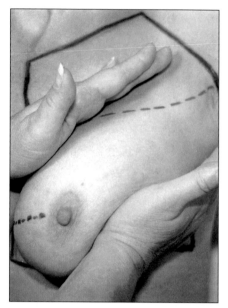

Figure 4.6 The breast is moved medially so that the nipple plane is now parallel with the *free margin* of the pectoralis muscle.

Figure 4.7 The plane of the nipple is parallel with the *free margin* of the pectoralis muscle - demonstrated with a patient.

simultaneous orientation of the compression paddle medially. Provided that the correct bucky angulation has been selected, the breast tissue will remain in this position, thus facilitating the visualization of the maximum amount of breast tissue on the image. An improper degree of angulation, particularly if the angle is too steep, can result in the omission of medial breast tissue on the resulting image (Figure 4.22). It will also result in unnecessary discomfort for the patient.

Once again, the degree of angulation is determined by the *free margin* of the pectoralis muscle as it forms the front of the axilla. When the breast is elevated and supported in this position, the nipple will be in line, or parallel with the free muscle margin. The result will be the inclusion of the maximum amount of breast tissue with the greatest possible degree of patient comfort (Figure 4.21). A critical factor here is that the pectoralis muscle must be relaxed. When compression is applied parallel to these loose, flexible muscle fibers, more tissue can be pulled away from the chest wall with the least amount of discomfort for the patient.

The method to determine the degree of angulation is simple. The patient's arm is elevated at 90 degrees to her thorax. This, in essence, simulates the position of the arm and shoulder for the MLO projection. The bucky should be aligned parallel to the *free margin* of the pectoralis muscle that forms the front of the axilla.

Because the pectoralis muscle extends from the area below the humeral head, forms the front of the axilla, and then crosses the thorax, inserting into the lateral aspect of the sternum, it is apparent that the orientation of this muscle will vary with body habitus. As the relationship of these anatomical components changes, so will the appropriate angulation for the MLO view. Specific attention should be placed on the length of the patient's thorax. A patient with a long thorax will require a steeper degree of angulation (Figure 4.9), while a patient

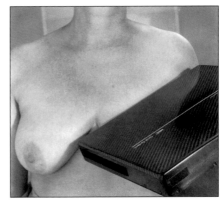

Figure 4.8 The bucky should be angled parallel to the free margin of the pectoralis muscle that forms the front of the axilla. From here, follow the muscle as it crosses the thorax to insert into the lateral aspect of the lower third of the sternum.

with a short thorax will need a lesser degree of angulation (Figure 4.10). The average muscle angle will fall between 45 and 55 degrees, with deviations of 5 to 10 degrees in either direction to accommodate changes in muscle orientation with varied configurations of the thorax area.

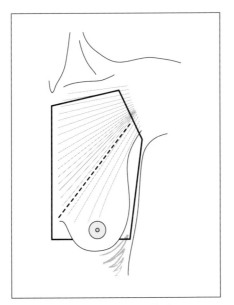

Figure 4.9 Approximately 60 degree angulation (steeper) due to an elongated thorax.

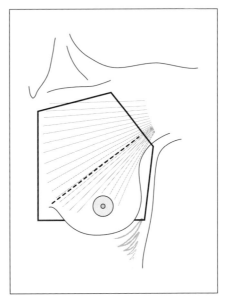

Figure 4.10 Approximately 40 degree angulation (less steep) due to a short thorax.

It is important to avoid selecting the bucky angle on the basis of overall body habitus. While generalizations may sometimes be correct, there are many exceptions. Taller patients often do require a higher degree of angulation (closer to 60 degrees), as their overall body habitus is elongated. Their legs, as well as their thorax are longer. However, a tall patient may have very long legs and a shorter, more average thorax. This patient will require average angulation (closer to 50 degrees), instead of the steeper angulation that would normally be appropriate for a tall patient. Also, a short patient may have an unusually long thorax and will therefore require steeper angulation than one would select based on her general body stature. The angle must always be chosen on the basis of the relationship of the pectoralis muscle to the thorax, not by the overall height of the individual.

The weight of the patient is not considered an important factor in this evaluation as an increase or decrease in weight will not change the basic relationship of the muscle to the thorax. Obviously, significant variations in weight, i.e. extremely thin or obese patients will require individual positioning considerations and options.

c. Clinical Image Evaluation of the Pectoralis Muscle

Mammographically, the pectoralis muscle serves as an anatomical landmark from which clinical images can be evaluated for the inclusion or exclusion of breast tissue. While it is only visualized on approximately 30% of all CC views, its presence on the MLO is mandatory.

i. MLO Criteria

For the MLO view, specific criteria should be used to evaluate the overall image based on the radiographic characteristics of the pectoralis muscle. Examining four individual factors will determine if breast tissue had been adequately visualized; it will also provide valuable information for repeat views should the basic criteria not be met initially.

The pectoralis muscle on the MLO should be visualized as follows:

- From the axilla down to the level of the PNL
- Wide margin at the axilla
- Convex in appearance
- Radioluscent appearance

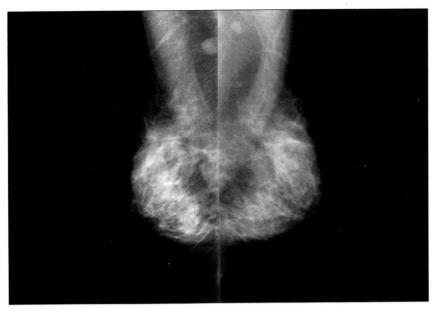

Figure 4.11 The criteria for visualizing pectoralis muscle is fulfilled by these MLO views.

ii. CC Criteria

The pectoralis muscle on the CC should be visualized as follows:

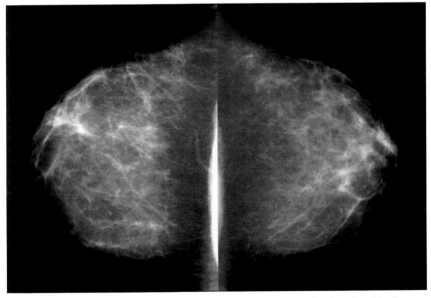

Figure 4.12 On a CC view, the pectoralis muscle is generally visualized in the central to medial aspect of the breast.

- On approximately 30% of all CC views
- Generally located in the central to medial aspect of the breast

While visualization of the pectoralis muscle is essential in the evaluation of the MLO view and its specific appearance is an indication of proper positioning, this is not true of its appearance on the CC view. Because the CC view is performed across (rather than parallel to) the alignment of the pectoral muscle, it will naturally be more difficult to image the muscle on this view. Improved positioning techniques that include elevation of the IMF (Figure 4.15), pulling the breast tissue onto the receptor with both hands (Figure 4.43), and the use of dependent positioning (available with some mammography equipment) will certainly improve the chances of demonstrating the pectoralis muscle on the CC view. Another consideration that is frequently overlooked is the general status of the pectoralis muscle itself. Where minimal muscle development is evident due to poor physical condition, demonstration of this structure on the mammogram can be very challenging. In other situations, when the pectoralis is tight, rigid and / or well developed, it may be very difficult to image muscle on the CC view because of its solid status. When the pectoralis muscle is loose and relaxed, it is far easier to pull it forward, away from the chest wall and thus image it on the film. Visualizing the muscle on the CC view may not actually indicate that *more* breast tissue has been imaged. Its presence simply confirms that breast tissue has been included back to the chest wall. Complete visualization of the breast tissue on the CC view can be confidently accomplished even when muscle is not imaged by evaluating the Posterior Nipple Line (PNL).

3. Posterior Nipple Line (PNL)

Although the posterior nipple line is not actually an anatomical structure of the breast or the patient, it is an important consideration in mammography positioning and in the analysis of the resulting images. The PNL is a landmark that represents the alignment of the nipple to the chest wall. It can also be referred to as the *axis of the nipple*. A young, developing woman's PNL will be almost perpendicular to the chest wall (Figure 4.13). As a woman ages and supportive fibrous structures atrophy, the axis of the nipple will change. The breast tends to droop, with the nipple pointing in a more downward position. As a result, the PNL, or the axis of the nipple, will also angle in a more downward position (Figure 4.14); this creates the potential for superimposition of inferior breast structures.

The goal of mammography is to visualize the breast completely and clearly. The PNL can influence both of these factors. Mammography positioning for

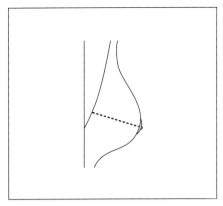

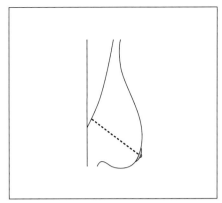

Figure 4.13 The PNL is elevated properly for the MLO view.

Figure 4.14 The PNL is not elevated properly for the MLO view. Sometimes this may be difficult, depending on the size and weight of the breast.

both the CC and the MLO views should include elevating the PNL so that it is perpendicular to the chest wall.

When positioning for the MLO view, the inferior border of the breast is elevated so that the breast is held in an *up and out* position. When the breast is positioned properly, the PNL should be as close to perpendicular to the thorax as possible; this may be particularly difficult with a large, heavy breast. However, every effort must be made to elevate the breast properly to minimize superimposition of inferior breast structures. The PNL also serves as a reference point for clinical image evaluation; the pectoralis muscle should be visualized down to this level on the MLO projection.

Positioning for the CC view again requires that the mobile inferior border of the breast be elevated. It is recommended that the breast be moved superiorly to its *maximum height of natural mobility*. An easier way to accomplish the proper position is to simply elevate the breast until, as with the MLO, the PNL is perpendicular to the chest wall (Figure 4.15). This, along with a number of other positioning factors, will help to ensure complete visualization of breast tissue for this view.

The length of the PNL is measured on the CC and MLO views to determine if adequate tissue has been imaged on the mammogram. On the MLO view, the PNL is extended back from the nipple, perpendicular to the anterior margin of the pectoralis muscle. Note: this line is perpendicular to the muscle, NOT to the edge of the film. In the majority of cases (when the PNL is perpendicular to the pectoralis muscle), the PNL on the MLO view will point slightly down-

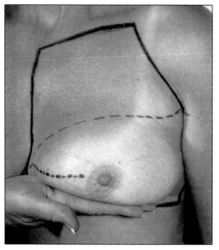

Figure 4.15 For the CC view, the breast is elevated until the PNL Is perpendicular to the chest wall.

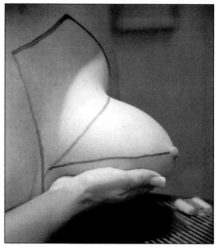

Figure 4.16 Elevating the breast until the PNL is perpendicular to the chest wall will help to ensure complete visualization of breast tissue for this view.

ward, following the natural contour of the breast tissue (Figures 4.13 and 4.17). This is easily understood, considering the natural angle or slope of the pectoralis muscle to which the PNL must be perpendicularly aligned. A linear measurement is made from the nipple to the point that the PNL intersects the muscle or when it reaches the edge of the film (whichever comes first).

On the CC view, the PNL measurement is made from the nipple to the edge of the film, regardless of whether muscle has been imaged. These two measure-

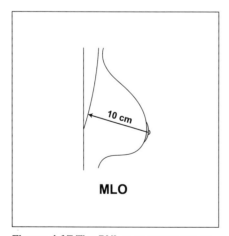

Figure 4.17 The PNL measurement on the MLO view.

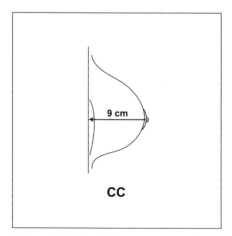

Figure 4.18 The PNL measurement on the CC view.

ments are then compared. Adequate tissue is considered to be imaged when the CC measurement is within 1.0 cm of the MLO measurement.

4. Glandular Breast Tissue

Breast tissue is distributed throughout the perimeter of the breast. The distribution varies, with the majority of breast tissue extending into the upper, outer quadrant. Imaging the breast using the two standard views will not always ensure visualization of all breast tissue for every patient. Because of variations in breast size and shape, there are times when it may be difficult for the technologist to include all the breast tissue on the MLO and CC views.

It should be noted that studies have shown that all components of the overall criteria for inclusion of breast tissue are rarely met 100% of the time using the standard, 4 view mammogram (Bassett, LW Radiology 1993; 188:803-806). While our primary goals are to achieve excellence in positioning and to image all the breast tissue, there are factors beyond our control that may prohibit the achievement of ideal images with every patient. Difficult body habitus and the lack of patient cooperation are two of the major inhibiting factors that mammographers frequently encounter. These challenges will be addressed in the following material.

C. POSITIONING PROBLEM SOLVING UTILIZING THE BREAST MAP

1. The Mediolateral Oblique - MLO View

There are numerous anatomic landmarks that help us to evaluate the MLO view while positioning the patient and critiquing the clinical images. These landmarks are helpful in determining whether the maximum amount of breast tissue has been included. Their exclusion can help us to evaluate and correct causative positioning problems.

a. Clinical Evaluation of the MLO

In order to ensure maximum inclusion of breast tissue, the technologist and radiologist should consider the following criteria:

- inclusion of maximum amount of breast tissue within the perimeter of breast margins (Figure 4.19)
- breast supported up and away from thorax (not drooping) and as close to perpendicular to the chest wall as possible (Figure 4.13)

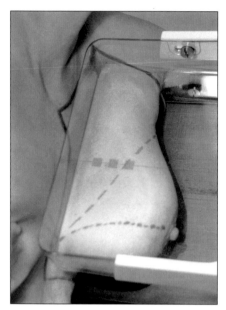

Figure 4.19 Include the maximum amount of tissue within the perimeter of the breast on the image.

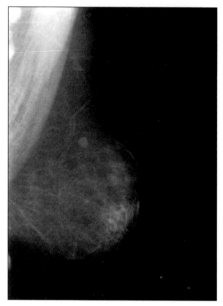

Figure 4.20 Clinical image reflecting the inclusion of the maximum amount of tissue within the perimeter of the breast.

- visualization of retroglandular fat
- inframammary fold open
- nipple in profile
- visualization of pectoral muscle:
  - included from axilla to PNL
  - wide margin at axilla
  - convex configuration
  - radioluscent appearance

b. Problems with the MLO View

Problems 1 to 5 deal with inadequate visualization of the pectoral muscle; additional, miscellaneous problems follow afterward.

1 *What's Wrong?*

Muscle not visualized down to the PNL (usually IMF is also excluded).

What it means:

Medial and inferior breast tissue could be excluded.

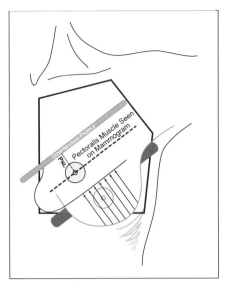

Figure 4.21 The proper degree of angulation supports (and therefore images) more of the medial breast tissue.

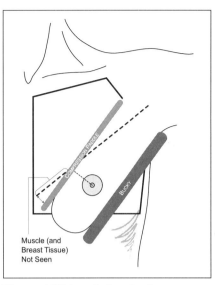

Figure 4.22 Angulation that is too steep will not support the medial, inferior breast. Breast tissue and pectoralis muscle in this area will not be visualized on the clinical image.

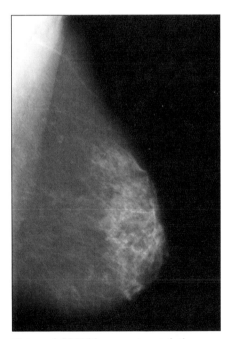

Figure 4.23 With correct angulation, the muscle is vusualized down to the PNL; more medial and inferior breast tissue will be included.

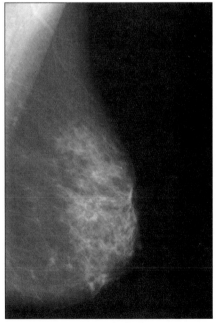

Figure 4.24 The angulation is too steep; muscle is not visualized down to the PNL and medial, inferior breast tissue could be excluded.

Corrective Action:

- Check degree of angulation - it's probably too steep (Figure 4.22). It should be parallel to the free, flexible margin of the pectoralis muscle that forms the anterior border of the axilla (Figure 4.21).
- Breast must be mobilized medially until nipple is parallel with free muscle margin (Figure 4.7).
- Patient must be facing machine with both feet, hips, and shoulders.
- Make sure breast tissue has been pulled away from chest wall.
- Compression paddle must be adjacent to sternum and ribs; be sure patient has not leaned away (Figure 4.37).

2 What's Wrong?

Pectoralis muscle is radiopaque (should be radioluscent).

What it means:

Medial and lateral breast tissue are superimposed over pectoral muscle which may subsequently obscure proper visualization of breast structures. This could result from improper compression; optimal visualization of anterior breast tissue will be compromised as well.

Corrective Action:

- Check for adequate compression of superior, lateral area of breast.
- Encourage patient to relax her shoulder and chest muscles.
- Make sure corner of the bucky is placed properly in the axilla - should be just anterior to (but not including) the latissimus dorsi muscle (Figure 4.30).
- Check technique selection.
- Check AEC (photocell) position.

3 What's Wrong?

Muscle is concave rather than convex in appearance.

What it means:

Breast tissue may be excluded by failing to mobilize the breast properly. The muscle must be relaxed.

Corrective Action:

- Make sure patient's shoulder is relaxed forward and down.
- Check height of bucky - it may be too high.
- Shoulder, elbow, arm, and hand must be relaxed; elbow should be bent behind the receptor.

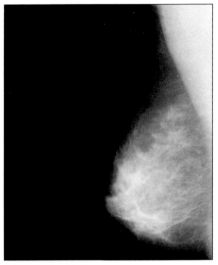

Figure 4.25 The pectoralis muscle is radiopaque; information has been compromised in all areas of the clinical image due to inadequate compression.

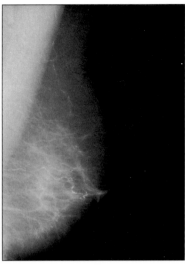

Figure 4.26 The pectoralis muscle is radiopaque; poor image quality is evident once again.

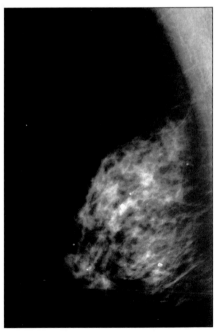

Figure 4.27 A concave contour to the pectoralis muscle indicates that the patient was not relaxed or the breast was not properly mobilized and compressed close to its fixed, medial border.

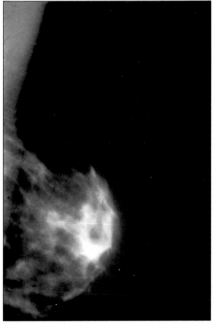

Figure 4.28 Again, a concave muscle configeration indicates that the patient was not relaxed, or the breast was not properly mobilized for the image.

4   What's Wrong?

Muscle appears with a narrow margin (vs. wide margin as it should appear) at the axilla and runs parallel to posterior margin of image down to PNL.

What it means:

Correct angle is chosen (indicated by visualization of muscle to PNL). However, posterior lateral and medial breast tissue could be excluded.

Corrective Action:

- Check placement of bucky in axilla - it may be too far forward in the axilla (Figure 4.31). It should be just anterior to latissimus dorsi muscle, in the posterior part of the axilla.
- Make sure breast is mobilized medially.
- Make sure shoulder is rolled forward and down.
- Make sure patient does not lean away as compression is applied.
- Check to make sure the compression paddle is adjacent to the sternum and the medial border of the breast (Figure 4.19).

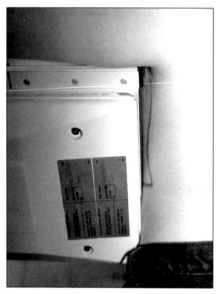

Figure 4.29 The corner of the bucky is too far forward in the axilla; the patient may have leaned away from the receptor before the compresssion paddle secured her position. Note how much lateral tissue has been excluded from the image.

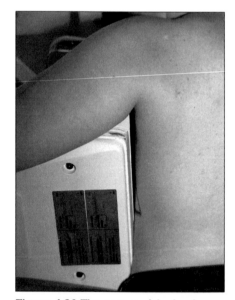

Figure 4.30 The corner of the bucky should be located just anterior to the latissimus dorsi muscle, in the posterior part of the patient's axilla.

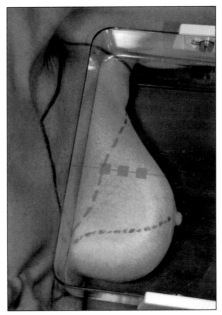

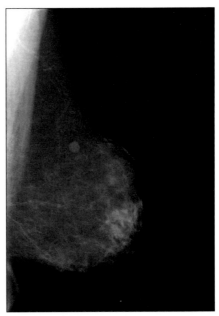

Figure 4.31 The corner of the bucky is not placed deep enough into the patient's axilla. Compare this picture with Figure 4.19, which demonstrates the correct position of the bucky in the patient's axilla.

Figure 4.32 The clinical appearance of an image when the corner of the bucky is not positioned deep enough in the patient's axilla. A narrow muscle shadow is seen along the edge of the film (compare to Figure 4.20).

5 What's Wrong?

Too much pectoral muscle.

What it means:

A well developed pectoral muscle could inhibit proper compression and visualization of anterior breast tissue. There should be good separation of anterior structures; motion should not be evident.

Corrective Action:

- Do additional MLO focusing on compression and visualization of anterior breast tissue.

 The pectoralis muscle is an important anatomical landmark that is used both to position the patient and to evaluate the clinical images.

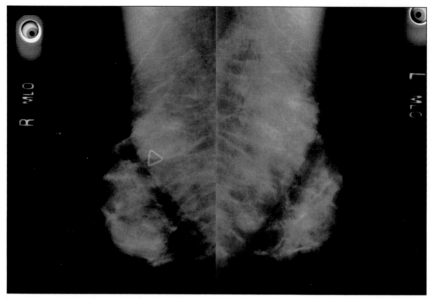

Figure 4.33 An overdeveloped pectoralis muscle can interfere with adequate evaluation of breast tissue. The palpable lesion on the R MLO view is difficult to see through the muscle tissue.

Other problems with the MLO:

6   What's Wrong?

Anterior breast drooping on the film (the camel's nose) reference (Figures 4.14 and 4.34)

What it means:

Possible superimposition and poor visualization of inferior and anterior breast tissue.

Corrective Action:

- Ensure that breast is supported *up and out* during the compression process.
- Try to position the nipple and PNL as close to *perpendicular to the chest wall* as possible (Figure 4.13).
- The technologist's hand must be drawn out in the direction of the nipple rather than down, toward the patient's feet. If the hand is withdrawn in a downward direction, it frequently pulls breast tissue down with it.

If the breast shape, prominent axillary tissue and/or pectoralis muscle inhibits adequate compression of the anterior breast, an anterior compression view should be performed (as described in Problem #5).

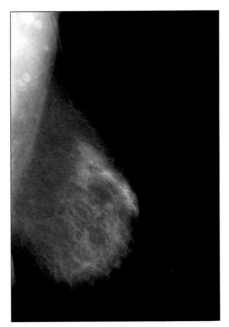

Figure 4.34 The anterior breast tissue is *drooping*; this is the classic *camel's nose* appearance.

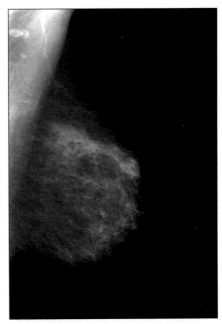

Figure 4.35 With correct support as compression is applied, the breast will maintain its *up-and-out* position for the MLO view.

7 What's Wrong?

Inadequate visualization of the IMF.

What it means:

Without visualization of the IMF it is not certain that all the posterior, inferior breast tissue (particularly the medial area) has been included.

Corrective Action:

- Check patient position - she must be facing machine with both feet, hips, and shoulders facing forward.
- Check degree of angulation - it may be too steep and therefore not supporting the breast medially (Figure 4.22).
- Check to make sure the compression paddle is adjacent to the sternum and *over* the IMF; the medial and inferior borders of the breast should be included in the LIQ (Figure 4.19).
- Elevate the breast with the "up-and-out" maneuver.

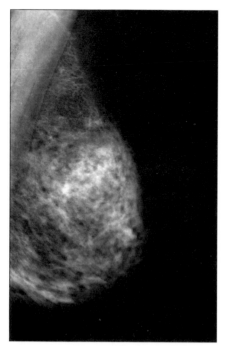

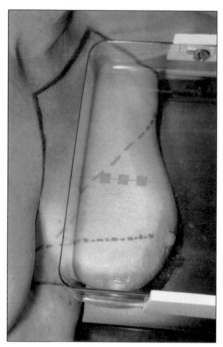

Figure 4.36 The IMF is not visualized; often posterior, inferior, medial breast tissue has also been excluded from the image.

Figure 4.37 Without adequate support, the breast will droop on the MLO view. Superimposition will be evident in the IMF area.

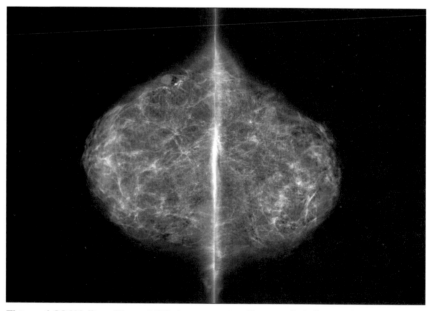

Figure 4.38 Well positioned CC views; pectoralis muscle is imaged on these views approximately 30% of the time.

2. The Craniocaudal - CC View

a. Clinical Evaluation of the CC

In order to insure maximum inclusion of breast tissue, the technologist and radiologist should consider the following criteria:

- Visualization of central, subareolar and medial aspects of the breast.
- Visualization of pectoral muscle on approximately 30% of cases.
- PNL must measure within 1.0 cm of PNL measurement on the MLO.
- Retroglandular fat visualized behind glandular breast tissue.

b. Problems with the CC

1 What's Wrong?

Failure to visualize adequate breast tissue compared to the MLO view (PNL measured on the CC should be within 1.0 cm of the PNL measured on the MLO).

What it means:

Possible exclusion of breast tissue.

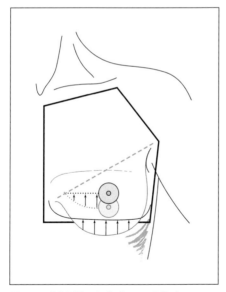

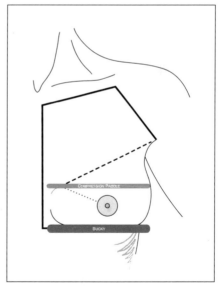

Figure 4.39 The inferior mobile breast border is moved superiorly so the PNL is perpendicular to the thorax.

Figure 4.40 When the breast is not properly elevated, the PNL is not perpendicular to the chest wall and it is unlikely that superior posterior breast tissue, including the medial aspect of the pectoralis muscle, will be imaged.

Corrective Action:

- Be sure that the IMF is elevated properly (the PNL should be perpendicular to thorax, Figure 4.15). Improper elevation will potentially exclude superior tissue. This positioning error can also lead to failure to visualize pectoralis muscle on the CC when it could otherwise be imaged.

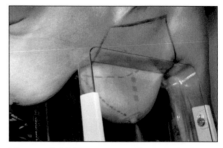

Figure 4.41 The pectoralis muscle is more likely to be imaged when the PNL is perpendicular to the chest wall.

- Breast should be pulled onto bucky with both hands (Figure 4.43).
- Check patient position - be sure she has not pulled back.
- Bring patient's head forward and around side of face shield and tube head, on the medial side of breast being imaged.
- Check that compression paddle is directly adjacent to the rib cage (Figure 4.41 and 4.122).

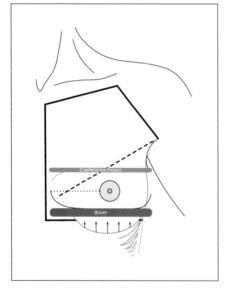

Figure 4.42 The PNL is perpendicular to the chest wall when the breast is properly elevated; there is greater likelihood of visualizing pectoralis muscle in the central-to-medial portion of the breast.

2 What's Wrong?

Pectoral muscle not visualized on approximately 30% of all CC views.

What it means:

Possible exclusion of breast tissue.

Corrective Action:

- Be sure that IMF is elevated properly (the PNL should be perpendicular to thorax) (Figures 4.39 and 4.42). Improper elevation will potentially exclude superior tissue (Figure 4.40). This positioning error may also be the reason for failure to visualize pectoralis muscle on the CC view.
- Breast should be pulled onto bucky with both hands (Figure 4.43).
- Check patient position - be sure she has not pulled back.

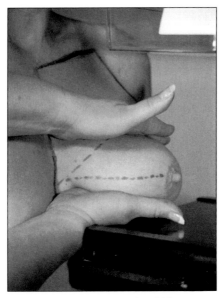

Figure 4.43 The breast should be pulled onto the bucky with both hands.

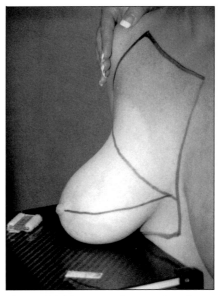

Figure 4.44 Improper breast elevation will miss the opportunity to visualize posterior tissue and pectoralis muscle on the image. Compare with Figure 4.16 showing correct elevation.

- Bring patient's head forward and around side of face shield and tube head, on the medial side of breast being imaged.
- Check that compression paddle is directly adjacent to the rib cage (Figure 4.41 and 4.122).

3 *What's Wrong?*

Inadequate lateral breast tissue visualized; glandular tissue extending off edge of film on lateral side of the image (Figure 4.46)
and / or
There is an area of concern in the posterior lateral aspect of the breast that is not visualized.

What it means:

Possible exclusion of breast tissue.

Corrective Action:

- Using hand that is anchoring top of the breast, pull lateral breast tissue forward while the compression is applied. Make sure medial breast is not sacrificed during this maneuver, but now also attempt to include more lateral glandular breast tissue.

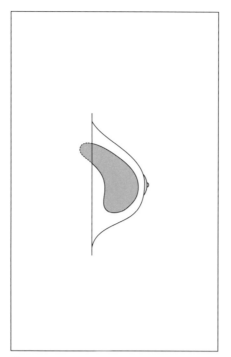

Figure 4.45 Glandular tissue extends laterally, beyond the edge of the film.

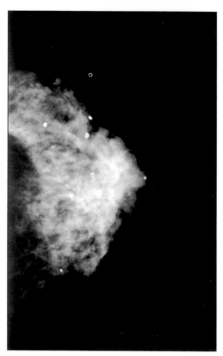

Figure 4.46 Clinical image demonstrating glandular tissue extending laterally, beyond the edge of the film.

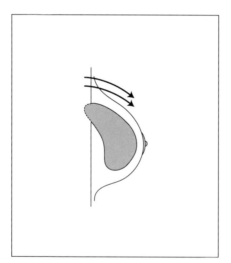

Figure 4.47 The lateral, mobile border of the breast should be pulled forward, onto the receptor as compression is applied.

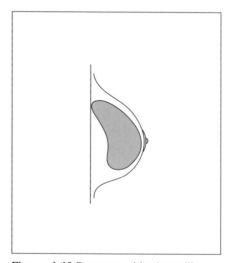

Figure 4.48 Proper positioning will help to include all lateral glandular breast tissue on the CC image.

- Perform an Exaggerated Lateral Craniocaudal View - XCCL.
- An Axillary Tail View - AT (formerly Cleopatra view) can be performed for better visualization of axillary tail, however, note: this view does not provide true lateral or medial orientation to the nipple and should not be used for localization purposes (Figure 4.67).

4 What's Wrong?

Inadequate medial breast tissue visualized
and/or
Area of concern in medial breast.

What it means:

Possible exclusion of medial breast tissue and incomplete visualization of medially located *mass* (could be medial insertion of pectoralis muscle, but must be proven).

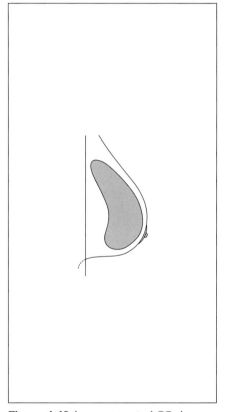

Figure 4.49 An exaggerated CC view (lateral) will image the posterior border of the lateral glandular breast tissue.

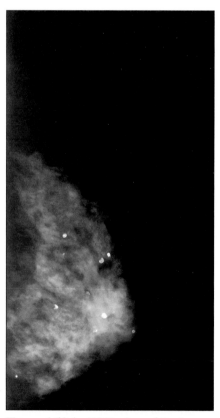

Figure 4.50 An XCCL view of the image in Figure 4.46 showing the posterior border of the lateral glandular breast tissue.

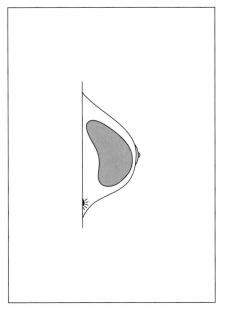

Figure 4.51 A questionable *mass* is seen in the medial aspect of the breast.

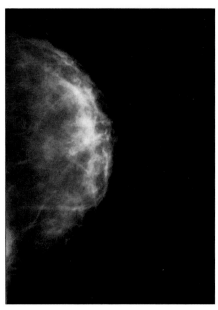

Figure 4.52 Clinical image demonstrating a questionable medial *mass*.

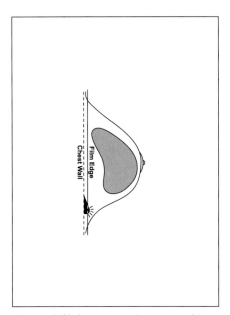

Figure 4.53 A suspected *mass* could simply be the medial insertion of the pectoralis muscle. The medial, posterior margin of the pectoralis muscle may not be seen on the film.

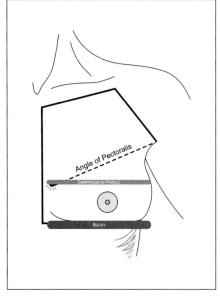

Figure 4.54 Breast MAP illustrating the deep medial *mass* as the insertion of the pectoralis muscle near the sternal border.

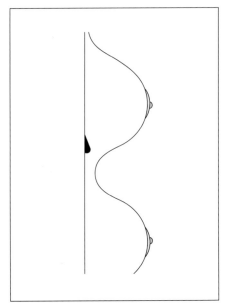

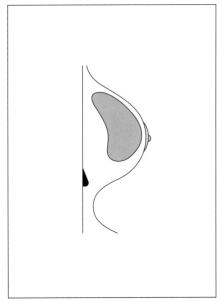

Figure 4.55 CV view, with the breasts centered symmetrically on the bucky. Manual technique will be required for this exposure. This image verifies insertion of pectoralis muscle versus a *mass*.

Figure 4.56 CV view, with the breast off-centered to allow the AEC device to be utilized for the exposure.

Corrective Action:

- Make sure patient's ribs (medially, adjacent to sternum) are resting against receptor (Figure 4.41 and 4.122).
- Make sure opposite breast is draped over corner of bucky (Figure 4.41).
- Patient's head should be brought forward and around the face shield and tube head on the medial side of the breast being imaged.
- Check that compression paddle is directly adjacent to rib cage (medially) (Figure 4.41 and 4.122).
- Perform a Cleavage View (CV) (Figures 4.55 and 4.56).

The majority of unacceptable clinical images are a result of failure to include adequate breast tissue. Many of these errors can be eliminated by utilizing the breast MAP to correlate positioning techniques with the patient's anatomy.

D. APPLYING THE BREAST MAP TO ADDITIONAL MAMMOGRAPHIC VIEWS

Additional views are occasionally required for a variety of reasons. The selection of additional views can be divided into specific categories, according to need.

Category 1: Views that Image Areas not Included on the Standard Views and that Provide Orientation Information

Category 2: Views that Counteract Superimposition and/or *Triangulate* an Area of Concern Seen Only on One Standard View

Category 3: Views Used to Detail and/or Provide Clarification of an Area of Concern

Category 4: Views Used for Mammography of the Difficult Patient

***Note:** Refer to page 173 in Section III of this Chapter for a list of mammography views and their standard abbreviations.

1. Views that Image Areas not Included on the Standard Views and that Provide Orientation Information

a. Views for Specific Areas of Breast Tissue Not Seen on Standard Views

There are times when a portion of breast tissue may not be included on the two standard mammography images. When this occurs, the technologist can determine which additional view should be done by asking and answering the following questions:

- *What part of the breast needs to be visualized?*
- *In which projection?*
- *Which view will accomplish this?*

The answers to these questions will direct the technologist to the most appropriate view to demonstrate the area in question. An example would be as follows:

On the MLO view, all positioning criteria were met. However on the CC view, a portion of glandular tissue was missing laterally; there was an area of concern close to the lateral edge of the film. Using this situation, ask and answer these three questions:

- *What part of the breast needs to be visualized?* ... Lateral
- *In which projection?* ... Craniocaudal
- *Which view?* ... XCCL

This category can also give the technologist and radiologist additional information that will be helpful to accurately locate an area of concern in the breast. Therefore, these views will also provide true orientation to the nipple for localization purposes.

b. Views that Provide Lateral / Medial Orientation to the Nipple or PNL

The following views will provide true lateral and medial orientation to the PNL (and the nipple) when an area of interest is not seen on the CC view:

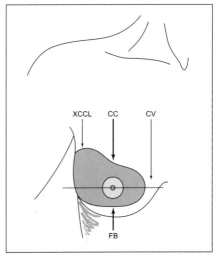

Figure 4.57 Views that demonstrate lateral / medial orientation to the nipple.

View	Target Area	Figure Reference
XCCL	lateral posterior tissue (in craniocaudal plane)	4.49
CV	medial posterior tissue (in craniocaudal plane)	4.55 and 4.56
FB	superior tissue	4.58
FBXCCL*	superior lateral posterior tissue	4.59
FBCV*	superior medial posterior tissue	4.60
Lumpogram	high superior tissue	4.62 and 4.63

*Note: These views are not included on list of views in ACR/CAR manuals. They are, however, creative ways of imaging difficult areas of the breast.

c. Views that Provide Superior /Inferior Orientation to the Nipple or PNL

Lateral mammography views will provide true superior and inferior orientation to the PNL (and the nipple):

- Lateral views can be accomplished by directing the beam from Medial to Lateral (ML) or from Lateral to Medial (LM). Lateral views are valuable for a number of reasons:

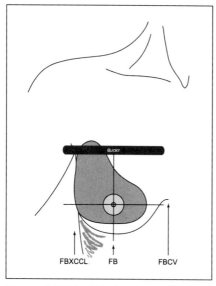

Figure 4.58 The FB view and variations, for improved visualization of superior breast tissue.

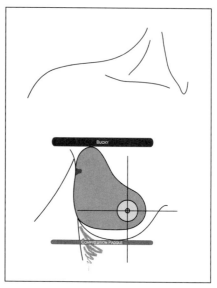

Figure 4.59 The FBXCCL view demonstrates high, superior, lateral areas of concern.

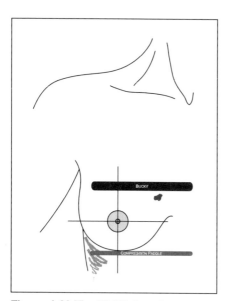

Figure 4.60 The FBCV view demonstrates high, superior, medial areas of concern.

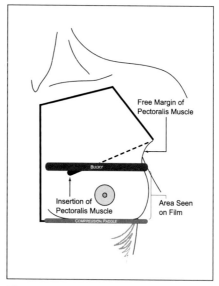

Figure 4.61 The FBCV view can be used to verify pectoralis muscle insertion.

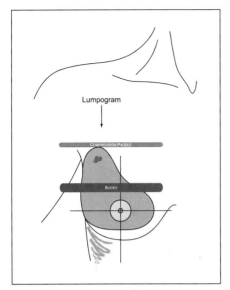

Figure 4.62 A lumpogram (anterior view) for high, superior masses.

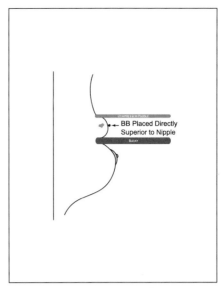

Figure 4.63 A lumpogram (lateral view) for superior areas of concern.

- To provide another projection of structures that may be superimposed on the MLO view.
- As an alternate view for patients who cannot be imaged with a MLO or a LMO view (those requiring a wheelchair or stretcher; difficult body habitus).
- To triangulate an area of concern seen on the CC and MLO views.
- To demonstrate the effect of gravity on air/fluid levels in the breast. This is important with pneumocystography and with milk of calcium (sediment *pools* in the bottom of microcysts, forming a *cup-like* appearance on a lateral view; area is vague and *smudgy* on the CC and unclear on the MLO due to a layering effect).

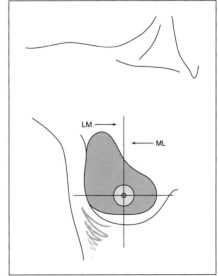

Figure 4.64 Views that provide true superior and inferior orientation to the nipple.

- To provide the shortest direct route to a lesion for a needle biopsy or needle localization procedure; for this application, the projection that will position the biopsy paddle closest to the area of concern must be used (ML for a medial lesion and LM for a lateral lesion).

The LM view should be the primary choice for a lateral projection except when a localization or biopsy procedure is being performed for a medial lesion. There are many reasons for recommending the LM projection:

1. More lateral breast tissue will be included due to utilization of the mobile lateral border of the breast when positioning.

2. Positioning a LM projection is much easier because there is *nothing in the way* of the compression paddle compared to the ML projection where the technologist must deal with the opposite breast, the ribs, the sternum, and the patient's abdomen. The potential to lose medial tissue is much higher when the compression paddle must maneuver around all these *obstacles*.

3. The position of the image receptor will facilitate improved visualization of the posterior medial breast tissue; this is often the most difficult area of the breast to image. The maximum amount of medial tissue will be imaged if the edge of the bucky is offset slightly toward the opposite side of the sternum, pressing into the breast that is not being imaged (Figure 4.66). This bucky placement will help ensure that the width of

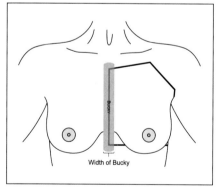

Figure 4.65 The bucky has been positioned improperly, directly over the mid-sternum; posterior, medial tissue will not be included on this image.

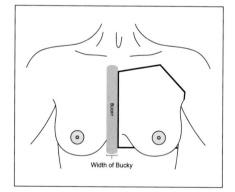

Figure 4.66 The bucky has been properly *off-set* toward the opposite breast; all the posterior, medial breast tissue will be included on this image.

the bucky does not obscure medial breast tissue on the side that is being imaged as in Figure 4.65.

4. The MLO view provides superior detail for lateral breast tissue, due to its proximity to the image receptor. Conversely, the LM view provides superior detail for medial breast tissue, again due to the location of the image receptor. This will provide the radiologist with the opportunity to now see the medial breast in better detail. Medial posterior breast tissue is often the most difficult area of the breast to image; it is also the area with the highest potential for exclusion on mammography images.

5. A conventional, logical protocol would automatically assume that a ML view is the best projection for a lesion seen in the lateral tissue on the CC projection. This projection would provide improved detail of the area of concern due to it's proximity to the image receptor. However, other considerations may influence this choice. First, the possibility exists that lateral tissue may actually move somewhat closer to the receptor on a lateromedial projection due to the mobility of lateral breast tissue. Second, and from the opposite perspective, positioning the lesion away from the receptor may be advantageous by providing a slightly magnified effect on the image; magnification technique is frequently used to investigate abnormalities.

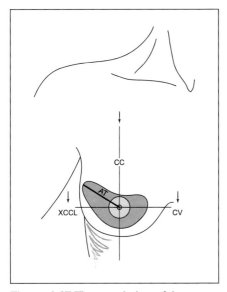

Figure 4.67 The angulation of the beam for the AT view will not provide true medial / lateral or true superior / inferior orientation to the nipple.

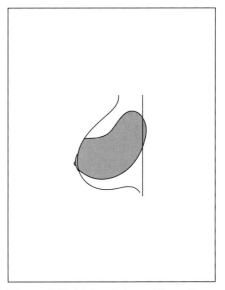

Figure 4.68 A lateral view of the axillary tail area.

Axillary Tail

The AT view will not provide information regarding medial or lateral orientation of a lesion relative to the nipple; it simply provides the opportunity to accomplish focal compression of the tissue in the axillary tail area. It can also be helpful when prominent superior and lateral breast tissue is present. It is sometimes impossible to *see behind* the lateral, glandular tissue on the CC view. An XCCL will visualize more lateral tissue (Figure 4.49), but it will not include superior tissue that is oriented obliquely toward the axilla. When an abnormality is located in this area, the AT view will provide an additional, alternate projection of this tissue. Note that the AT view is usually performed with a 25-30 degree angulation. If the CC is imaged at 0 degrees and an average MLO is imaged at 50-55 degrees, the AT view would be almost exactly half way between the MLO and the CC view. While it does provide valuable additional information, it cannot be used for orthogonal (a view that is 90 degrees different) localization of a lesion relative to the nipple because of the tube angulation.

2. Views that Counteract Superimposition and/or Triangulate an Area of Concern Seen Only on One Standard View

The LM view and Rolled CC views are very useful and may have some advantages compared to spot compression views (with or without magnification) when an area of interest is seen on only one view and there is a low degree of suspicion that the area of interest is, in fact, a real lesion. These views can be accomplished quickly and without the additional time and effort needed to change the equipment set up for spot compression or magnification views. This will also help to minimize patient anxiety; she will perceive little change from her routine images. If the area of concern persists after performing the LM view or the Rolled CC view, by triangulation you will be able to determine where to look for it on the view where it was not initially seen.

a. Triangulation Made Easy

(Based on an article published by Sickles, EW. Practical Solutions to Common Mammographic Problems: Tailoring the Examination. AJR 1988; 151:31-39.)

When you see an area of concern on the MLO view that is not demonstrated on the CC view and you want to:

    a) prove it is real versus superimposition of structures, and

    b) locate it on the CC view,

the first question that must be answered will be: Is it real?

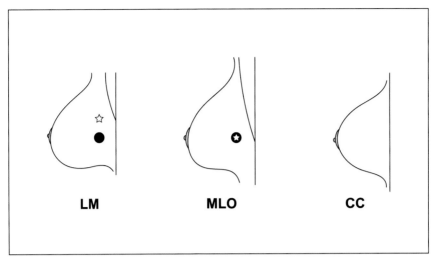

Figure 4.69 The use of the LM view to counteract the superimposition of structures. If it *goes away*, it was most likely superimposed breast tissue.

This may be accomplished by performing a LM view. If the area of concern was not real, but simply superimposed structures, it will *disappear* (Figure 4.69).

If it is real and persists on the lateral image, compare its location on the LM view to its location on the MLO view. This will help to determine where it will be located on the CC view.

1. Line up the films on the view box in the following order, from left to right: LM - MLO - CC (or right to left: CC, MLO, LM*).

   *TIP: This is easy to remember - the films must be hung in the sequence they are done:
   CC, first ... MLO, second, ... and LM, last.

2. Make sure all the nipples are pointing in the same direction, and are at the same level on the viewbox.

3. Draw an imaginary line through the area of concern on the LM, then through the same area of concern seen on the MLO view. Extend this line into the CC view, and it will *point* to the area where the lesion is located (Figure 4.70). Knowing the general location of the abnormality allows you now to focus on additional views that will demonstrate this area more thoroughly. For example: XCCL for lateral lesions, CV for medial lesions, FB for central areas.

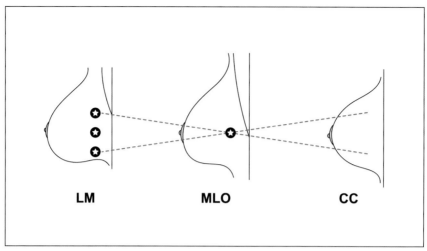

Figure 4.70 The use of the LM view to *triangulate* an area of concern not seen on the CC view. If it *remains* on the LM view, note the direction the area of concern *moved*. When comparing the LM to the MLO, it will *point* to the area of the breast you should focus on for the CC or variation of the CC view.

b. Rolled CC Views

A roll view can also be used in the same way a lateral view is used in the above circumstances. If an area of concern is seen on the CC view but not on the MLO view, first one must determine if the area of concern is, in fact, real. Perform a rolled CC view. If the area is again seen on this image, then one can determine where to look for it on the MLO or the LM view. If it *disappears*, it was simply superimposed tissue and no further views will be required (Figure 4.71).

If the area of concern persists on the rolled view, it is in fact real; this image should now be compared to the standard CC view. Note the direction the area of concern has *moved* on the roll view.

- If it moved medially compared to its location on the CC view, and the top of the breast was rolled medially (as is generally recommended - see below), it can be determined that the area of concern is located in the superior part of the breast (since this tissue was rolled medially). The technologist will now focus on the superior aspect of the breast for the MLO or the LM view (Figure 4.72, Example A).
- If the area of concern moved laterally compared to its location on the CC view, and the top of the breast was rolled medially, it can be determined that this area is located in the inferior aspect of the breast (since this tissue moved laterally for the image). The technologist will now focus on the inferior aspect of the breast for the MLO or the LM view (Figure 4.72, Example B).

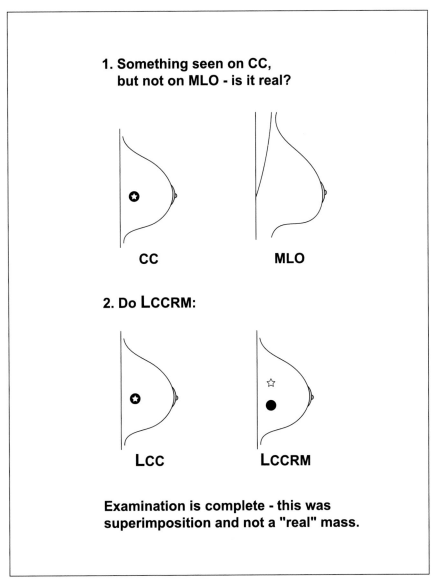

**1. Something seen on CC,
but not on MLO - is it real?**

CC   MLO

2. Do LCCRM:

LCC   LCCRM

**Examination is complete - this was
superimposition and not a "real" mass.**

Figure 4.71 The use of the rolled CC view to counteract the superimposition of structures.

The *direction* of the rolled view (lateral or medial), always refers to the direction that the superior tissue (*immediately beneath the compression paddle*) was rolled. This view will be labeled:

RCCRM - R (right breast) **CC** (view) **R** (rolled) **M** (medially)

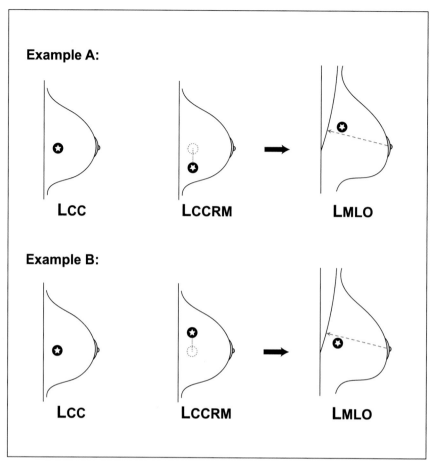

Figure 4.72 The use of the rolled CC view to *triangulate* an area of interest seen only on the CC view.

It is recommended that the Rolled CC view be performed rolling the superior tissue medially. There are three reasons for this protocol.

1. The lateral border of the breast is mobile and the tissue will therefore be more easily moved toward the medial aspect of the breast.

2. The standard CC positioning is performed with the technologist standing on the medial side of the breast being imaged. In this position, it will be very easy to pull her hand out to the side, medially, rolling tissue and maintaining its rolled position as she moves out of the way of the compression paddle.

3. The majority of glandular breast tissue is located in the U.O.Q., making it statistically more probable that an abnormality will be located in the

superior, lateral breast tissue. Rolling superior tissue in a lateral direction will often superimpose a lesion over additional dense glandular tissue. The exception would be a suspected abnormality located in the far lateral aspect of the breast as seen on the original CC view. In these cases, it is recommended that the superior breast tissue is rolled laterally to increase the likelihood of positioning the area of concern tangentially in the subcutaneous fatty tissue, where visualization would be superior. In the majority of cases, however, a medially rolled CC view is superior in spreading out glandular tissue and clarifying superimposed structures.

3. Views Used to Detail and/or Provide Clarification of an Area of Concern

This category provides information that is important in order to clarify or to better define a specific area in the breast. These views minimize the superimposition of structures on the radiographic images.

The most common views used to clarify areas of concern are:
- Spot Compression - to minimize adjacent tissue superimposition
- Spot Compression with Magnification - to improve visualization of microcalcifications and borders of masses
- *Open* Magnification - to provide a generalized view of a large area of concern, or for difficult to *spot* areas.
- Tangential View - to verify the dermal location of microcalcifications; also to minimize superimposition with palpable abnormalities (Figure 4.79)

a. Spot Compression Views

Spot compression views are used to minimize adjacent tissue superimposition. It is important not to *cone-down* (collimate), limiting the image to only the area of concern when performing spot views. The ability to visualize some of the surrounding breast tissue will provide valuable orientation information for the radiologist. Also, with tightly coned views, if the area of concern has been *missed* and the lesion is located just beyond the edge of the coned compression device, the radiologist may be misled into believing that the abnormality was only superimposed tissue that was eliminated by focal compression when in fact the abnormality may have been eliminated from the image by *coning* it off.

If only one projection is requested, go back to the view on which the abnormality is best seen. If it is seen equally well on both views and the radiologist has only asked for one view, the CC projection will be the easiest to duplicate your positioning and to stabilize the breast in the identical, original position.

Three measurements are made on the film, regardless of the projection that will be used.

1. How far *Posterior* to the nipple the area of concern is, using the PNL as your reference.
   Note: For posterior lesions in very large breasts, it is easier to measure how far *Anterior* the area of concern is from the chest wall, using the PNL as your reference.

2. The next measurement will be made from the CC, MLO or LM/ML as follows:
   CC: How far *Medial* or *Lateral* the area of concern is from the PNL.
   MLO or LM/ML: How far *Superior* or *Inferior* the area of concern is from the PNL.

3. The last measurement is made by extending the above *line* (#2), measuring from the area of concern to the skin.

Simple forms (on post-it notes) can be made for this purpose (Figure 4.73). It is not recommended that the technologist take the film into the room with the patient. This may increase anxiety and prompt difficult questions from the patient. (See Patient Relations Chapter.)

Important:
Before transferring the *measurements* from the film to the patient for spot compression views, the technologist must simulate compression of the breast, using her hand. This will provide greater accuracy in locating the area since the original measurements were taken from a film in which the breast was well compressed.

Spot/Mag Measurements

RIGHT   LEFT

CC   MLO   LM   ML

_____ POSTERIOR / ANTERIOR _____

_____ MED / LAT   SUP / INF _____

_____ SKIN _____

Figure 4.73 Sample to make *post-it* notes for spot film measurements.

b. Spot Compression with Magnification Views

Magnification can and should be used with spot compression to clarify an area of concern. This technique is known to improve visualization of microcalcifica-

---

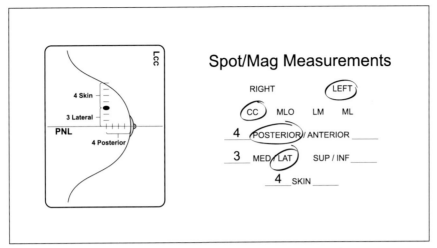

Figure 4.74 Sample measurement for CC view - anterior area of concern.

tions and to better delineate borders of irregular masses. The images can be performed in one or both mammography projections. It is often preferable to do a magnification view in the LM versus the MLO projection ... this will provide true superior/inferior orientation to the nipple as well as verify the existence of milk of calcium.

Note: Many times the radiologist may request a spot mag view in two projections. This may be important to provide additional information that will be of great value in analyzing an abnormality.

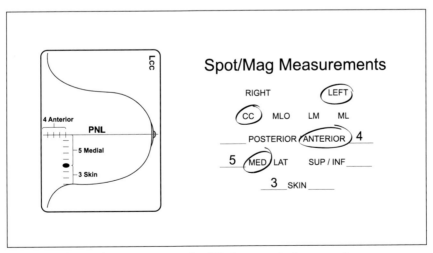

Figure 4.75 Sample measurement for CC view - posterior area of concern.

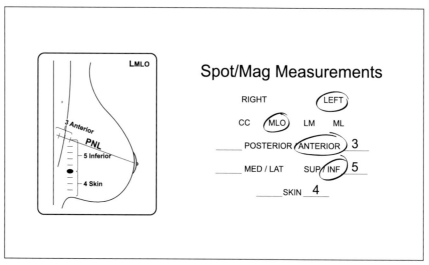

Figure 4.76 Sample measurement for the MLO view.

c. Open Magnification Views

Open magnification views can be performed with full-film exposure to provide a large field of view. This technique is utilized for improved visualization of multifocal areas of calcifications and for large, diffuse abnormalities within one segment of a breast. It can also be useful for visualizing areas that may otherwise be difficult to image due to their location, i.e. just behind the nipple. The retroareolar tissue is frequently very difficult to compress with a small spot compression paddle; also, localized compression in this area may cause unnecessary discomfort for the patient. A larger paddle, particularly the modern variety that *tilts* (to secure anterior tissue) will be much more successful for compressing this area for localized views.

d. Tangential Views

Tangential views are used for two individual purposes: to verify the existence of dermal calcifications and to minimize superimposition when imaging palpable abnormalities.

i. Tangential views of the skin

A *skin localization* must be performed to *find* the location of the suspected dermal calcifications BEFORE a tangential view is done. The following technique should be used:

1. Determine in which quadrant the calcifications are located by studying the 2 screening images.

2. Using the localization breast map (Figure 4.77), choose the appropriate view that will position the biopsy paddle closest to the area of concern.

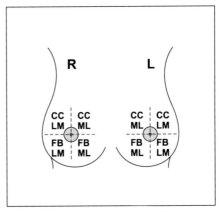

Figure 4.77 The Localization Breast Map.

3. Using the biopsy paddle with alpha-numeric coordinates, position the hole(s) so that it is centered directly over the approximate location of the calcifications (Figure 4.78). Complete the exposure, making sure that you do not release compression (override the auto compression release if your mammography unit has this feature). It is best to seat the patient for these views, as she will have to wait, with her breast compressed, while the film is being developed.

4. After developing the film ... with the patient's breast still compressed, mark the location of the area of concern using the biopsy coordinates.

5. Place a BB on the patient's skin to mark this location; release the compression.

6. Draw an imaginary line from the BB to the nipple.

7. Rotate the C-arm to position the bucky parallel to this line (Figure 4.79). Note: Alternately, the patient or the breast may be turned or rotated to create this same alignment.

8. Perform a tangential image using this projection.

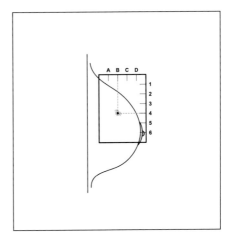

Figure 4.78 The location of the area of concern is determined using the alpha-numeric legends on the biopsy paddle. This lesion is located at coordinates *B - 4.*

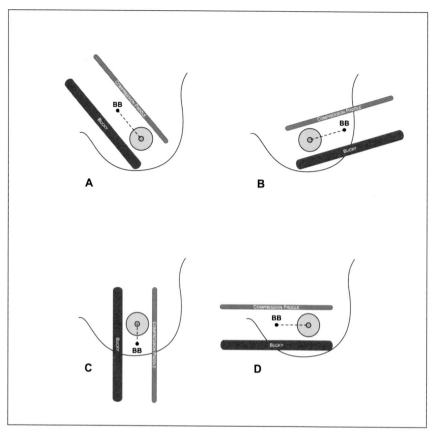

Figure 4.79 The C-arm is angled so that the bucky will be parallel to the line connecting the BB marker and the nipple.

ii. Tangential views for palpable masses

    1. A lead BB marker is placed on the palpable mass.

    2. Repeat steps 6-8 as described above.

4. Views Used for Mammography of the Difficult Patient

The last category of additional views consists of views that help position patients with a difficult body habitus or patients who present challenges because they are confined to a wheelchair or a stretcher.

The following views are helpful in these situations:

- LM - as a second image of the breast tissue when it is not possible to perform a MLO or a LMO
- LMO - as an alternative to the standard MLO view
- FB - as an alternative to the standard CC view
- SIO - as an alternate oblique projection (rarely used)

Refer to the detailed description regarding mammography of the difficult patient in Section III of this chapter.

E. CONCLUSION

The Breast MAP, again, has been designed to help the technologist understand the relationship between the anatomy *seen* on the patient and the anatomy seen on the film. These areas serve as anatomical landmarks, similar to those used in conventional radiography, from which the technologist can correct any potential positioning problems. Just as the technologist would not cone off part of the anatomy on any other body part that she is imaging, she will learn not to *cone off* or exclude any breast tissue during the positioning process by identifying the anatomical structures of the breast. She will then use these same anatomical structures in evaluating the resulting clinical images. As the technologist becomes familiar with these principles, she will be able to avoid positioning errors before they ever occur.

In addition to the anatomical factors that have been discussed, there are obviously a number of additional important considerations that also relate to the clinical appearance of a mammogram. Correct film receptor size, adequate compression, appropriate technique selection and photocell placement must be carefully considered because they all affect the clinical image. However, *the majority of unacceptable films that are produced in clinical practice are due to poor positioning techniques that result in failure to include adequate breast tissue on the image.* Many of these errors can be avoided or easily corrected with a clear understanding of breast and patient anatomy and how they relate to the step-by-step positioning of the patient for clinical images.

POSITIONING FOR MAMMOGRAPHY

SECTION II:
A TECHNOLOGIST'S APPROACH
TO MAMMOGRAPHY

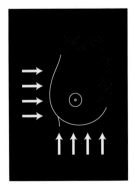

SECTION II:
A TECHNOLOGIST'S APPROACH TO MAMMOGRAPHY

SECTION II:
A TECHNOLOGIST'S APPROACH TO MAMMOGRAPHY

A. INTRODUCTION

The mammography technologist must never lose sight of the importance of her contribution as a member of the breast health care team. One of the most critical aspects of early detection, and therefore improved survival, is the quality of the mammogram. The knowledge and the skills required to properly position the patient and her breast combined with attention to optimal imaging and exposure techniques is one of the most difficult yet critical components of breast cancer detection. Meticulous attention to these details is the cornerstone of quality mammography. This responsibility lies in the hands of the mammography technologist. The quality of the mammography examination impacts the early detection of breast disease, which impacts the initiation of early intervention and treatment. This, in turn, impacts patient survival. Quality mammography saves lives.

The knowledge and the skills required to properly position the patient and her breast combined with attention to optimal imaging and exposure techniques is one of the most difficult yet critical components of breast cancer detection.

There are a number of factors and considerations that are important for the technologist to understand and incorporate into her positioning protocol in order to consistently produce images of high quality. This section of the positioning chapter is dedicated to describing an assortment of issues that impact the technique of mammography.

B. POSITIONING CONSIDERATIONS

1. General Overview

It is standard practice to examine both breasts, even though only one may be of concern. The breasts are essentially symmetrical, that is, they are *mirror images* of each other. From woman to woman, they are also as individual as a person's fingerprints.

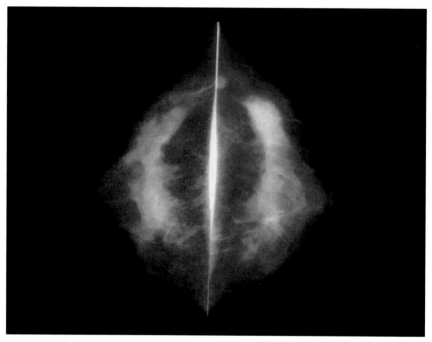

Figure 4.80 Comparing the troublesome breast to the *normal* breast helps to detect abnormalities; this is important since every woman's breasts are as individual as her fingerprints.

The value of comparing the troublesome breast and the *normal* breast to facilitate the detection of subtle abnormalities is obvious. This process of comparison is also conducive to a thorough examination - a must in view of the insidious nature of breast cancer and the well documented benefits of preclinical detection. After the initial examination of both breasts, supplementary views and ancillary modalities can be pursued according to the unique parameters of each individual situation. Examinations of young women (under the age of 30 years) should be limited in nature; the radiologist should direct the mammography examination according to the woman's clinical presenta-

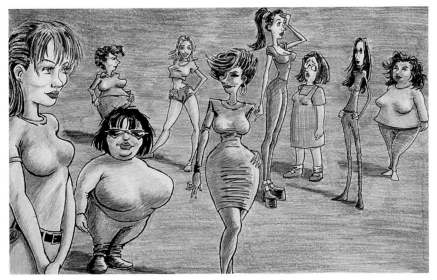

Figure 4.81 Breasts, like women, come in all shapes and sizes; the accompanying body habitus also presents positioning challenges.

tion and concerns. Mid-cycle is generally the best time to perform mammography in the best interest of patient comfort and therefore cooperation.

It is important to understand that mammography cannot be performed in a stereotyped manner; it must be tailored to each patient with attention to their individual body habitus, breast tissue, and clinical presentation. The ultimate goal must be to demonstrate all of the breast tissue. Considering the variability in size and shape of the breast, it is also extremely important to establish a standard method of positioning for mammography to ensure that all patients will receive a thorough, high quality examination.

 It is important to understand that mammography cannot be performed in a stereotyped manner; it must be tailored to each patient with attention to their individual body habitus, breast tissue, and clinical presentation.

It is critical to image ALL of the breast tissue. In some cases, this may require additional views or supplementary projections.

Using a standard positioning protocol, consideration must be given to the breast size and shape and to the contour of the adjacent thorax when performing the mammography examination. The role of the mammographer is to skillfully position the patient in order to include and visualize as much breast parenchyma as possible on each projection.

It is critical to image ALL of the breast tissue. In some cases, this may require additional views or supplementary projections. These views should always be undertaken after the initial mammography examination has been performed. Occasionally, overlapping sections may be required for some breast sizes and shapes. Many abnormalities occur in the axillary tail. A complete study must demonstrate this area on at least one projection (Figure 4.67).

A poorly performed mammogram is more detrimental for a woman than not having mammography at all. It can provide false reassurance, when in fact an unsuspected abnormality may simply not have been included on the images. The diagnosis of breast disease may be delayed one or two years, until it is time for the patient's next routine examination; this woman would miss the opportunity for early detection and treatment.

The mammography examination is limited only by the skill and ingenuity of the mammography technologist.

2. Nipple Profile

The nipple is the most important external reference point on the breast. It is used as a landmark to measure and plot the location of areas of interest in the breast in order to efficiently communicate this information to other members of the health care team. Therefore, it is ideal to image the nipple tangentially to the x-ray beam on the mammogram.

The mammography examination is limited only by the skill and ingenuity of the mammography technologist.

In general, the nipple is imaged in profile on the majority of mammography images. While at least one profile image of the nipple and retroareolar tissue for each breast is both desirable and advantageous, the primary goal of demonstrating all of the breast tissue must remain the first priority. On a standard mammography examination, never sacrifice tissue coverage in order to image the nipple in profile. Also, in the event that the nipple will not be profiled, it should be marked with a lead BB marker or it should be noted on the patient's requisition so that it will not be mistaken for a mass on the mammogram. An additional image with the nipple *in profile* can also be performed.

On a standard mammography examination, never sacrifice tissue coverage in order to image the nipple in profile.

3. Breast Mobility

The superior and medial breast margins are firmly attached to adjacent anatomical structures; therefore, the breast cannot be moved away from these areas. Tissue will be excluded from the mammography image when the compression paddle moves past these borders before it captures and compresses the *mound* of the breast. Therefore, it is very important to fully utilize the mobile lateral and inferior breast margins to move breast tissue toward the fixed borders so that the compression paddle will capture tissue as close as possible to these immobile margins. Refer to page 85 (Breast Mapping) for detailed information on the mobile borders of the breast and how they impact mammography positioning.

Far more tissue will be visualized if the technologist utilizes breast mobility to lift and maneuver the breast while positioning the patient. Elevating the breast for the CC projection will include more superior tissue. Also, lifting the lateral tissue medially and superiorly for the MLO projection will include more medial tissue. The degree of breast mobility that a patient exhibits is highly individual; the literature suggests a range of 1 - 8 cm of tissue mobility.

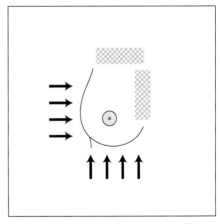

Figure 4.82 The superior and medial breast margins are fixed; breast mobility is accomplished with the mobile inferior and lateral breast margins.

4. "Up-and-Out" Maneuver

The *up-and-out* maneuver utilizes breast mobility. This positioning technique is used with all full-breast images. The goal is to elevate the breast until the Posterior Nipple Line (PNL) is perpendicular to the chest wall; this will also position the breast parenchyma perpendicular to the chest wall (Figures 4.13 and 4.16). The technologist will then need to gently pull tissue *out*, away from the chest wall, and stabilize it on the receptor with her hands until compression is in place to secure this position. This technique is extremely effective in eliminating the tissue superimposition that is frequently noted when the breast is allowed to droop. Also, when breast parenchyma is positioned perpendicular to the chest wall with the *up-and-out* maneuver and the patient is relaxed,

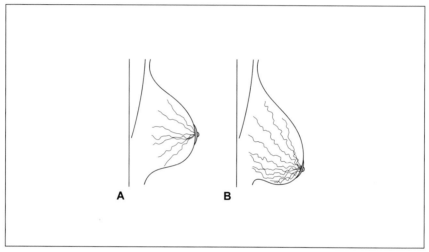

Figure 4.83 When the breast is supported with the *up-and-out* maneuver (A), compression will separate tissue in a radiating, spoke-like fashion from the axis of the nipple. Visualization and evaluation of the breast parenchyma will be maximized. If the breast is allowed to droop (B), superimposed tissue can easily *hide* abnormalities; adequate tissue evaluation will not be accomplished.

 When breast parenchyma is positioned perpendicular to the chest wall with the up-and-out maneuver and the patient is relaxed, glandular tissue is in an ideal position to maximize the effects of compression, separating tissue in a radiating, spoke-like fashion from the axis of the nipple.

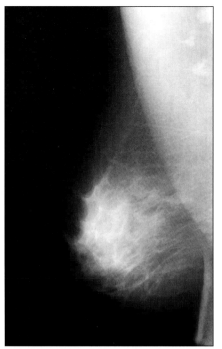

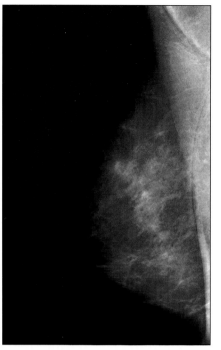

Figure 4.84 This examination illustrates the results of releasing the breast before the compression paddle has secured its position; the tissue slips back and folds against the chest wall. The opportunity to visualize posterior tissue near the chest wall is lost and superimposition of structures is evident.

Figure 4.85 Another example of tissue superimposition and folds that occur when the breast is not supported until the compression paddle has secured its position on the image receptor.

glandular tissue is in an ideal position to maximize the effects of compression, separating tissue in a radiating, spoke-like fashion from the axis of the nipple.

Therefore, proper compression begins with the technologist's hands, as she positions the breast for each projection, supporting it with her hands until the compression paddle is in place, exerting enough pressure to maintain this position for the x-ray exposure (Figures 4.129 and 4.130).

The flat surface of the compression paddle will then distribute breast tissue more evenly over the surface of the film, reducing tissue thickness and minimizing the overlapping of anatomical structures. However, it is the technologist's hands that first create the desired breast position for each mammography view. Allowing the breast to droop or letting go of the breast before the compression paddle has secured its position will result in superimposition of breast structures on the mammogram and possible *loss* of breast tissue on the film. This frequently requires repeat exposures or additional views for tissue clarification. Care should be exercised to avoid wrinkles or skin folds; these also result in tissue overlap and images must be repeated when folds occur in glandular areas.

5. Patient Relaxation

While performing the mammography examination it is important to encourage the patient to relax her muscles in the shoulder and thorax area. This will facilitate maximum maneuverability of the breast as the technologist positions each projection. This also allows the breast to

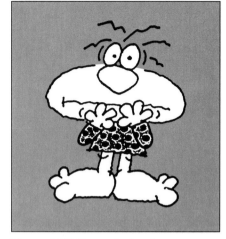

Figure 4.86 The majority of our patients are very anxious; it is important to encourage them to relax before beginning the examination.

be gently pulled away from the chest wall to include more tissue on the images. Patient relaxation is the single most important factor in patient positioning; it is essential for a successful examination. In fact, if the patient is relaxed and her shoulder and chest muscles are loose, every other positioning step will fall into place with amazing ease.

6. Patient Positions

Mammography can be performed with the patient recumbent, seated, or standing. Some equipment manufacturers have developed multipurpose chairs that facilitate both seated and recumbent patient positioning. Unless there is urgency due to a worrisome clinical presentation, consideration should be given to postponing a routine mammogram for a patient who is temporarily confined to a wheelchair or stretcher. The quality of the mammography

Mammography can be performed with the patient recumbent, seated, or standing. Some equipment manufacturers have developed multipurpose chairs that facilitate both seated and recumbent patient positioning.

examination will be superior when the numerous positioning obstacles inherent with these patient positions have been eliminated.

In a screening setting, when large volumes and rapid throughput are essential, the standing position is necessary for a number of reasons. First, it is very efficient from the perspective of throughput volume. Second, it facilitates the intricate physical interaction between the patient and the technologist during mammography positioning. Finally, the retraction of folds from the inframammary area is easily accomplished with this patient position.

Although the preferred method of positioning requires both the patient and the technologist to be standing, it may occasionally be necessary to position the patient while she is seated. This would apply to patients with physical impairments and to those who may be ill or feel unsteady. The seated position will maintain stability and minimize motion problems; this is also the best choice from the standpoint of patient safety. However, the seated patient is more challenging to position for mammography. The technologist assumes a heavier burden in the form of cumbersome working conditions and awkward body postures in order to compensate for restricted patient mobility. While maneuvering the patient and the chair, she needs to utilize proper techniques of body mechanics in order to avoid excessive strain on her back, shoulders, neck, arms, and lower extremities. A focus dedicated to minimizing repetitive stress injury and to pre-

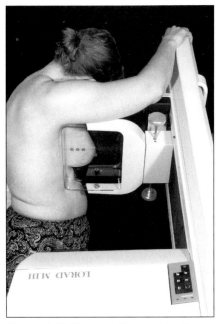

Figure 4.87 The standing position is the ideal patient position for performing mammography examinations.

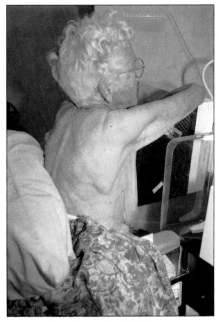

Figure 4.88 Occasionally it is necessary to perform a mammogram on a seated patient.

serving the physical well-being of the mammography technologist is very important. Refer to Chapter 11 for detailed information on this subject. Erect positioning minimizes the back strain and fatigue that can develop with the repetitive motions of patient positioning. It also facilitates efficient guidance of the patient into various positions during the process of mammography positioning.

7. Limitations of Mammography

It is important to be aware that mammography may experience limitations with:

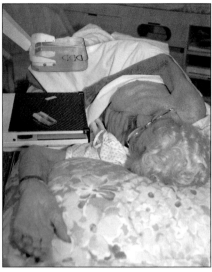

Figure 4.89 If necessary, a mammogram can also be performed on a recumbent patient.

- Dense breast tissue
- Chest wall lesions
- Juxtathoracic breast tissue (blind areas)

8. Blind Areas

The mediolateral oblique (MLO) view demonstrates more breast tissue than any other mammography projection because it maximizes breast mobility relative to the pectoralis muscle. However, the fact that it is difficult to demonstrate the entire breast on one single projection is also a true statement. This is primarily due to the fact that the breast follows the natural curvature of the rib cage, and our image receptors are not curved, but instead have straight edges. This results in *Blind Areas* that we must be aware of when performing and interpreting mammography examinations. Although recent improvements in positioning techniques have enabled us to include more tissue in these blind areas, the potential for exclusion still exists and must be in the forefront of the mammographer's thoughts as she positions her patient.

Erect positioning minimizes the back strain and fatigue that can develop with the repetitive motions of patient positioning.

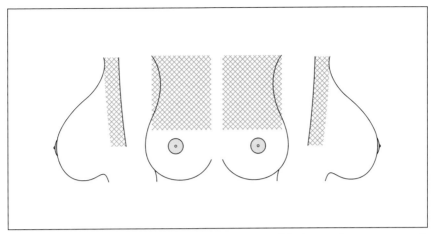

Figure 4.90 When the breast is compressed for the CC view, unless correct positioning techniques are used, the superior/posterior portion of the breast tissue may not be imaged completely.

9. Breast Compression

The value and benefit of adequate breast compression during mammography cannot be overemphasized. The skill of consistently obtaining correct compression for mammography is a critical factor affecting image quality; it must never be neglected or trivialized. A brief discussion with the patient regarding the importance of taut compression should occur before the examination begins. Visual aids such as posters or examples of mammograms with and without adequate compression are extremely valuable to clearly present this information to the patient and gain her cooperation. An informed, relaxed and

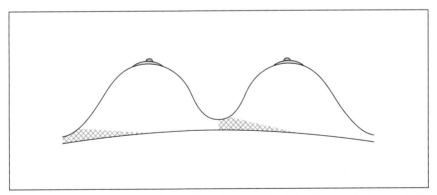

Figure 4.91 Also for the CC view, either the posterior/lateral or posterior/medial tissue may not be included, depending on the alignment of the patient's thorax to the plane of the receptor. This occurs as a result of the curved contour of the rib cage and the straight edge of the image receptor.

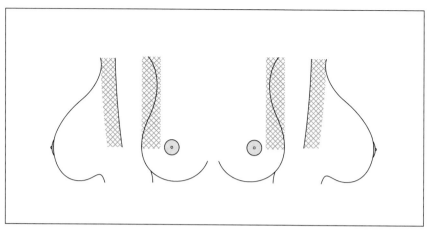

Figure 4.92 With a lateral view, the posterior/lateral tissue may not to be imaged.

cooperative patient will tolerate compression more readily; this is important to the success of the examination.

Our goal with mammography is to achieve compression that is taut, or at maximum, less than painful. Taut compression has been achieved when a gentle tapping of the breast with one finger does not indent the tissue. This degree of compression is rarely painful. However, individual patient tolerance is highly variable and must be acknowledged. Taut compression will:
- Separate overlapping structures
- Visualize more posterior tissue by gently pulling the tissue away from the chest wall

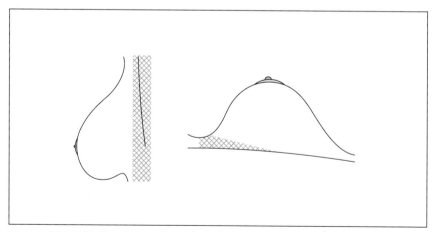

Figure 4.93 With the oblique projection, the posterior, medial, inferior area of the breast has the greatest potential for exclusion on the image.

The value and benefit of adequate breast compression during mammography cannot be overemphasized. The skill of consistently obtaining correct compression for mammography is a critical factor affecting image quality; it must never be neglected or trivialized.

- Provide a uniform film density
- Reduce scatter, improving contrast
- Reduce unsharpness
- Reduce radiation dose

Compression should always be applied gradually, allowing the patient time to adapt to the pressure; it is important to observe the patient's reaction as you proceed. Manual compression is available on all modern mammography equipment; it can be applied much more gently and gradually and should be used as soon as the patient appears uncomfortable.

While the mammography technologist is aware of the value and the need for taut breast compression, there are two patient factors that cannot be overlooked or ignored. First is the degree of compressibility of the individual woman's breast tissue. The overall breast tissue thickness of a basically fatty breast can be reduced significantly with breast compression. This same degree of thickness reduction may be impossible to achieve with a dense glandular breast or with a breast containing a large mass or multiple cysts. The second

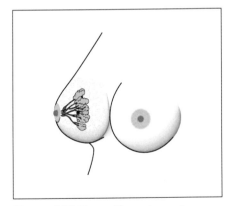

Figure 4.94 Normal breast parenchyma can easily hide lumps and other breast abnormalities.

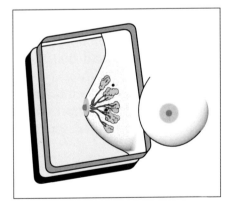

Figure 4.95 Breast compression spreads out the breast tissue; lumps and other abnormalities are much easier to detect.

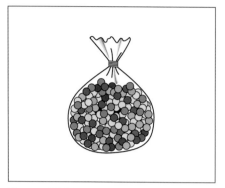

Figure 4.96 An uncompressed breast can be compared to a bag of marbles. It is difficult to see individual marbles (lumps) when they are all clustered together.

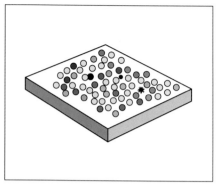

Figure 4.97 Spreading the marbles out on a flat surface (like breast compression) allows us to clearly examine each marble (lump) individually.

factor is the individual tolerance of the woman. Once the patient understands the benefits of taut compression, she is usually cooperative and tolerant of the discomfort. Using these two variables as guidelines, the mammographer should work toward achieving a level of compression that is taut; at its maximum level, it should be less than painful.

10. Pain and Mammography

Despite the popular tendency to associate pain with mammography examinations, the great majority of patients report that their examination was uncomfortable, but very tolerable. Unfortunately, many women are misled by insensitive remarks and jokes about breast compression and/or the personal, although exaggerated experience of a well-meaning friend or relative. When some women share what may have actually been a painful experience, they often do not understand that this may have been an unusual and isolated experience, and that it is based on their personal perception of pain. All of these factors may consequently influence the patient's thoughts about mammography, specifically about compression. These women arrive for their examination with a preconceived expectation of great discomfort and a high level of anxiety.

An informed, relaxed and cooperative patient will tolerate compression more readily; this is important to the success of the examination.

a. Classification of Breast Pain

Breast pain is one of our patient's most common complaints. It is important to be aware that breast pain is not related to the size of a woman's breasts; large and small alike exhibit the same potential for breast pain and discomfort. While this symptom is often an influential factor that encourages women to pursue mammography, at the same time it can also be the most common reason for reluctance to comply with this examination. The perception of pain, in general, is highly subjective and uniquely individual in nature; breast pain is no exception.

The types of breast pain that women experience can be categorized as either true physical pain or as perceived pain, related to a high level of anxiety.

i. Physical Pain
True physical pain can be further divided into a number of categories.

> *The perception of pain, in general, is highly subjective and uniquely individual in nature; breast pain is no exception.*

A. Pain Related to Mammography
This category of breast pain is of primary interest and focus for the mammography technologist. As a rule, mammography should not be painful. The exception would be the patient who presents with large, tense cysts and the patient who may be tender as a result of recent surgical procedures. However, the great majority of pain that is associated with mammography is a result of excessive tension on the patient's skin. It is important to attempt to leave some *loose* skin along the chest wall for the compression paddle to stretch out as breast compression is applied; patient relaxation and loose, flaccid muscles in the thorax area will help to achieve this goal. Another contributing factor is the elasticity of the skin on the breast; this is variable from patient to patient and will affect the amount of compression the woman can tolerate before the pressure becomes uncomfortable. At the onset of breast compression, if the compression paddle encounters skin that is already stretched tight, without fail, the patient will experience discomfort very early and adequate compression will be impossible to accomplish. The technologist can alleviate a great deal of her patient's discomfort by ensuring that the skin is relaxed and loose along the plane that the compression paddle encounters as compression

begins. This will only be accomplished with proper positioning techniques that take full advantage of beast mobility and with patient relaxation.

While many patients note discomfort where the corners of the bucky meet their ribs or their axilla, this is seldom interpreted as truly painful.

Refer to the discussion that follows on *Pain During Mammography Examinations* for additional information.

The great majority of pain that is associated with mammography is a result of excessive tension on the patient's skin.

B. Pain Related to the Breast

Breast pain is usually categorized as either cyclical or non-cyclical in nature. Cyclical breast pain occurs as a result of hormonal fluctuations. Although this type of pain usually becomes prominent in the pre-menstrual phase of a woman's monthly cycle, other cyclical patterns of breast pain have also been reported. These breasts are frequently nodular in nature and the pain may be described as *heaviness* and/or *tenderness to the touch*. Although fluid retention during this part of a woman's cycle is not responsible for breast pain, it can make it appear worse because of the accompanying heaviness of the breast tissue. If these symptoms are pronounced, mammography is generally avoided during this period of time.

Breast pain that is unrelated to the menstrual cycle is classified as non-cyclical and occurs in both pre- and post-menopausal women. When confined to the breast tissue only, this pain is experienced as varying degrees of a dull *ache*, *sensitivity*, and/or *tenderness to the touch*; this tenderness may be general in presentation, or it may be localized to a specific area (or areas).

Frequently, however, the pain women experience during mammography arises from adjacent musculoskeletal structures, specifically the ribs and chest wall. This pain is commonly described as a *drawing* and/or *burning* sensation. Although this may occur along the lateral side of the breast, the most common site for musculoskeletal pain is medially, along the sternal border. Many women in the age group that is routinely screened with mammography have developed a type of arthritis known as costochondritis; this affects the junction of the ribs medially along the sternum. Unfortunately, this anatomical area

The elasticity of the skin on the breast is variable from patient to patient and will affect the amount of compression the woman can tolerate before the pressure becomes uncomfortable.

coincides with the edge of the compression paddle at the onset of compression for the MLO view. Pressure in this area will be very uncomfortable for these women. Therefore, many times the pain a woman reports during mammography arises from discomfort along her medial rib cage rather than from the breast tissue itself. Also, arthritic changes in the neck area may create pinched nerves that will radiate pain down into the breast and chest area, much the same way that pain from a pinched nerve in the lower spine radiates down the legs. Phlebitis in the breast tissue (Mondor's syndrome) can also be very painful. A thickened cord can frequently be palpated and the patient experiences tenderness and a drawing sensation in this area. All of these conditions contribute to tender, sensitive breast tissue even before we begin to position the patient for a mammogram.

ii. Perceived Pain (related to anxiety)

Many women are very anxious about mammography examinations. Their underlying emotion is fear, which may be a result of the anticipated discomfort, the uncertainty of the results of the mammogram, and/or the loss of control associated with the examination.

Frequently, their anxiety reflects their unspoken *self-diagnosis* of breast cancer. It is very helpful for the technologist to point out that most breast pain is not a result of breast cancer, in fact, it seldom indicates serious disease at all. Hearing this information from a *breast* health professional can be very comforting and may bring about an immediate sense of relief. However, it is important for the technologist to encourage the patient to discuss any concerns she may have about her breasts, including pain, with her physician.

One of the more critical factors required for successful mammography positioning is a relaxed patient. In an anxious state, the muscles subconsciously

Frequently the pain women experience during mammography arises from adjacent musculoskeletal structures, specifically the ribs and chest wall.

become tense. These patients are frequently very stiff and rigid; this posture is extremely counterproductive when attempting what should be easy and comfortable breast positioning. Furthermore, because this manifestation is subconscious in nature, the patient is often unaware of her rigid demeanor and may easily become frustrated by the technologist's repeated requests for her to relax during the examination. Refer to the chapter on *Patient Relations* for more information and suggestions on this aspect of mammography pain.

It is important that the technologist first acknowledge and then address the pain her patient is experiencing; the patient's feelings must be validated. Despite the technologist's interpretation of the situation, the fact remains that *perception is reality* and, to the patient, at this moment in time, the pain is very real. Then, by questioning the woman, the true source of the pain should be determined. If an adjustment of the bucky or the patient position can alleviate the problem, this can be quickly and easily accomplished; at the same time, the patient's confidence and comfort level may improve significantly, having noted the technologist's caring and compassionate approach.

 It is important that the technologist first acknowledge and then address the pain her patient is experiencing; the patient's feelings must be validated.

b. Pain During Mammography Examinations

During the mammography examination, when a woman experiences extreme discomfort or pain or when she clearly indicates *That's enough ... stop* or *Stop - I cannot tolerate this* as compression is applied, the technologist must discontinue the examination immediately and then inquire if this degree of discomfort is normal or quite unusual for the patient. Should the technologist continue, saying *Hang on - just hold your breath* or *Just a minute ... just a minute* and quickly complete the exposure, she is, in essence, ignoring and therefore trivializing the patient's request. This approach is unacceptable; it violates any trust that has been established between the patient and the technologist.

Again emphasizing the critical nature and the importance of compression (that has already been discussed at the onset of the examination), the technologist should clearly communicate that without a *reasonable* degree of compression, the examination will be inferior and the results may be misleading, providing false assurance because the breast tissue has not been adequately assessed. The definition of *reasonable* compression is variable and individual; it will need

The examination should not proceed without the consent of the patient. A bad experience, where the woman has not been a willing participant, may discourage this patient from ever returning for future examinations.

to be assessed by the patient and the technologist in each individual situation. If at all possible, and provided that an urgent clinical symptom is not involved, the examination may be postponed until the discomfort subsides. Every effort should be made to accommodate this patient on short notice, at a time when her breasts are less tender, perhaps soon after her next period begins. At this point during the current examination, a decision must be made: the examination will be delayed until conditions improve; or the examination will proceed, knowing and understanding that it will be very uncomfortable, perhaps even painful. This decision must be made by the woman; the technologist's only role is to provide her with honest and accurate information that she must then evaluate. The examination should not proceed without the consent of the patient. A bad experience, where the woman has not been a willing participant, may discourage this patient from ever returning for future examinations. Refer to the chapter on *Patient Relations* for additional information and suggestions regarding patients who can tolerate little or no breast compression.

Whatever the source, the mammographer must be compassionate and supportive of any patient who experiences discomfort during her mammography examination.

It is good practice to document cases of excessive discomfort on the patient's records for the benefit of the interpreting radiologist and for reference with future examinations.

Patient relaxation is the single most important factor in patient positioning; it is essential for a successful examination.

Manual compression is available on all modern mammography equipment; it can be applied much more gently and gradually and should be used as soon as the patient appears uncomfortable.

C. TECHNICAL CONSIDERATIONS

1. Automatic Exposure Control (AEC) Placement for Mammography Imaging

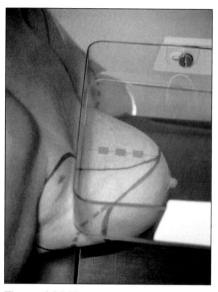

Figure 4.98 The selected AEC cell position is critical to the optical film density of the image.

The use of automatic exposure control (AEC) devices for mammography provides consistency in optical density for mammography images and minimizes the need for frequent repeat exposures due to incorrect film density. The AEC device terminates the exposure when it has received the amount of exposure that will produce the programed optical film density on the developed image. This precise selection is based on the exposure *information* that the AEC device receives during the exposure. Therefore, consistently obtaining the desired optical film density is dependent on the location of the AEC (under the breast) for each image. For all standard, full-image views, the AEC device should be placed under glandular breast tissue; this is usually located behind the nipple, in the retroareolar area. Underexposured images will result from positioning the AEC device under posterior fatty tissue.

The position of the AEC devise is critical for spot compression films. Often these images are focused on clarifying a mass or superimposed glandular tissue. The AEC must be positioned directly under the area of concern in order to produce an adequate optical density to demonstrate this glandular tissue. Otherwise, the optical density may be selected on the basis of adjacent fatty tissue and the film may need to be repeated.

For all standard, full-image views, the AEC device should be placed under glandular breast tissue; this is usually located behind the nipple, in the retroareolar area.

The position of the AEC device is critical for spot compression films.

Technique charts should be posted for the technologist to refer to when it is necessary to select a manual exposure technique. This will be required for mammography of breasts with implants and for some very small breasts.

2. Spot Compression Views

When spot compression films are required to clarify tissue detail in a specific area of the breast, a smaller size of compression paddle should be used. These paddles provide improved focal compression in a localized area; this is very effective in spreading out superimposed structures.

The size of the image field can be collimated in a number of ways:

1. To include only the area of the small compression paddle (Figure 4.101). While restricting the size of the image field will help to control scatter and improve resolution minimally, the clear, unexposed area of the film will transmit light from the view box when the images are mounted for interpretation. The high intensity of light emitted by bright mammography view boxes diminishes the visual acuity of the interpreter; this is detrimental to the perception of subtle detail on the mammogram. Masking will alleviate this problem but it is cumbersome and inconvenient to use (consider turning masks with the emulsion out to reader - this will reduce glare). In general, the scatter control accomplished by closely collimating a coned spot image is considered minimal and negligible for the small film size that is used for mammography.

2. To include an area slightly larger than the size of the compression paddle. Landmarks and adjacent structures are very helpful to visualize on the image; they help to orient the interpreter and to confirm the location of an abnormality in the breast.

3. The entire film can be exposed, as with a standard mammogra-

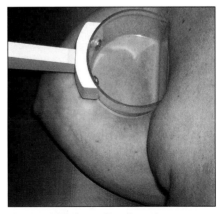
Figure 4.99 A smaller size of compression paddle will provide improved focal compression.

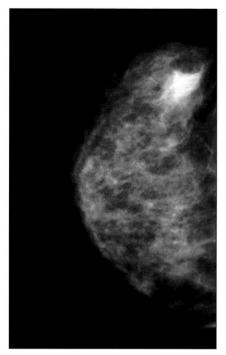

Figure 4.100 CC image with an area that requires focal compression.

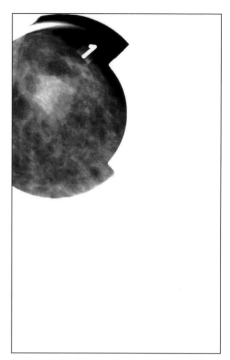

Figure 4.101 Spot compression with tight collimation; the clear area of the film will transmit light from the view box when these images are viewed.

phy image. Many facilities choose this option, even when only a small area of the breast has been compressed for a spot compression view because the detrimental effects of the additional scatter are considered negligible and the improved viewing conditions, without the need for masking, are extremely advantageous (Figure 4.103).

3. Systems Used to Communicate Location in the Breast

There are two systems that can be used to communicate the location of a mass or an area of interest within a breast: the *Quadrant* system and the *O'clock* system.

 Radiopaque markers indicating laterality and position must be placed adjacent to the axillary tissue on each mammography image

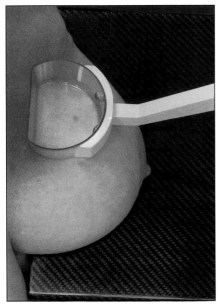

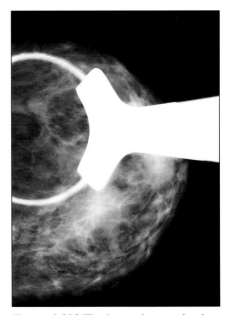

Figure 4.102 The breast is compressed with a small compression paddle.

Figure 4.103 The image is completely
exposed. Adjacent structures will provide orientation information and, because the image is completely
exposed, it will not present viewing
problems during interpretation similar
to the image in Figure 4.101.

a. Quadrant Division of Breast Tissue

To facilitate communication, the breast is frequently divided into four *Quad-
rants*; the division is based on nipple location. Reference will be made to this
classification throughout this text.

U.O.Q.	=	Upper, Outer Quadrant	=	A
L.O.Q.	=	Lower, Outer Quadrant	=	B
L.I.Q.	=	Lower, Inner Quadrant	=	C
U.I.Q.	=	Upper, Inner Quadrant	=	D

b. O'clock Division of Breast Tissue

A second communication system utilizes the face of a clock to plot locations
in the breast; this designation is also based on nipple location.

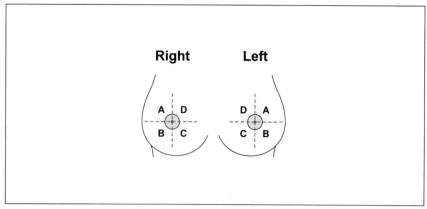

Figure 4.104 The quadrant division of breast tissue, based on nipple location.

4. Examination Identification

The American College of Radiology (ACR) and the Canadian Association of Radiology (CAR) Mammography Accreditation Program(s) (MAP) require that each mammography image has permanent identification that includes:

- Facility name
- Facility location
- Patient name (First and last)
- Patient identification number (medical record number, social security number, date of birth)
- Date
- Radiopaque markers indicating laterality and projection
- Technologist identification
- Cassette/screen identification

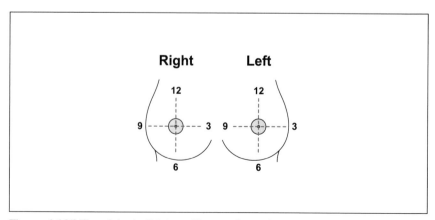

Figure 4.105 The o'clock division of breast tissue, based on nipple location.

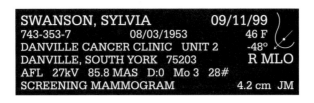

SWANSON, SYLVIA	09/11/99
743-353-7 08/03/1953	46 F
DANVILLE CANCER CLINIC UNIT 2	-48°
DANVILLE, SOUTH YORK 75203	R MLO
AFL 27kV 85.8 MAS D:0 Mo 3 28#	
SCREENING MAMMOGRAM	4.2 cm JM

Figure 4.106 A sample of image identification information that is stamped on each film.

- Mammography unit number
- A permanent, flashed I.D. system (rather than labels) is strongly recommended
- Also recommended are a separate date sticker and technical factors.

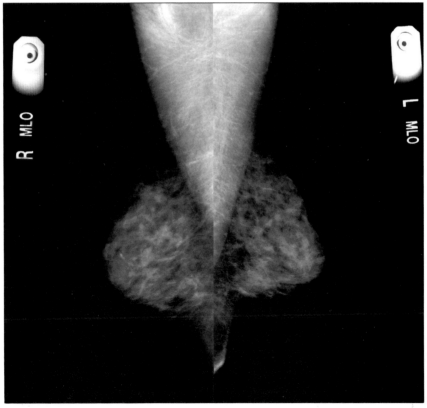

Figure 4.107 Lead markers indicating laterality and position are placed on the axillary side of the image.

5. Labeling Codes for Mammography Positioning

The standard labeling codes for mammography images are outlined below:

Laterality

    Right   ....R*

    Left   ....L*

Projection / Position

    Craniocaudal CC

    Mediolateral Oblique   ....MLO

    Lateral

        Lateromedial   ....LM

        Mediolateral   ....ML

    Spot Compression

    Magnification   ....M*

    Exaggerated Craniocaudal XCCL

    Cleavage CV

    Axillary Tail   ....AT

    Tangential   ....TAN

    Roll

        Rolled Lateral   ....RL†

        Rolled Medial   ....RM†

        Rolled Superior ....RS†

        Rolled Inferior.......................................RI†

    From Below

    Caudocranial   ....FB

    Lateromedial Oblique   ....LMO

    Superolateral to Inferomedial Oblique ....SIO

    Implant Displaced   ....ID†

* Used as a prefix before the projection.

E.g. RMMLO = Right Magnification MedioLateral Oblique

† Used as a suffix, after the projection.

E.g. LCCRS = Left CranioCaudal, Superior Tissue Rolled Superior

Note: Radiopaque markers indicating laterality and position must be placed adjacent to the axillary tissue on each mammography image (Figure 4.107 and Figure 4.120). In order that they do not distract the interpreting radiologist, they should be placed near the edge of the film rather than directly adjacent to the breast tissue. They should be clear and legible without being overly large and distracting. As well, they should be positioned so as to be legible from overhead. The standard labeling codes (abbreviations) that have been developed should be used to promote universality between facilities.

D. THE TECHNOLOGIST / PATIENT INTERACTION

1. Introduction

The mammography technologist spends more time with the patient and has the most intimate interaction with the patient during the process of mammography positioning than any other individual in a facility. For this reason, the mammographer must always be prepared to deal with a variety of issues during the examination:

- comments regarding misconceptions about mammography (mammograms cause cancer, compression ruptures tumors, compression spreads disease);
- information presented in (often misleading) articles in the media; and last, but not least
- patient anxiety and fear. Patients experience fear in many ways.

First are the physical considerations: How much will the compression hurt? How long will my breasts be compressed? Will I be bruised? How much radiation will I be exposed to? Will the radiation cause permanent damage?

There are also many emotional issues: My breasts are too small or too large or just plain embarrassing! My breasts are so lumpy - will they be able to tell if something is wrong?

What if they find cancer? Will they tell me the truth? Are they using the most modern technology? I hope they are competent! Should I get a second opinion, just to be sure?

Many patients rely on the mammography technologist to dispel these concerns. Their overall experience and impression of the examination as well as their

 Many patients rely on the mammography technologist to dispel their concerns. Their overall experience and impression of the examination as well as their willingness to return for future mammograms is directly related to the quality of their interaction with the mammography technologist.

willingness to return for future mammograms is directly related to the quality of their interaction with the mammography technologist.

A detailed and comprehensive description of the patient/technologist interaction can be found in the chapter on *Patient Relations*.

2. Patient Preparation

Patient care and preparation truly begins at the time the mammography appointment is scheduled. A professional manner with a friendly and courteous attitude will enhance the patient's confidence and comfort level with the facility. Unless there is urgency in booking the examination, the patient's breasts will be less tender and she will tolerate compression much more readily if the examination is scheduled during the week following her menses. The patient should be told to wear a two piece outfit so that when she disrobes to the waist, she will still be partially clothed and therefore feel more comfortable during the examination.

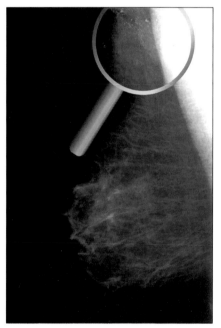

Figure 4.108 Deodorant can mimic microcalcifications on a mammogram. The patient needs to thoroughly remove her deodorant before having a mammogram.

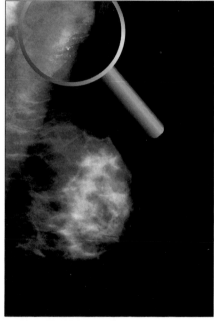

Figure 4.109 Again, body powder and deodorant must be removed before performing a mammogram.

Always review the patient's previous images when they are available before you begin an examination.

She should also be told to avoid the use of deodorant, body powders, oils, and creams (especially those containing zinc oxide) in the breast and chest area on the day of her examination. Although studies have shown that the ingredient in antiperspirants that mimics calcifications is aluminum chlorhydrate, it is best to avoid all skin products and deodorants in general.

An inquiry should be made regarding previous mammography examinations so that they may be obtained prior to her appointment, particularly if they are current and were done after the onset of clinical symptoms. Finally, the patient should be given an approximate indication of the length of time that her appointment will take in order that she can schedule the appropriate time period into her day. More time will be needed if there is a clinical concern that may require additional images or adjunctive modalities, such as ultrasound. Also, if the patient has breast implants, is confined to a wheelchair or has any other condition that may require extra time, she should be prepared for a longer appointment.

The more prepared the patient is when she arrives in your facility, the greater the chance that she will be more relaxed and comfortable for the mammogram.

3. Previous Examinations

Always review the patient's previous images when they are available before you begin an examination. This will alert you to specific conditions (implants, unusually dense tissue) and may encourage you to select the most appropriate exposure technique at the onset of the examination.

4. Greeting the Patient

Greet the patient using both her first and last name; take a moment to plan your

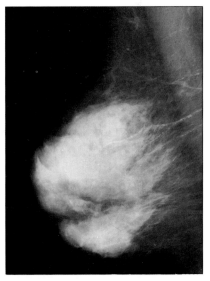

Figure 4.110 Reviewing previous films will alert the technologist to particularly difficult conditions before the examination begins.

pronunciation with difficult names. As you proceed with the examination, use the patient's last name unless she has given you permission to call her by her first name. In the x-ray room introduce yourself and tell her that you are the technologist that will be taking her images. Stress the importance of her participation in the mammogram, indicating that a partnership between the two of you is the most successful approach. Maintain a professional atmosphere under all circumstances. Try to present a light, pleasant ambience, despite the personality that your patient may present; worry, fear, and apprehension can dramatically alter a person's disposition.

Stress the importance of the patient's participation in the mammogram, indicating that a partnership between the two of you is the most successful approach.

5. Documentation

a. Clinical Symptoms and History

Documentation of the patient's history and present condition is frequently incorporated into a standard questionnaire. The following is a sample of questions that are frequently asked:

- Is this her first examination or has there been a previous mammogram? Where? When?
  (This inquiry may be made at the time the appointment if made. The films can then be obtained prior to the examination.)

- Is this a routine examination or is there a specific clinical symptom or concern?
  Document details of clinical symptoms.
  Record any clinical symptoms and information the patient discloses relating to the mammogram. There are two distinct categories of clinical information that require attention.

- First is the detailed description of conditions, symptoms or abnormalities that is reported and described by the patient herself. This may be much more detailed and sometimes even conflicting with the clinical data provided on the requisition by the referring physician. Always clearly document the patient's description, using quotations to reiterate her words, for example: *Patient describes lumpiness in the L.I.Q.*; or *Patient reports burning pain in the retroareolar area.*

- Second, marking palpable lumps and masses with a lead BB marker also requires attention. The patient should be asked to point out the palpable lump. The technologist can then attach the BB marker to her skin in the area indicated by the patient. Some technologists ask the patient to position the BB on the correct area herself. A notation should then be made on the requisition or chart, *BB marker on skin over area indicated by patient.* It is important to understand that although many technologists will palpate a patient's lump to correlate its location and characteristics to the appearance on the mammogram, in most cases they have not been officially trained and certified to perform a clinical breast examination. While some technologists may be very proficient at this task, the fact remains that unless they are qualified in clinical breast evaluation (as physicians are) it is inappropriate to comment on or record their personal impression of the clinical component of the examination. Having said this, another sensitive issue may arise. While positioning the patient for the mammogram, the technologist may notice a lump or some other obvious abnormality that the patient appears unaware of; this information must be passed on to the radiologist. Verbal communication is the best way to inform the radiologist, but if they are not *on site*, a note describing the finding could be attached to the patient's file. When the radiologist is available, they may elect to personally perform a breast examination on this patient to confirm this important clinical information.

Document details of clinical symptoms.
Record any clinical symptoms and information the
patient discloses relating to the mammogram.

- Is there a family history of breast cancer?
  Pay particular attention to first degree relatives: mother, sister, daughter.
  Who? and at approximately what age was she diagnosed?
  Was it unilateral or bilateral?
  Also note any paternal family history.

- Menstrual status and reproductive history:
  At what age did she first menstruate?
  When did the last menstrual period begin?

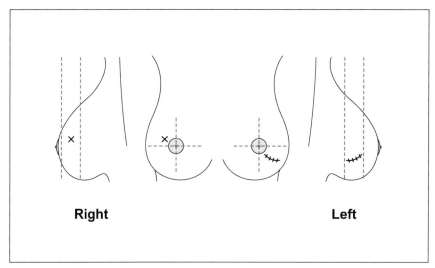

Figure 4.111 Indicate on a diagram any scars from previous biopsies. Indicate the presence of large moles that may be visualized on the mammogram (mark with a lead BB or other opaque marker on the patient's skin) and any other physical findings that the radiologist should be aware of.

If past mid-cycle, any chance of pregnancy? (If the woman is actively trying to get pregnant or is unsure if she may be, it is appropriate to postpone the mammogram until she begins her next period, especially when there is no urgent clinical concern.) See note on shielding that follows.

- How many children has she given birth to?
- How many did she breast feed?
- Is she now, or in the past has she been on birth control pills or any other hormone preparation? How long?

- What other medications is she currently taking?

- Is she wearing any deodorant, body powder, oil, talc, or cream in the breast area? If so, have her wash thoroughly. Powder and deodorant can mimic calcifications on a mammogram.

b. Visual Inspection

- Perform a visual inspection of the breast and anterior chest wall. Draw, on a diagram, any scars from previous biopsies. Indicate the presence of large moles that may be visualized on the mammogram (mark with a lead BB or other opaque marker on the patient's skin) and any other physical findings that the radiologist should be aware of. Note the condition of the skin along the inframammary fold. With large, pendulous breasts, heat and moisture are regularly trapped in this area. Often these women apply creams and/or powders to this area to alleviate the constant irritation they experience. As a result, the skin in this area becomes very thin and fragile and is susceptible to breaking during mammography positioning. Refer to Helpful Hints *k* following the description for CC positioning for information on practices that will minimize trauma to this area. It is advantageous to address this issue with the woman during the visual inspection and before positioning begins; this will establish mutual acknowledgement of the skin condition and any breaks in the skin that may already be present. Any obvious skin deterioration in this area should be documented on the patient's chart before the examination begins. Gloves should be available for the technologist to wear for these occasions.

- Any recent change in breast size or shape?
- Any skin changes?
- Nipples: If inverted, is this new or not? How long?
  Any discharge? Both sides or one? What color? Does it discharge spontaneously or must it be extracted by pressure in the nipple area?

If the patient has filled out the history sheet without your assistance, it is a good idea to briefly review the information with her before you proceed to the mammography unit and move on to the technical details of the examination. Check that she has documented scars from previous breast surgery accurately. Fine, linear lead scar markers may be used to identify scars on mammography images; they are used at the discretion of the interpreting radiologist.

Always encourage the patient to perform regular breast self-examination as part of her personal breast health program. Brochures and pamplets should be available for the patient to read and take with her when she leaves your office. Also, many sites will have a video on Breast Self-Examination (BSE) playing in the waiting area. This serves a dual purpose: it refreshes the woman's memory regarding the details of BSE; and it can serve as a distraction as she sits in the waiting area.

 Always encourage the patient to perform regular breast self-examination as part of her personal breast health program.

6. Patient Shielding

In the event that a patient requests a lead apron or thyroid shield, it is important that these items are available for her examination. While the x-ray beam is restricted to the size of the receptor and scatter radiation is not considered to be significant, much less harmful at the low energy levels used for mammography imaging, it is important to respect the patient's concerns and provide for her accordingly. While local legislation may present a unique and individual policy on this matter, it is generally accepted that shielding is neither necessary nor warranted with current mammography practice. Rare exceptions would include the pregnant woman or the woman who is actively trying to get pregnant and who requires a limited mammography examination because of an urgent clinical concern.

You may want to clean the surface of the image receptor, the compression paddle and the face shield in the presence of the patient.

7. Equipment Preparation

Prepare the mammography equipment before you remove the patient's gown. Program the patient's information into the identification system and briefly check the technical settings on the control panel; last minute delays due to improper equipment settings are unacceptable when the patient is compressed and prepared for the exposure. Be sure your film markers are nearby and readily available. You may want to clean the surface of the image receptor, the compression paddle and the face shield in the presence of the patient. Many women appreciate this personal, visual confirmation that the equipment is sanitary before positioning begins.

Many facilities attempt to warm the surface of the image receptor for the patient's comfort before positioning begins. Electric heating pads on a very low setting may be used provided the equipment manufacturer has no objections. *The use of heating pads should always be verified with the equipment manufacturer in order to avoid inadvertently damaging the bucky and/or the grid.* An alternate suggestion that works very well is a large pad filled with gel, fiber, beans, etc. that can be heated in a microwave oven. These pads are very effective for safely warming the surface of the equipment that the breast will contact; they will need to be reheated every few hours.

Before beginning to position the patient for the mammography examination, always provide a brief description of the steps involved in order to prepare her for the procedure. This will help the examination to flow along smoothly without interruption once you begin.

8. Explaining the Procedure

Before beginning to position the patient for the mammography examination, always provide a brief description of the steps involved in order to prepare her for the procedure. This will help the examination to flow along smoothly without interruption once you begin. Many women forget parts of the examination, or they may have consciously chosen to block out this information. A new patient should be given a more detailed description because this is her first personal experience.

Always inquire if the patient has any questions or concerns that you can address before you begin the examination. Inform her of the number of films that you will take and prepare her for the possibility that additional views may be needed, describing that these are frequently required to clarify overlapping breast tissue. Advance warning of this possibility is extremely important should the patient need to be recalled for more images; her anxiety may not be as high, knowing this is a common occurrence.

The rationale for breast compression and the manner in which it will be applied should be included in your discussion. A poster that visually communicates these principles is very helpful. You may want to demonstrate the way the compression paddle moves so the patient is prepared for this movement and the noises she will hear. Avoid using terms such as *squeeze, pinch,* or *hurt*; words like *snug, tight,* and *uncomfortable* would be better choices. Be sure to emphasize the brief period (a matter of seconds) that the final, taut compression will be applied. Always apply compression gradually, allowing the patient time to adapt to the pressure. Invite her feedback as you proceed; this allows

Always inquire if the patient has any questions or concerns that you can address before you begin the examination.

---

the patient to feel that she has maintained some control in the situation. Manual compression is available on all modern equipment; it can be applied much more gently and gradually and should be used as soon as the patient appears uncomfortable.

Throughout the examination, maintain an attentive and caring attitude. Handle the patient and her breast gently, to acknowledge the sensitivity of the examination, but firmly, to control the positioning process. A confident, assured approach will be comforting for the patient. Eye contact with the patient is very helpful to assess her tolerance as you proceed and to distract her from becoming excessively anxious. Light conversation is also helpful to alleviate anxiety and to provide timely distraction as compression is applied. Try to convey an awareness that you have devoted your undivided attention and focus to her from the moment that compression is applied. Do not be distracted by a knock on the door or a ringing telephone. These measures are invaluable in alleviating the patient's anxiety and in developing an atmosphere of confidence and trust.

Having covered the above variety of imaging considerations, we are now ready to proceed with the mammography examination.

 Throughout the examination, maintain an attentive and caring attitude. Handle the patient and her breast gently, to acknowledge the sensitivity of the examination, but firmly, to control the positioning process.

POSITIONING FOR MAMMOGRAPHY

SECTION III:
MAMMOGRAPHY PROJECTIONS / VIEWS

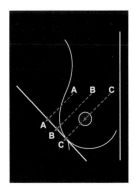

SECTION III:
MAMMOGRAPHY PROJECTIONS / VIEWS

The following views / projections will be described in this text:

Throughout this text, the term <u>view</u> has been used interchangeably with the term <u>projection</u> because mammography images are frequently viewed from a similar perspective to the beam projection used to produce the image.

SECTION III:
MAMMOGRAPHY PROJECTIONS / VIEWS

A. STANDARD MAMMOGRAPHY VIEWS

1. Craniocaudal View

(CC View, Cephalocaudal View)

 FOcus Medial, central and retroareolar breast tissue; lateral tissue can often be completely visualized as well.

Over the years, considerable variability has been noted with the CC view (projection). The potential for variability arises from the discrepancy that exists between the curved contour of the rib cage and the straight edge of the image receptor (Figure 4.112 B).

NOTE:
Early positioning practices for the CC view emphasized the lateral portion of the breast (Figure 4.112 C). The axillary tail (also referred to as the Tail of Spence) extends laterally and obliquely from the breast parenchyma of the U.O.Q. into the axilla. This is directly responsible for the fact that the largest percentage of breast parenchyma is located in the U.O.Q. This is also why, statistically, cancer occurs most frequently in the U.O.Q. of the breast. Therefore, it seemed both logical and desirable to rotate the patient slightly to consistently image more of the lateral, high risk breast tissue on the CC view. The downside of this practice was that medial breast tissue was often sacrificed on the CC image. Because very few breast cancers occur in the medial breast tissue, this protocol was considered acceptable by the mammography community for many years. An awareness of the mammographic *blind* areas adjacent to the rib cage and the fact that medial tissue has the greatest potential

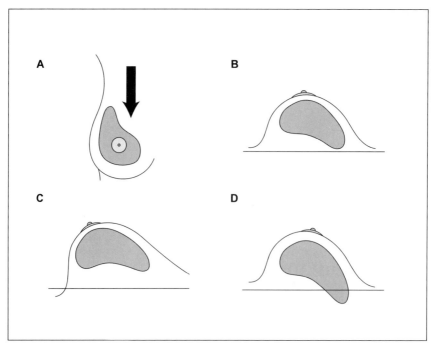

Figure 4.112 Line Diagram Representing Positioning for the CC View. Diagram B illustrates an ideal CC view of the breast with the nipple centered; medial tissue is included and the majority of lateral glandular tissue is also visualized. Diagram C incorrectly illustrates lateral breast emphasis (at the expense of medial tissue) to focus on lateral glandular tissue. Diagram D incorrectly illustrates medial breast emphasis at the expense of lateral tissue.

for exclusion on the MLO view did not raise serious concern because, statistically, breast cancer does not commonly occur in the medial breast tissue.

Two factors eventually encouraged mammographers to reconsider their positioning protocols. First, when mammography screening programs were introduced for asymptomatic women, it became apparent that in order to optimize mammography, and consequently, the ultimate goal of breast screening, *all of the breast tissue* had to be imaged using only the two standard screening views (CC and MLO). Second, clinically occult cancers in the medial breast were frequently not visualized on a mammogram. Occasionally a subtle hint of abnormality deep in the medial tissue on the CC view led to a cleavage projection that demonstrated an obvious carcinoma. It became clear that the CC view needed to image medial tissue to complement the MLO view that focused on lateral tissue and the upper, outer quadrant of the breast. Together, these two views will image all of the breast tissue for a complete examination.

This protocol has replaced traditional practices and is now the basis of our current positioning techniques.

PROCEDURE

A. The Short Version:

1. Select the appropriate receptor (film) size.

2. Place the correct film marker on the axillary side of the receptor.

3. Have the patient face the mammography unit, with her shoulders and chest muscles relaxed.

4. Standing on the opposite side of the patient, elevate the breast until the PNL is perpendicular to the chest wall or to its maximum height of natural mobility.

5. Position the receptor to support the breast in this position.

6. Using both hands, gently pull breast tissue forward, away from the chest wall, onto the receptor. The patient's medial ribs should be adjacent to the image receptor.

7. Drape the opposite breast over the corner of the receptor.

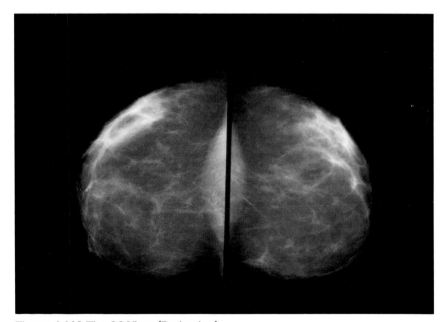

Figure 4.113 The CC View (Projection)

8. With your arm around the patient's back, rest your hand on her shoulder. Gently pull skin up, just above the clavicle. With your front hand firmly anchoring the breast position on the receptor, pull lateral breast tissue forward.

9. Apply compression, sliding your hand out toward the nipple as the paddle reaches the breast tissue.

10. Select the appropriate AEC cell position.

11. Smooth out any skin folds and wrinkles.

12. Ask the patient to stop breathing - expose the film - release the compression immediately.

B. The Long Version: Everything You Wanted to Know ... and More ...

1) Select the appropriate receptor (film) size.

2) Place the correct film marker on the axillary (lateral) side of the receptor.

3) Have the patient remove high heels and any other footwear that is not stable and solid; only flat shoes with a traction sole should be allowed. Also remove large earrings, jewellery, and scarves from the neck area. Small pendants or chains can simply be swung around the patient's back. Glasses should also be removed. If you anticipate problems with the patient's hair overshadowing the image, you may offer her an elastic band to keep long hair off the shoulder area; for short hair, bobby pins or clips can be used to control stray hair.

4) The patient should approach the mammography equipment, facing the unit, and stopping about half a step back from the image receptor. Her hands should be resting comfortably at her sides rather than clasped together in front of or behind her body. Turn her body slightly medially to align her breast with the image receptor. Her feet should be slightly separated for better balance. It is recommended that the technologist stand on the opposite side of the patient from the side being imaged, with her arm around the patient to maintain control and to gently guide the patient into position. This facilitates observation of the breast being positioned, especially the medial tissue and the PNL; it also allows the technologist to maintain eye contact with the patient during the examination The patient's shoulder and arm obstruct vision when the technologist stands on the same side as the breast being imaged.

5) If the patient is standing very straight and tall with her shoulders drawn back, lean her forward slightly from the waist so that the rib cage directly

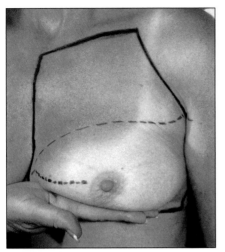

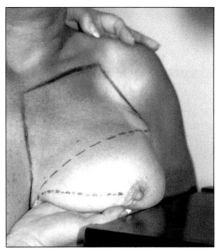

Figure 4.114 Turn your hand to support the weight of the breast with the palm of your hand; the lateral border of your hand should remain firmly anchored to the rib cage along the inferior margin of the breast and your palm should be parallel to the receptor.

Figure 4.115 Adjust the image receptor to the height that will comfortably support the breast in this position when you remove your hand.

above the breast *mound* is perpendicular to the receptor. Then encourage her to relax and *slouch* her shoulders forward and down.

6) Place your front hand flat against the patient's ribs directly under the breast being examined and slide it upward, elevating the breast until the PNL is perpendicular to the chest wall. Turn your hand to support the weight of the breast with the palm of your hand. The lateral border of your hand should remain firmly anchored to the rib cage along the inferior margin of the breast and your palm should be parallel to the receptor. Adjust the image receptor to the height that will comfortably support the breast in this position when you remove your hand; it may appear somewhat high until your hand has been removed. The patient should still be standing about half a step back from the receptor; when she leans forward against it, she will feel comfortable and stable.

7) Instruct the patient to turn her head toward you and ask her to loosen and relax the muscles of her neck, shoulders, and thorax. With your free hand on top of the breast, have the patient lean forward until the edge of the receptor contacts the rib cage along the lateral border of your lower hand; the breast should be centered on the image receptor, perhaps allowing some additional room on the axillary side where

more tissue may be present. Using both hands, *gently but firmly* pull breast tissue away from the chest wall onto the receptor, sliding your lower hand out while firmly anchoring the superior tissue with your upper hand. Again reminding the patient to relax her shoulder muscles, bring your free hand over the hand on the superior tissue and secure this tissue, gently pulling it away from the chest wall as you carefully remove your lower hand. The medial ribs should be resting firmly against the image receptor. Ideally, the nipple should be centered on the receptor and pointing directly away from the chest wall; neither medial nor lateral deviation should be evident. Check that the patient's feet remain flat on the floor; she should not stretch up on her toes because of the height of the image receptor.

8) Lift the medial corner of the op-posite breast and drape it over the corner of the image receptor (Helpful Hints *d*). If the patient tends to lean away from the unit, encourage her to bring her head forward, around the side of the face shield (Helpful Hints *e*). Again, bring your arm around the patient's back, resting your hand on top of her shoulder to ensure that it remains down and relaxed. At this point, the PNL should be parallel to the receptor and per-pendicular to the chest wall, with the nipple in profile in the major-ity of cases. This, however, is not a positioning criterion; including as much tissue as possible is the primary goal (Helpful Hints *c*).

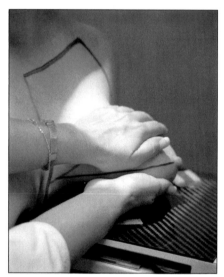

Figure 4.116 Using both hands, gently but firmly pull breast tissue away from the chest wall onto the receptor.

9) On the same side that you are positioning, the patient's arm should be relaxed by her side. If she needs to hold onto the mammography unit for stability, she should do so with her opposite hand. Immediately prior to applying compression, *gently but firmly* wrap the fingers of the anchoring hand around the lateral tissue and pull as much tissue forward as possible; the shoulder must be relaxed to facilitate this maneuver. Do not rotate the patient's thorax - her ribs must remain firmly adjacent to the edge of the receptor on the medial side.

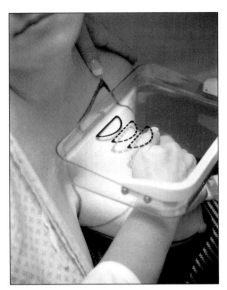

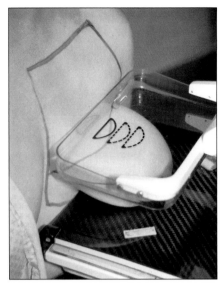

Figure 4.117 Gently but firmly wrap your fingers around the lateral tissue and pull as much of this area forward as possible.

Figure 4.118 The breast was not adequately elevated for this CC view. Note how much superior breast tissue has been excluded from the image compared to Figure 4.117.

10) Using the fingers of the hand resting on the patient's shoulder, carefully pull loose skin upward, just above the clavicle. As the compression paddle contacts the rib cage, just below the clavicle, gradually let this skin go as you feel tension on the skin with the continued downward movement of the compression paddle. This practice relieves excessive tension on the skin in the neck and shoulder area, which many patients find extremely uncomfortable during the final stages of compression for the CC view (Helpful Hints *e*). As well, the free skin that you release improves mobility of the compression paddle as it passes along the anterior chest wall, immediately above the breast.

11) Apply compression *gradually* while continuing to draw tissue away from the chest wall (Figure 4.117); withdraw your anchoring hand toward nipple as the compression paddle contacts the superior breast tissue. Instruct the patient to resist the temptation to pull her shoulder back to accommodate the compression paddle as it passes by the axillary area. This is a natural reaction that will result in loss of tissue on the image. Gentle pressure from the arm around the patient's back is used to maintain her forward position and control any subconscious tendency to lean back as compression is applied.

12) Place the patient's opposite hand on the handlebar (Helpful Hints *j*). When you remove your arm from around the patient's back, this will provide security and help the patient remain steady for the exposure. This also helps the patient to keep her ribs forward, resting firmly against the compression paddle and therefore more posterior tissue will remain in the field.

13) The breast should be compressed until the tissue is *taut* (*firm to the touch*); at maximum, it should be *less than painful*. Compression should be applied as gradually as necessary, according to the comfort level and tolerance of the patient. The manual compression control should be used during the final stages, as this allows the compression to be applied much more gradually and gently; the patient will find this much more tolerable. Just before the final, full compression is achieved, be sure that film markers are in place and all skin folds, etc. have been corrected. Any delay or hesitation is unacceptable once taut compression has been applied.

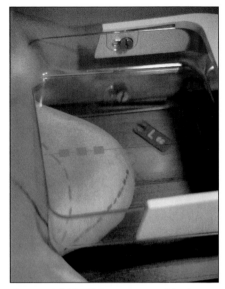

Figure 4.119 With proper positioning techniques, the pectoralis muscle will be imaged over the central to medial breast tissue on the CC view.

14) Select the appropriate Automatic Exposure Control (AEC) cell (photocell) position.

15) Ask the patient to stop breathing (Helpful Hints *l*). Complete the exposure and release the compression immediately.

HELPFUL HINTS

a) The face shield is designed to keep the patient's head, ear, chin, etc. out of the image field on the medial side of the breast being imaged. The technologist may remove the face shield during positioning if the patient has limited neck movement and she finds the position of the face shield creates excessive neck strain. Unfortunately, the patient will have a natural tendency to relax her neck and perhaps lean into the image area; therefore, the technologist must check that a shadow from

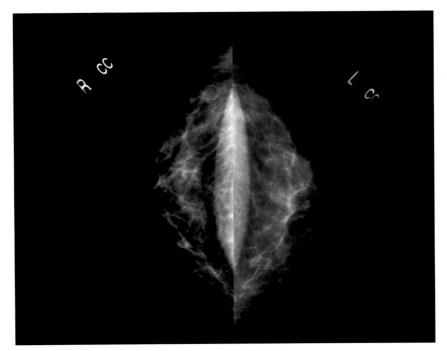

Figure 4.120 Well positioned, symmetrical CC views.

the patient's head, ear, chin, etc. is not over the breast tissue just before she exposes each image.

b) Small lead BB markers may be placed on the patient's nipples *before* positioning begins. This provides a definitive indication of nipple location to facilitate measurements that may be taken from the images to indicate the location of an area of interest. Accurately locating the nipple on a mammogram has become increasingly difficult (even with the aid of a bright light) as the optical density of our images has increased and as the contrast of our films has improved dramatically.

c) *NEVER sacrifice breast tissue to project the nipple in profile and / or centered on the standard views.* The primary goal of mammography is to image all of the breast tissue. In the majority of cases (unless the patient presents with an unusual nipple location) the nipple will be projected in profile when correct positioning techniques have been followed. Should this not be the case, the film can be marked *Nipple not in profile* and an additional anterior view with the nipple in profile can then be performed. Many radiologists will accept an examination (without requiring additional views) in which the nipple is profiled on one of the two standard views. A lead BB is very helpful to mark the nipple when it will not be projected in profile; this eliminates the possibility that it may be mistaken for a lesion on the mammogram.

d) The purpose of draping the opposite breast over the corner of the image receptor is to facilitate complete imaging of the posterior, medial breast tissue (Figure 4.122). Even a *small* breast can cause the patient to be pushed away from the bucky (Figure 4.121). Lifting a portion of the opposite breast onto the receptor relieves skin tension that would otherwise pull posterior tissue off the surface of the receptor on the medial side of the breast being imaged. There is an art to the process of draping. The corner of the opposite breast should never be superimposed over the medial tissue of the breast being imaged. In general, the breasts can be gently separated on the image receptor in such a manner that the extreme medial tissue will be imaged free of superimposition (Helpful Hints *j*).

e) Many patients experience discomfort related to tension in the neck area as compression is applied. Frequently this is due to excessive tension on the skin; refer to step # 10 in the detailed CC positioning description

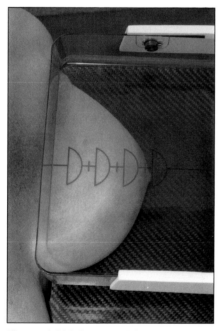

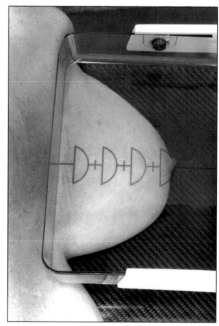

Figure 4.121 Careless CC positioning: The opposite breast is not draped over the corner of the bucky and the superior tissue was not pulled onto the receptor.

Figure 4.122 Improved CC positioning: Medial tissue is now adequately covered and far more superior tissue has been included. The AEC cell position confirms how much more tissue has been imaged.

for information on how to alleviate skin tension. In addition, encourage the patient to bring her head around the side of the x-ray tube, turning her face slightly toward the breast being imaged and resting her cheek against the face shield. This may also relieve tension in the neck area; at the same time, it will help to keep posterior and medial tissue pulled forward onto the image receptor during breast positioning. If the patient still experiences discomfort as compression is applied, have her drop her chin down and ask her to consciously relax and loosen her neck muscles.

f) A small fold of tissue from the abdomen is sometimes seen resting on the image receptor, under the medial breast tissue. When this happens, air will be trapped between the receptor and the inferior breast tissue; visually, the inferior, medial corner of the breast will appear slightly raised, rather than lying flat on the image receptor (Figures 4.123 and 4.124). A black, triangular shaped shadow (trapped air) will be imaged in the medial tissue, adjacent to the chest wall on the mammogram. To eliminate this problem, place your free hand on the patient's abdo-

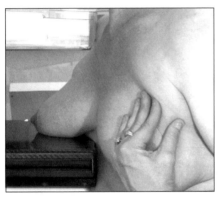

Figure 4.123 A small fold of tissue from the abdomen is sometimes seen resting on the receptor, under the medial breast tissue.

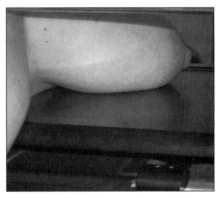

Figure 4.124 A close up view of Figure 4.123. Note the corresponding clinical image in Figure 4.125.

men just below the bucky and *gently pull tissue downward*. You will see the fold disappear and the inferior surface of the breast will be now be resting flat on the receptor. Instruct the patient to avoid leaning back as you perform this maneuver.

g) If a shadow from the patient's shoulder is superimposed over the breast tissue, a number of tactics may be used to eliminate this appearance:
  ▪ Encourage the patient to relax her shoulder and drop it down
  ▪ Rotate her hand outward

- Have the patient bend her elbow, resting her hand on her abdomen
- Ask the patient to gently roll her shoulder back, being very careful that lateral tissue is not drawn away during the process.

h) To eliminate the shadow of excess tissue that may project from above the compression paddle over the posterior tissue beneath the compression paddle, gently experiment with a variety of shoulder positions, taking care that no lateral tissue slips out from beneath the compression paddle.

i) *Do not attempt to smooth out folds and wrinkles until compression is nearly complete.* Minor skin folds will often compress out as pressure is applied to the breast tissue. To eliminate wrinkles under the compression paddle along the chest wall, approach the breast from the side and gently slip your index finger between the breast and the paddle to smooth the skin. While this must be addressed before full compression has been applied, sufficient pressure must be in place in order to achieve the skin tension that is necessary to successfully manipulate folds and wrinkles. Most folds can be eliminated in this fashion. Pulling on the tissue in the shoulder area or above the compression paddle frequently results in loss of tissue on the final image.

j) When the patient grasps the handlebar with her opposite hand, her arm may inadvertently

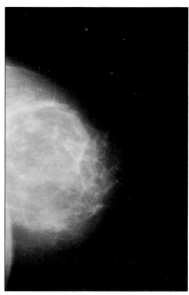

Figure 4.125 A clinical image demonstrating the presence of a small tuck of tissue under the medial side of the breast. Note the dark shadow immediately anterior to the tissue fold; this represents free air trapped between the breast and the receptor. Tissue detail is sacrificed in this area.

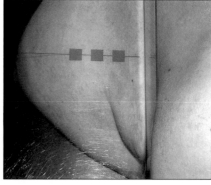

Figure 4.126 Minor folds and skin wrinkles will compress out as compression is applied to the breast. When a fold remains, slip one finger between the compression paddle and the breast to gently smooth out the tissue.

press the opposite breast medially, superimposing breast tissue in the cleavage area. If this occurs, gently rotating her elbow away from her body will relieve excess pressure on the opposite breast and allow the overlapping to be cleared in the medial tissue. With large, pendulous breasts that will resist resting on the corner of the image receptor as a result of the weight of the remaining breast tissue, use the opposite arm to support the weight of this breast beside the bucky in order to successfully accomplish breast draping.

k) The skin in the inframammary area is often very thin and fragile with large-breasted women. During the mammography examination, the skin in this area may break and bleed. Lift and manipulate these breasts with care. You may want to wear gloves when this area appears very fragile or when the skin is already broken. To minimize trauma to this area, avoid multiple breast adjustments once you have placed the breast on the image receptor. Also, instruct the patient that she should avoid pulling away from the receptor immediately after the exposure when the compression releases; instead, she should carefully lift her breast off the image receptor before she steps back. Most women are acutely aware of the compromised condition of their skin in this area and they appreciate the technologist's care and concern in this matter.

l) Respiration should be suspended for the x-ray exposure. It is preferable to simply instruct the patient to stop breathing for a moment; if she appears short of breath, it is advisable that you warn her a few moments ahead of time. Asking her to *hold her breath* will encourage her to inhale; her ribs will move and positioning may change slightly. With slim patients, where draping of the opposite breast has been difficult to accomplish, this minimal movement is enough to sacrifice the breast position.

m) Kyphotic patients are very difficult to image in the CC projection. Refer to the section on *kyphotic patients* for detailed information regarding the best way to image these patients.

n) For very small breasts and for men with well developed pectoral muscles, rotate the C-arm 180 degrees and perform a From Below (FB, reverse CC) View. This is an excellent option. The image receptor will be in contact with the superior breast tissue and the compression paddle will contact the inferior breast surface.

o) For very large breasts, that must be imaged in sections or *pieces*, it is important to proceed in a logical, organized manner. Refer to the section on *large breasts* for additional information regarding this subject.

---

2. Mediolateral Oblique View

(MLO View, Oblique View)

 The entire breast with emphasis on the U.O.Q. and the axillary tail.

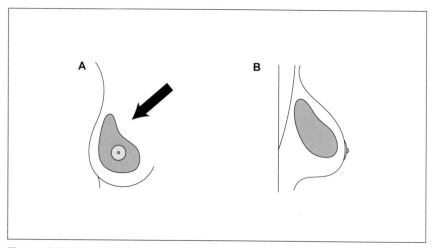

Figure 4.127 The MLO View (Projection)

The MLO view demonstrates more breast tissue than any other single mammography projection. It may be used alone, for a limited mammography examination with young patients. It also provides a second view of lesions seen in the CC projection.

The term oblique refers to the *axis of the plane of compression* rather than to the patient position. The MLO projection is designed to take advantage of the anatomical relationship of the breast on the pectoralis major muscle. This muscle is most easily compressed parallel to its long axis. With this principle in mind, aligning the image receptor parallel to the pectoralis muscle and directing the central ray perpendicular to it will maximize the process of gently pulling the breast tissue away from the chest wall and onto the image receptor. Also, the greatest amount of breast tissue possible should be demonstrated with the least amount of discomfort for the patient.

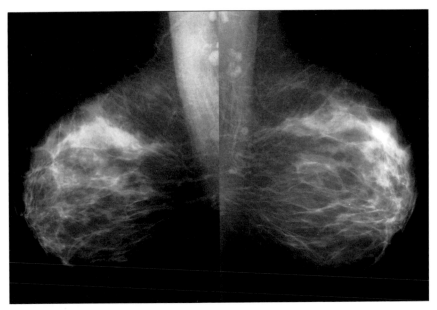

Figure 4.128 Clinical images in the MLO projection

PROCEDURE

A. The Short Version

1. Select the appropriate image receptor (film) size.

2. Place the correct film marker on the axillary side of the receptor.

3. Select the correct C-arm angulation based on the patient's body habitus. The angulation will vary, on average, between 45 and 55 degrees; patients with a long thorax will need higher angulation (closer to 60 degrees) while patients with a shorter thorax will need lower angulation (closer to 45 degrees).

4. Turn the patient's thorax about 45 degrees to the image receptor; her shoulders and chest muscles must be relaxed.

5. Adjust the height of the receptor so that the corner of the bucky is located halfway between the top of her shoulder and the axillary crease or approximately at the height of the sternoclavicular joint.

6. Place the patient's hand on the handlebar and bend her elbow behind the bucky.

7. Gather up as much lateral and inferior tissue as possible, lifting the breast medially and superiorly. Lift her shoulder, placing the corner of

the bucky into her axilla at the same time that you place her breast on the receptor.

8. Gently pull breast tissue forward and away from the chest wall with both hands.

9. Support the breast up and away from the chest wall as compression is applied.

10. When the compression paddle has passed the sternum, rotate the patient medially and turn her feet, hips, and shoulders straight ahead.

11. Complete the compression.

12. Clear the IMF.

13. Ask the patient to stop breathing - expose the film - release the compression immediately.

B. The Long Version: Everything You Wanted to Know ... and More ...

1) Select the appropriate image receptor (film) size.

2) Place the correct film marker on the axillary side of the receptor.

3) Have the patient remove high heels and any other footwear that is not stable and solid; only flat shoes with a traction sole should be allowed. Also remove large earrings, jewellery and scarves from the neck area. Small pendants or chains can simply be swung around the patient's back.

4) The patient should approach the mammography equipment, facing the unit, and stopping about half a step back from the image receptor. Her hands should be resting comfortably at her sides rather than clasped together in front of or behind her body. Her feet should be slightly separated for better balance. The technologist should be standing on the opposite side of the patient from the side being imaged. As positioning begins, the technologist will stand very close to the patient, with her sternum in contact with the arm resting along the patient's opposite side. The technologist's back arm will be used to reach behind the patient, providing support and guidance in the upper thorax area; her front hand will be used to lift and position the breast that is being imaged. Maintaining this very close proximity allows the technologist to completely control the patient's position; it should also provide a sense of security to the patient who may be nervous or very anxious.

5) Determine the appropriate C-arm angulation (Helpful Hints *a*) and rotate the C-arm to this position.

6) Have the patient drop both shoulders down, to a natural, relaxed position. Adjust the height of the image receptor so that the corner is located halfway between the top of the shoulder and the axillary crease below, or approximately to the level of the sternoclavicular joint.

7) Turn the patient's body until her feet are pointing towards you at about 45 degrees to the image receptor. Reaching behind the patient, help her to raise her arm 90 degrees to the thorax and, with the elbow bent, rest her hand loosely on the handlebar (Helpful Hints *d*). *Grasping* the bar tightens the muscles which will result in less breast tissue being imaged and much more difficulty in guiding the patient into position.

8) With your front hand along the lateral / inferior breast, gather up and gently draw as much breast tissue as possible away from the chest wall, elevating it medially toward the sternum. Your back hand can also help to move lateral tissue forward at the same time. It is very important that the patient's shoulder and thorax muscles be relaxed in order to successfully draw the maximum amount of breast tissue possible away from the chest wall for this image (Helpful Hints *c*).

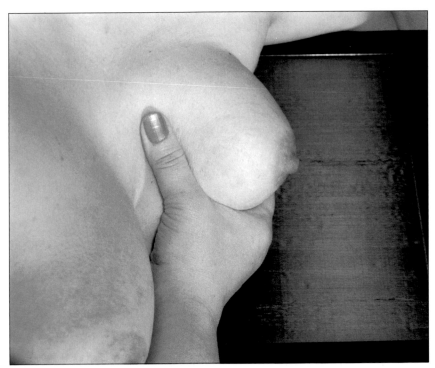

Figure 4.129 Using the up-and-out maneuver, gather up as much breast tissue as possible, elevating it medially toward the sternum.

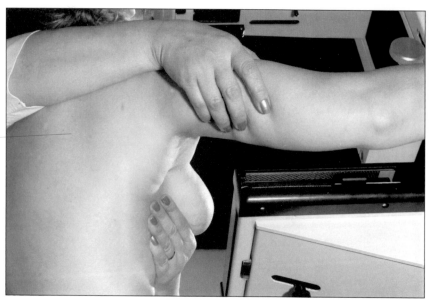

Figure 4.130 A posterior view: after the breast tissue has been gathered up with the up-and-out maneuver, the patient's axilla is stretched over the corner of the bucky as her breast is positioned on the image receptor.

9) Reminding the patient to relax her shoulder once again, with your back hand guiding the upper humerus, roll her shoulder forward. If all the positioning steps have been properly performed at this point, one smooth motion will now complete the positioning for this view. Using your arm along her back, lean the patient slightly forward and down; her ribs will now contact the bucky as you position her breast on the image receptor while simultaneously easing her shoulder forward as much as possible to stretch her flaccid axilla over the upper edge of the receptor; the breast should be placed on the image receptor at the same time the axilla is stretched forward and the elbow is bent and relaxed behind the receptor. Place your hand on the patient's shoulder to maintain its forward and down position. As the compression begins, secure the tissue immediately in front of the clavicle with your fingers. Your body contact with her thorax will stabilize the patient's position as you proceed.

10) With your front hand, continue to support the breast up and away from the chest wall with your thumb in front and fingers behind, gently pulling tissue forward. *A quick visual check should now find that the anterior margin of the clavicle (where your fingers are located), the posterior breast tissue along the sternum and ribs, and the inframammary area*

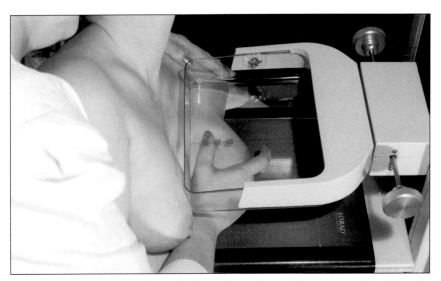

Figure 4.131 An anterior view: the breast is resting on the receptor; the elbow is now bent behind the bucky.

are all aligned and parallel with the edge of the compression paddle. If this is not the case, pressure from your arm on the patient's back or from your body against the patient's side can correct the upper and lower alignment, respectively. Again, the patient must be relaxed and loose to allow you to move her breast and body in this manner.

11) Remind the patient to keep her shoulder and thorax muscles loose and relaxed and slowly begin compression. When the compression paddle passes the sternum, rotate the patient forward and down with pressure from your arm behind her back; this will roll the deepest medial tissue forward, into the image field. At the same time, ask the patient to turn her body so that her feet, hips, and shoulders are now facing the machine. As the paddle approaches your thumb, slip your fingers out from behind the breast, securing the position of the inferior tissue with your thumb and the heel of your hand. The upper corner of the compression paddle should pass immediately below the head of the humerus and in front of the clavicle as the remainder of the paddle captures tissue along the rib cage, adjacent to the sternum. As the paddle contacts the patient's tissue to secure the position of the breast, remove your front hand, sliding it out in the direction of the nipple and continuing to pull tissue forward as you leave. The fingers securing the tissue near the clavicle can also be used to pull axillary tissue forward as compression is applied. If the compression paddle has secured the

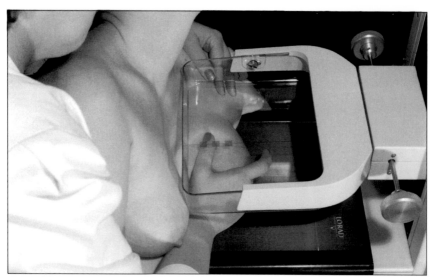

Figure 4.132 The technologist rolls the patient's shoulder forward and down; note the width of the axilla along the superior margin of the bucky compared to Figure 4.131, before this shoulder maneuver.

tissue adequately, the breast should not fall or droop when you release your hand.

12) Slide the index finger of your front hand between the receptor and the patient's breast to feel for any tissue folds in the inframammary area. Superimposed tissue can easily be smoothed downward or gently pushed backward, off the surface of the receptor while your back arm applies pressure from behind to prevent the patient from leaning away. Folds from the upper abdomen can be successfully cleared from the inframammary area using this technique (Helpful Hints *i*). Failing to check this area and clear the tissue folds will result in a black triangular area being imaged along the inferior posterior margin of the breast. This appearance represents trapped air under the breast tissue; because the breast is rolled up along the skin fold, rather than lying flat on the receptor, the tissue in this area has not been imaged adequately. If the opposite breast is casting a shadow over the compressed breast, have the patient gently hold this breast back, out of the image with her free hand.

13) Select the appropriate AEC cell position.

14) Ask the patient to stop breathing. Complete the exposure and release the compression immediately.

HELPFUL HINTS

a) The correct angulation for the MLO view will generally vary between 40 and 60 degrees depending upon the patient's body habitus. To determine the correct angle, raise the patient's arm 90 degrees to her thorax to simulate the MLO position. The shoulder must be relaxed and not elevated. Observe the angle of the free margin of the pectoralis muscle as it forms the anterior border of the axilla. Follow this angle (that forms the *free margin of the axilla*) as it extends across the muscle fibers on the anterior rib cage. These fibers (and angle) will cross the thorax from the lateral, free margin of the axilla and extend medially, at an angle, toward the lower third of the sternum. It is this *angle* of the muscle fibers that determines the *angle* of the bucky. They must be parallel. Refer to *mammography angulation* in the previous section on Breast Mapping for additional information regarding this subject.

b) Correct angulation will be reflected on clinical images by the *length* of the muscle. A long muscle shadow, extending down to or beyond the PNL indicates that the selected C-arm angle was correct for the patient's body habitus (Figure 4.21). A short, often sharply angled muscle shadow that does not extend down to the PNL indicates that the C-arm angle was too steep for the patient's body habitus; medial posterior tissue will be excluded from these images (Figure 4.22).

c) *The importance of relaxation cannot be overemphasized.* This relaxation will be evident by a convex configuration of the pectoralis muscle on the MLO image. Loose, relaxed muscles will allow the breast to be pulled away from the chest wall, visualizing the most posterior tissue of the breast. A soft muscle will facilitate taut compression and separation of breast structures without undue discomfort for the patient. Finally, positioning of the breast and the patient will be accomplished with greater ease when the patient is relaxed. Also, fewer repeats and additional views will be required because the original images will be optimal from the perspective of positioning, compression, and technique. The time spent relaxing the patient and obtaining her full cooperation in this matter is invaluable. If this is not done properly during initial positioning, much more time will be consumed to bring the patient back into the room and set up once again for a repeat film.

d) When placing the patient's hand on the positioning handlebar, instruct her *not to grip the bar firmly*. This will tighten the muscles in her hand, arm and shoulder. A tight muscle will have a concave configuration on the mammogram; it may also cause the muscle to be radiopaque. The muscle must be radioluscent to insure visualization of medial and lateral breast tissue that may be superimposed on the pectoralis mus-

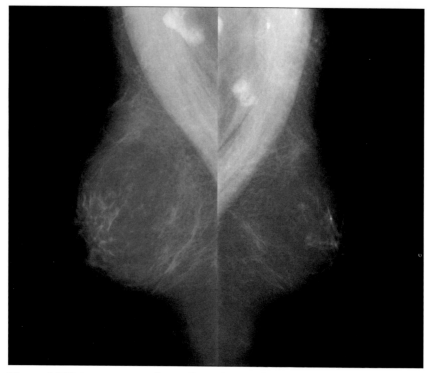

Figure 4.133 A convex muscle configuration confirms that the patient was re-laxed, the bucky was not elevated excessively (which would stretch the muscle and result in a straight or concave configuration) and the breast was properly mobilized toward the medial fixed border.

cle. She will need to relax this grip in order to proceed with successful and comfortable positioning. With patients who find it difficult to relax their hold, have them straighten their fingers and rest their entire hand on top of the handlebar.

e) The axilla should be lying flat on the image receptor, unless the latis-simus dorsi muscle (upper posterior shoulder area) has inadvertently been positioned in front of the bucky as well. If this is the case, gently ease it up and over the corner of the receptor, being careful not to allow the patient to roll her shoulder back, thereby losing pectoral muscle on the image.

f) The correct position of the corner of the bucky in the axilla will be reflected on clinical images by the *width* of the superior part of the pectoralis muscle. A wide margin along the top of the image indicates that the bucky is correctly located in the *posterior* part of the axilla, just in front of the latissimus dorsi muscle. A narrow margin along the top of the image indicates that the bucky is located too far forward in the patient's axilla; posterior tissue and lymph nodes may not be imaged on this film.

g) For patients with limited arm and shoulder mobility who cannot raise their arm to rest their hand on the handlebar, simply lift their axilla over the corner of the image receptor and allow their arm to hang freely behind the bucky. If the shoulder muscles can be relaxed somewhat, the MLO view will be very successful.

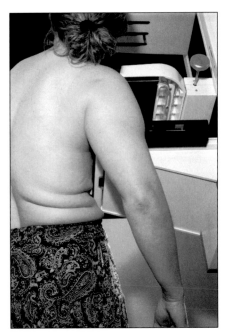

Figure 4.134 The arm can simply hang behind the bucky when the patient has limited arm and shoulder mobility.

h) Minor skin folds under the compression paddle in the axillary area can be eliminated by slipping one finger between the patient's skin and the compression paddle to gently smooth the skin. A fold along the undersurface of the axilla would need to be gently smoothed from beneath this tissue. When soft tissue from the arm is situated in front of the receptor along the upper edge, lift the patient's arm from behind and gently roll the excess tissue backward, to position it behind the receptor. *Be sure the patient's elbow is bent behind the bucky*; this will automatically position the majority of soft tissue from the arm behind the receptor.

i) Folding in the inframammary area is a common occurrence. As you clear the folds (as described in step # 12) be very careful not to lose tissue in this area. When a large, protruding abdomen creates overlapping, ask the patient to bend her hips back, away from the receptor. With minimal superimposition, perform the *knee-bend* maneuver: Have the patient bend the knee of the side being imaged, allowing her hip to drop down somewhat as her knee bends. This creates a *pull* in the inframammary area which will assist in smoothing out tissue folds.

j) The *knee-bend* maneuver (Helpful Hints *i*) is also extremely successful in helping the very tense, rigid patient to relax during positioning for the MLO view. Bending her knee breaks the rigidity of her stance and forces her to relax somewhat as she leans against the image receptor for support.

k) Occasionally inframammary tissue is not present after compression has been applied. When this happens, grasp the patient's hips and gently rotate them around, toward the front of the bucky, bringing some tissue

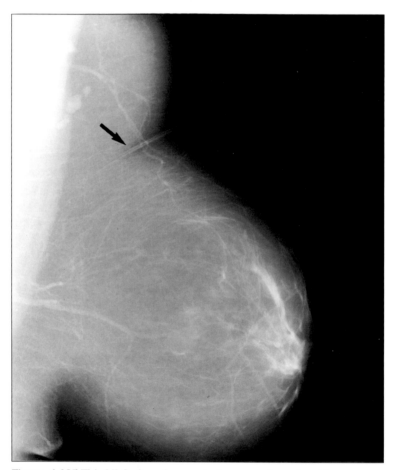

Figure 4.135 This MLO view demonstrates a number of problems. Note the folds in the inframammary area. The vertical fold (Figure 4.136) is due to excess tissue from the abdomen that has been pulled onto the receptor. Inserting one finger between the bucky and the patient will allow the technologist to smooth this fold out. The horizontal fold (Figure 4.136) is due to "drooping" of the anterior breast tissue. The breast was not supported adequately before it was compressed. Also note the fold that is evident in the axillary area (black arrow). This is frequently seen with large, heavy breasts. It is sometimes difficult to lift the breast enough to clear the IMF without creating a fold in the axilla.

forward onto the image receptor. Smooth this tissue to eliminate any skin folds in the area.

l) The thickness of the axillary tissue with a breast that is wide from side to side (a broad thorax) presents specific imaging difficulties for the MLO projection; this will be even more pronounced when the breast is also large. In particularly difficult cases, two views may be necessary: one for the posterior and axillary tissue (the anterior breast will not be well compressed; it may also be overexposed due to the thickness of the posterior tissue) and one for the anterior breast (with this tissue compressed optimally, the technique will also be improved). The anterior image should be performed with a lateral C-arm orientation. Refer to the section on *large breasts* for additional information.

m) With very large, pendulous breasts, it may be difficult to provide enough support to clear the inframammary tissue without creating folds in the axilla area (Figure 4.135). Small axillary folds can often be smoothed out after compression has been applied. When this is difficult to accomplish or the folds are large and prominent, two images may be required. In these situations, the technologist should first position for optimal axillary imaging on the standard MLO view (because the axilla and U.O.Q. are the primary focus of this projection). An additional film or a localized *spot* view to demonstrate the inframammary area free of

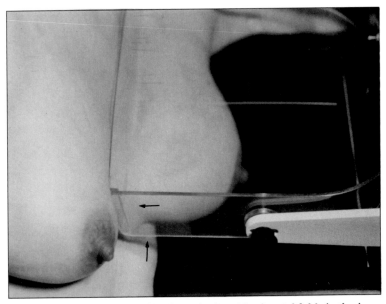

Figure 4.136 The effects of both vertical and horizontal folds in the inframammary area are illustrated here (Figure 4.135).

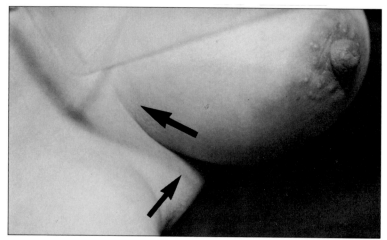

Figure 4.137 A close up view of vertical and horizontal folds in the inframammary area (Figures 4.135 and 4.136). The C-arm angulation is too steep for this patient. The inferior breast tissue would be supported better with lower angulation.

superimposition can then be performed (Figure 4.138). This image should be performed with a 90 degree C-arm orientation.

n) Occasionally a very high MLO view focused on the axilla may be required to image a deep axillary mass or to visualize abnormal lymph nodes. Positioning for this view will be identical to the standard MLO positioning; the emphasis will simply be on the superior axillary tissue.

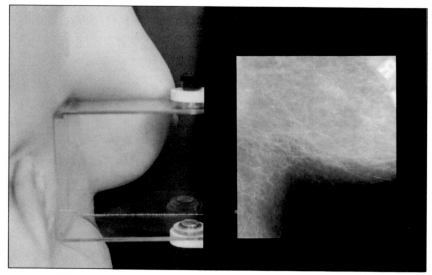

Figure 4.138 A 90 degree localized view can clarify tissue in the inferior breast when folding has been difficult to eliminate on the standard views.

This view is frequently confused with the axillary tail view although they are completely different projections. A high MLO view for the axillary region focuses on tissue that is much higher and deeper than the axillary tail area of the breast.

o) The following breathing technique may help to relax the pectoral muscles with a very tense patient: At the point when the compression paddle has just passed the sternum and is about to contact the breast tissue, instruct the patient to inhale slowly

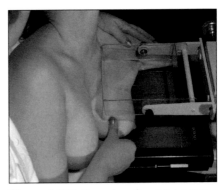

Figure 4.139 Occasionally a high MLO view, focused on the axilla, is required to image deep axillary tissue or abnormal lymph nodes.

and gently, without moving her shoulder, ribs, or breast tissue. The technologist must keep one hand on the patient's shoulder while the other firmly anchors the breast tissue on the image receptor. Then ask her to slowly exhale. Again, instruct her to inhale (as before) and then to gently exhale. As she exhales this time, slowly apply more compression. When she stops exhaling, instruct her to breathe out just a little more ... and again, just a little more ... each time easing the compression down further. This forced exhalation is extremely effective in relaxing

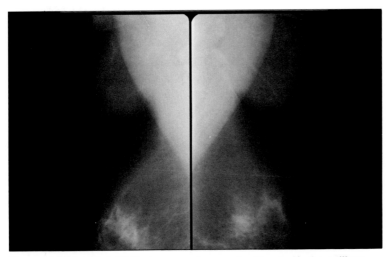

Figure 4.140 A high MLO view may be required to clarify the axillary area when accessory breast tissue creates excessive tissue overlapping on the MLO view.

the shoulder and pectoralis muscles. Allow the patient to take very shallow, gentle breaths while you clear any skin folds before you finally ask her to stop breathing for the exposure.

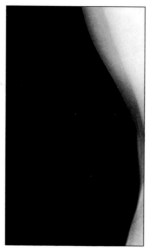

Figure 4.141 The MLO view is also used to image tissue remaining after a mastectomy, particularly if the patient develops clinical symptoms in this area.

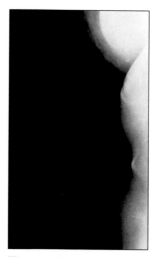

Figure 4.142 There is considerable variation in the amount of tissue that remains after mastectomy. A modified MLO view is much easier to image when there is more residual tissue.

The MLO view demonstrates more breast tissue than any other single mammography projection. It is designed to take advantage of the anatomical relationship of the breast on the pectoralis major muscle. This muscle is most easily compressed parallel to its long axis. With this principle in mind, aligning the image receptor parallel to the pectoralis muscle and directing the central ray perpendicular to it will maximize the process of gently pulling the breast tissue away from the chest wall and onto the image receptor.

B. SUPPLEMENTARY VIEWS

1. Modified Craniocaudal Views

a. Exaggerated CC View - Lateral

(XCCL View, Extended CC View - Lateral)

 FOcus Tissue in the extreme lateral aspect of the breast, not visualized on the standard CC view, just beyond the edge of the image receptor.

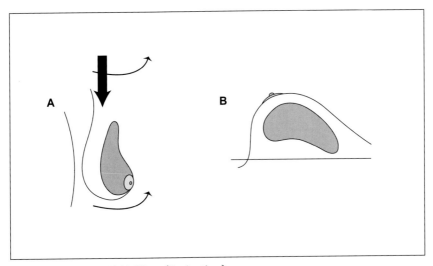

Figure 4.143 The XCCL View (Projection)

A small percentage of women have an abundance of glandular tissue that *wraps* laterally around the rib cage. This view is extremely successful in demonstrating the posterior margins of the lateral extensions of glandular tissue that may not be visualized on a standard CC projection due to the natural curvature of the rib cage in combination with a straight image receptor.

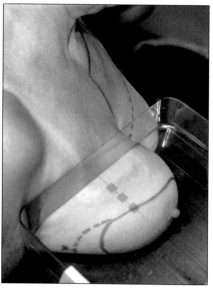

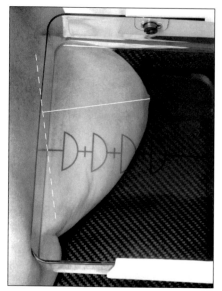

Figure 4.144 The patient is rotated to place the lateral tissue that "wraps" around the rib cage on the image receptor. The patient and breast remain in the same orientation that was used to image the standard CC view.

Figure 4.145 A superior view of the breast positioned for the XCCL view.

PROCEDURE

1) Place the correct film marker on the axillary side of the image receptor.

2) Begin positioning the patient as for the CC view. Rotate the patient's thorax to place the extreme lateral aspect of the breast onto the image receptor. Relax the patient's arm at her side.

3) Encourage the patient to relax her shoulder and consciously loosen the tissue in this area. Gently pull the lateral tissue forward as much as possible and secure this position on the receptor with your hand.

4) With your opposite arm around the patient's back, secure her position to ensure that she does not pull away from the receptor when the compression paddle passes her shoulder.

5) Apply compression, taking care to include the tissue that extends laterally, along the ribs. Very rarely, minimal C-arm angulation may be helpful to allow the compression paddle to pass by the head of the humerus.

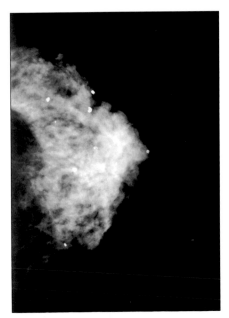

Figure 4.146 Lateral glandular tissue extends beyond the edge of the receptor in this CC view.

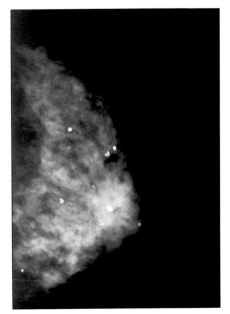

Figure 4.147 An XCCL view of the CC view in Figure 4.146 demonstrates the posterior border of the glandular tissue that was not visualized on this patient's routine examination.

6) Select the appropriate AEC cell position (usually the chest wall position).

7) Ask the patient to stop breathing. Complete the exposure and release compression immediately.

HELPFUL HINTS

1) You may find that a large spot compression paddle works well to position exaggerated views when the corner of the full 18 x 24 cm. compression paddle encounters the head of the humerus as it passes by the shoulder area.

2) As a rule, *angulation should not be used for exaggerated CC images.* This view is truly an extension of the standard CC projection. Therefore, breast tissue and the x-ray beam should remain in the same craniocaudal orientation. Angulation will orient the beam obliquely to the axillary tail rather than to the lateral extension of breast tissue, which is the true focus of this projection.

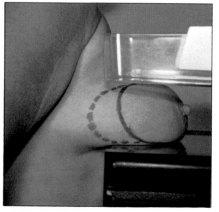

Figure 4.148 The posterior border of the lateral glandular tissue (marked with a broken line) is not imaged on this patient's routine CC view.

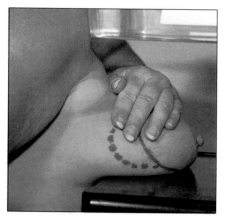

Figure 4.149 Rotating the patient (in the CC orientation) will bring this tissue onto the receptor for an XCCL view.

b. Cleavage View

(CV View, Valley View)

The extreme medial posterior tissue of both breasts; tissue anterior to the sternum.

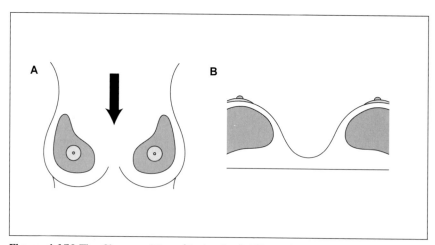

Figure 4.150 The Cleavage View (Projection), Bilateral examination

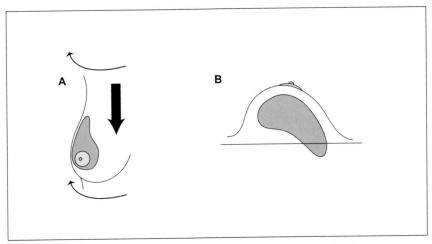

Figure 4.151 The Cleavage View (Projection), Unilateral examination

This projection is frequently used to verify that a suspicious medial *mass* is simply the point of insertion of the pectoralis muscle along the anterior chest wall.

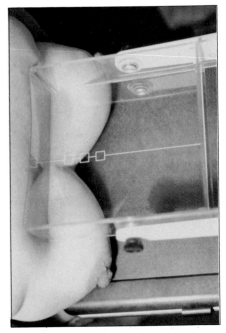

Figure 4.152 A patient positioned for a bilateral cleavage view.

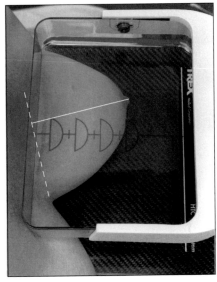

Figure 4.153 A patient positioned for a unilateral cleavage view.

PROCEDURE

1) Place the correct film marker on the axillary side of the image receptor.

2) The patient should be facing the mammography unit with her feet slightly separated for better balance.

3) Adjust the height of the image receptor to support the medial tissue of both breasts perpendicular to the chest wall.

4) Instruct the patient to relax her shoulder and chest muscles and lift both breasts onto the imager receptor, pulling as much medial tissue forward as possible. This is best done standing behind the patient, using your body to maintain the patient's forward position.

5) The patient's head should be turned to the side, usually away from the side of interest. The patient should hold the handlebars with both hands to keep her body forward, against the image receptor.

6) Ensure that the patient remains relaxed; if you are standing at the patient's side, keep one hand on the patient's back to prevent her from leaning away from the receptor.

7) Gradually apply compression using one hand to pull breast tissue forward while carefully guiding the compression paddle past the ribs and sternum.

8) Select the appropriate AEC cell position (usually the chest wall position).

9) Ask the patient to stop breathing. Complete the exposure and release the compression immediately.

HELPFUL HINTS

a) Place an R or L marker on the appropriate side of the receptor to indicate the breast being imaged; both markers can be used for bilateral examinations.

b) This exposure may be phototimed if there is enough tissue to cover the AEC device. Alternately, the cleavage may be offset slightly to include more tissue on the side of concern. Otherwise, a manual exposure technique must be set. For an average breast with very little cleavage tissue, one-quarter to one-third of the mAs used for the CC view would be a good starting point. The selected mAs will depend upon the quantity of tissue that will be imaged in this view as well as the density of this tissue. For a patient with an abundance of cleavage tissue,

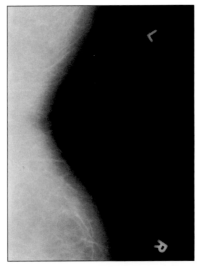

Figure 4.154 A bilateral examination of the cleavage view.

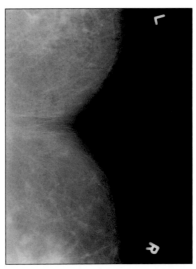

Figure 4.155 A bilateral cleavage view; these views often require a manual technique selection.

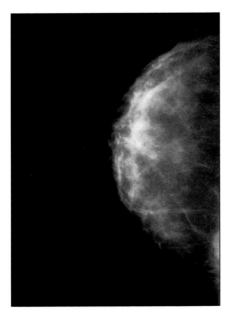

Figure 4.156 A cleavage view was performed to clarify the suspicion of a medial mass in this patient's breast.

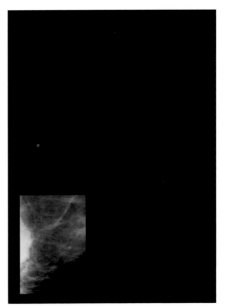

Figure 4.157 This coned cleavage view of the examination in Figure 4.156 confirmed that the suspicious mass was simply the medial insertion of the pectoralis muscle.

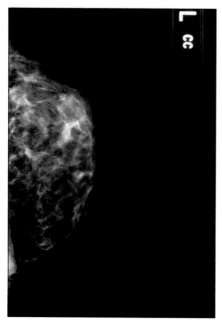

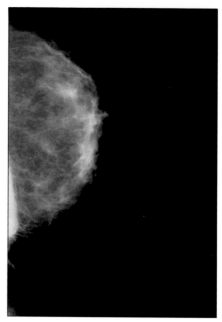

Figure 4.158 The medial insertion of the pectoralis muscle is clearly demonstrated on this patient's cleavage view.

Figure 4.159 The muscle on this patient's cleavage view is very pronounced compared to that seen in Figure 4.158.

especially if it is dense in nature, the exposure will have to be increased and may approach the full CC technique.

c) There is *great variation* in the quantity of tissue that will be imaged with this view. This projection may be very difficult to accomplish with thin, small-breasted women.

d) To relax the superior tissue more, have the patient roll her shoulders forward just before compression is applied.

e) Very large, pendulous breasts may be difficult to keep in position on the image receptor for this view. In these cases, the larger film size may provide improved support and stability.

 Patient relaxation is the single most important factor in patient positioning; it is essential for a successful examination.

c. From Below View

(FB View, Reverse CC View, Caudocranial View)

 FOcus | Identical to the CC View, with emphasis on the superior breast tissue (due to the location of the image receptor).

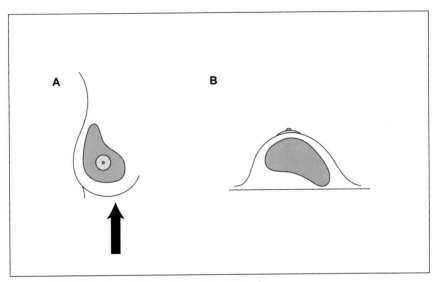

Figure 4.160 The From Below View (Projection)

The FB view is the exact opposite of the CC view. It will maximize tissue visualization for very small breasts, for male patients and for patients with severe kyphosis.

PROCEDURE

1) Rotate the C-arm 180 degrees; the x-ray tube will be located close to the floor.

2) Place the correct film marker on the axillary side of the image receptor.

3) Have the patient approach the unit, facing forward with one foot on either side of the tube head.

4) Have the patient bend forward slightly from the waist; if she finds it comfortable, she can rest her arm and head on the bottom of the image receptor.

5) With the patient's shoulders re-laxed down, place your hand flat against her ribs, directly under her breast and elevate the breast tissue until the PNL is perpendicular to the chest wall. Turn your hand to support the weight of the breast with the palm of your hand.

6) Adjust the height of the C-arm so that the superior surface of the breast will be in contact with the image receptor.

7) Gently pull tissue away from the chest wall. Have the patient lean forward; the receptor should contact the rib cage immediately above the breast.

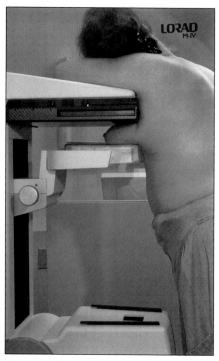

Figure 4.161 A patient positioned for the FB view.

8) Compress the breast tissue; the compression paddle will contact the inferior breast tissue. Slide your hand out in the direction of the nipple as the compression paddle secures the breast tissue.

9) Have the patient hold the handle-bars for support. Gently tip the patient's hips slightly back, to eliminate any superimposition along the posterior margin of the image.

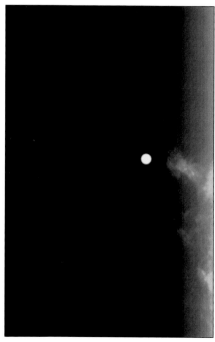

Figure 4.162
This FB view was performed on a mastectomy patient. The lead BB marks an area where she detected a small, pea-sized lump that, with diagnostic work-up, was found to be malignant.

10) Select the appropriate AEC cell position.

11) Ask the patient to stop breathing. Complete the exposure and release the compression immediately.

HELPFUL HINTS

a) Watch for superimposition from gowns, belts, and protruding tissue from the abdomen.

b) This positioning may be used for patients with a prominent pacemaker. Pressure will not be applied directly on the pacemaker; the compression will be applied to the inferior surface of the breast and the thickness of breast tissue will provide a soft cushion between the compression paddle and the pacemaker.

c) The FB approach can also be used for exaggerated CC views and for cleavage views.

d. Roll View

(Rotated View)

 FOcus Any area where superimposition of breast tissue inhibits adequate tissue evaluation.

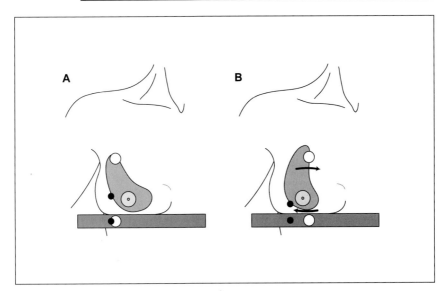

Figure 4.163 The Roll View (Projection)

Roll views are generally performed in the CC projection, although this technique can be used with any mammography view. When performing roll views, breast tissue can be rolled in a number of directions: RL - rolled lateral, RM - rolled medial, RS - rolled superior, and RI - rolled inferior. The resulting images will help to determine if an abnormality is located in the superior, central, or inferior part of the breast. On the rolled image, if the abnormality moves in the same direction the superior tissue was rolled, it is located in the superior third of the tissue; if it moves in the opposite direction, it is located in the inferior third of the tissue; if it remains relatively stationary, it is located in the central third of the breast.

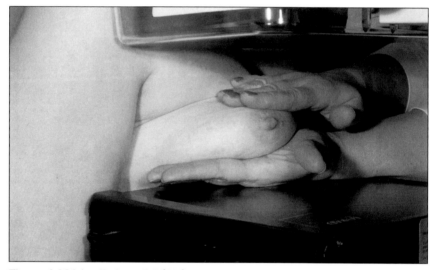

Figure 4.164 A rolled medial (RM) view is performed on this patient.

PROCEDURE

1) Place the correct film marker on the axillary side of the image receptor. Although this is not necessary if the correct film marker has been utilized, you may choose to include a small lead arrow on the image receptor, indicating the direction the superior breast tissue will be rolled for this view.

2) Reposition the patient for the same projection that demonstrated the objectionable superimposition. That is, if the superimposition is noted on the CC view, then use this same position for the rolled view. Most rolled views are performed in the basic CC position.

3) The majority of roll views are performed with a medial or lateral tissue roll. Begin to compress the breast; keep your hand in contact with the

superior tissue. As the compression paddle reaches your hand, slide your hand out to the side, rolling breast tissue toward you as you leave, just before the compression paddle contacts the patient's skin.

4) Alternately, hold the breast in the desired position with both hands (one above and one below the breast). Just before placing the breast on the image receptor, using both hands *roll* the breast tissue in opposite directions to achieve the desired direction of shift with the breast; carefully remove your lower hand as you position the breast on the receptor (Figure 4.164).

5) Complete the compression.

6) Select the appropriate AEC cell position.

7) Ask the patient to stop breathing. Complete the exposure and release the compression immediately.

HELPFUL HINTS

a) For improved tissue control with a medial or lateral tissue roll, the technologist should always stand on the side that the superior tissue is being rolled towards. Because rolled views are frequently performed in the CC position, the technologist will be standing on the medial side of the patient. With this position, it will be much easier to keep the tissue rolled correctly when she removes her hand, just as the compression paddle contacts the breast tissue.

b) If at all possible, avoid projecting the questionable structure(s) over dense, fibrous tissue; select the direction of roll that will image the tissue over a more fatty area of the breast. Because most glandular tissue is located in the U.O.Q. and most abnormalities are therefore found in the U.O.Q., it is recommended that the superior breast tissue be rolled medially for the CC roll view to avoid possible superimposition over more dense glandular tissue in the lateral breast.

c) It is desirable to avoid folds and wrinkles in the tissue as the roll is accomplished; this would again interfere with visualizing the structures clearly.

d) The breast should *spring back* into its natural, resting position when the compression paddle releases the tissue; if this is not apparent, the breast has not been rolled sufficiently for this view.

e) This view may also be used for triangulation purposes. Refer to pages 118 and 275 for a complete description of this procedure.

e. Lumpogram

FOcus Tissue situated very high on the chest wall, above the breast *mound* and immediately adjacent to the rib cage.

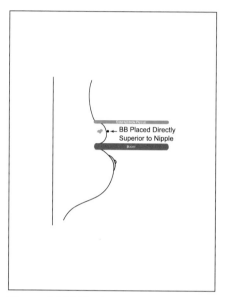

Figure 4.165 The Lumpogram View (Projection)

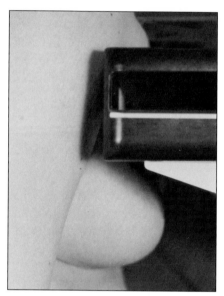

Figure 4.166 A patient positioned for a lumpogram view

Breast tissue is to some extent elastic, but with limitations. As the compression paddle moves down the rib cage to contact the superior surface of the breast, it may pass an area of interest that is located very high on the chest wall. Additional views will be required to demonstrate this area for the radiologist. The greater the degree of breast mobility for CC positioning, the more likely that deep superior tissue will be included on the standard CC image. When there is limited mobility of the IMF for CC positioning, the compression paddle will travel further down the rib cage to contact the superior breast tissue and there is greater opportunity for deep superior tissue to be excluded from the image. This view can be used to provide a CC projection of the superior breast tissue in this area.

PROCEDURE

1) Prepare the patient for the possibility that this positioning technique may be difficult and somewhat uncomfortable if she has tender breasts.

2) The correct film marker should be positioned on the axillary side of the image receptor.

3) Instruct the patient to relax her shoulder and chest muscles as much as possible. Gently but firmly pull forward loose tissue in the superior breast area.

4) Adjust the height of the image receptor to support this tissue. The bucky will be located above the level of the nipple.

5) With your hand, firmly hold the tissue on the receptor until the compression paddle is in place, securing the tissue in position for the x-ray.

6) Select the appropriate AEC cell position; this will be the cell adjacent to the chest wall in the majority of cases.

7) Ask the patient to stop breathing. Complete the exposure and release the compression immediately.

HELPFUL HINTS

a) Because the majority of the breast tissue will be located below the compressed area for the CC view, pressure to keep the patient close to the image receptor may be uncomfortable. This is especially true for patients with painful breasts.

b) Rotating the C-arm 180 degrees and performing this view with a FB projection is very successful. This approach secures the superior tissue in the field and takes better advantage of breast mobility than does a CC approach for this projection. Some professionals believe that the FB approach is more successful than the CC approach for imaging deep superior breast tissue.

c) When a palpable lump is present in the superior posterior tissue, it should be marked with a BB marker for these views.

d) If the volume of compressed tissue does not cover the AEC device, a manual exposure technique will need to be selected.

e) Since the nipple will not be imaged on this view, a lead BB marker can be placed on the skin in the area that will be imaged, directly above the location of the nipple on the breast. This will serve as a reference point and will help to determine how far medial or lateral an area of concern is, relative to the plane of the nipple.

2. Modified Oblique Views

a. Lateromedial Oblique View

(LMO View, Reverse Oblique View)

 The entire breast tissue, with emphasis on clarifying medial structures and lesions.

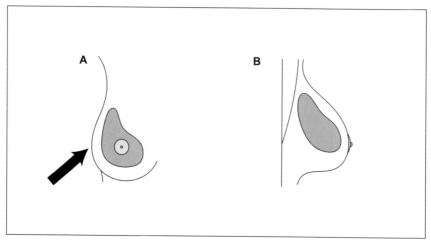

Figure 4.167 The LMO View (Projection)

The LMO view should be used any time that breast positioning or compression is difficult to accomplish with the standard MLO view. With difficult patients, or whenever physical limitations compromise optimal positioning, the LMO provides the best alternate projection for patient positioning; it demonstrates the same anatomical structures as the MLO view.

 The LMO view should be used any time that breast positioning or compression is difficult to accomplish with the standard MLO protocol. With difficult patients, or whenever physical limitations compromise optimal positioning, the LMO provides the best alternate projection for patient positioning; it demonstrates the same anatomical structures as the MLO view.

PROCEDURE

1) The C-arm can be positioned in a simple and efficient manner using the following protocol. Rotate the C-arm to a LM position for the side being imaged; this accomplishes the *LM* part of the *LMO* positioning. The last letter of the acronym LMO is an *O*, which represents the *O*pposite C-arm orientation - in other words, the C-arm will now move down (opposite direction compared to the MLO view). If the MLO was performed at 45 degrees, the LMO will be performed at 135 degrees (90 degrees plus 45 degrees). It is far easier to remember that *the average LMO angulation is 135 degrees*, and then adjust the angulation somewhat, according to your patient's body habitus.

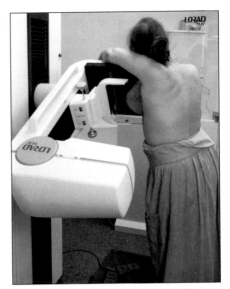

Figure 4.168 A patient positioned for the LMO view. The beam is directed in an inferolateral to superomedial direction.

2) Place the correct film marker on the axillary side of the image receptor.

3) Have the patient approach the mammography unit; her sternum should be close to, but not touching, the edge of the image receptor. Bend her elbow and rest her hand on the handlebar toward the opposite breast.

4) Adjust the height of image receptor to place the upper corner just inferior to the head of the humerus and immediately adjacent to the clavicle (approximately at the level of the sternoclavicular joint). This position should be ideal to include all of the breast tissue when the breast is supported up and away from the chest wall, with the medial surface resting on the image receptor.

5) The technologist should be standing behind the patient.

6) Ensure that the patient is as close as possible to the image receptor without actually touching it. Encourage the patient to relax her shoulder and chest muscles. Gently but firmly pull as much medial breast tissue as possible away from the sternum; lean the patient forward to rest the sternum against the image receptor. To include as much medial breast tissue as possible, always offset the edge of the receptor slightly toward the opposite breast. Support the breast up and away from the ribs with the medial tissue against the receptor.

7) Apply compression gradually, adjusting the shoulder if necessary, to allow the corner of the compression paddle to pass by the latissimus dorsi muscle. Rotate the patient toward the receptor to include all of the lateral tissue and the axillary tail on the image. Clear any folds from the inframammary area.

8) At this point, if the patient's arm overshadows the image field, you can gently place it over the edge of the receptor; positioning the arm up and over the receptor before compression has been applied will tighten the pectoralis muscle, inhibiting taut compression and limiting the inclusion of deep lateral tissue.

9) Select the appropriate AEC cell position.

10) Ask the patient to stop breathing. Complete the exposure and release the compression immediately.

HELPFUL HINTS

a) Positioning for this view is the exact reverse of the positioning used for the standard MLO view. Just as with the MLO view, the angulation of the C-arm will be determined by the patient's body habitus. However, *the beam will be directed from inferolateral to superomedial* (L.O.Q. to U.I.Q.). The positions of the x-ray tube and the image receptor will be reversed from their usual position for the standard MLO projection, placing the receptor parallel and adjacent to the pectoralis muscle.

b) This view may be utilized for patients with large, protruding abdomens; placing the image receptor against the medial tissue will assist in keeping excess tissue pushed back and out of the image. The U.O.Q. will not be optimally imaged, however, because it will not be located directly adjacent to the image receptor.

c) This additional view should be used routinely for patients with pectus excavatum since medial tissue will not be adequately demonstrated on their standard MLO view.

d) This positioning may be used as an alternate for the MLO view in imaging the augmented breast where a rigid fibrous capsule has developed around the implant, preventing its posterior displacement for ID views. The LMO projection maximizes breast mobility as the compression paddle encounters the lateral breast tissue, moving it toward the image receptor.

e) This projection better visualizes the surgical site for lumpectomy patients where the surgical incision is located in the medial breast tissue.

f) This position will be more comfortable for patients who have had recent heart surgery and patients with a pacemaker.

g) With kyphotic patients, when an MLO view is unsuccessful due to interference from the patient's neck and shoulder, LMO positioning will accomplish an improved oblique projection.

h) Improved compression can be obtained with this positioning for male patients who present with a solid pectoralis muscle.

b. Superolateral to Inferomedial Oblique View

(SIO View)

 Primarily the upper, inner breast quadrant; secondly, medial breast tissue in general.

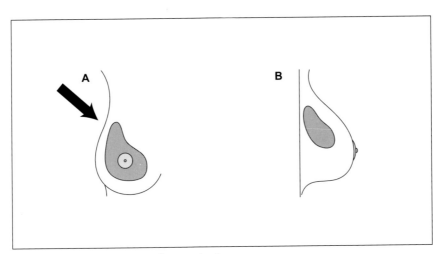

Figure 4.169 The SIO View (Projection).

This view is of limited value and therefore it is not frequently utilized for mammography. It may be used for kyphotic patients with pectus excavatum to better visualize the U.I.Q. and the L.O.Q. as a whole, because these general areas will be positioned parallel to the surface of the image receptor. At the same time, lesions and other abnormalities in the medial breast tissue will be imaged with improved resolution because they will be located directly adjacent to the image receptor.

PROCEDURE

1) Rotate the C-arm to approximately 45 degrees, to allow the upper medial tissue to rest comfortably against the image receptor. The receptor will not be parallel to the pectoralis muscle. The beam will be directed superolateral to inferomedial (U.O.Q. to L.I.Q.).

2) Place the correct film marker on the axillary side of the image receptor.

3) Adjust the height of the C-arm to allow the breast to be centered on the receptor.

4) Have the patient lean forward (not sideways); her medial breast tissue should be resting against the image receptor. Her hand should be resting on the handlebar with her elbow flexed.

5) Encourage the patient to relax her shoulder and chest muscles. Gently pull the breast tissue up and away from the chest wall.

6) Apply compression, gently easing the corner of the compression paddle past the latissimus dorsi muscle. Once compression is complete, raise the patient's arm up and over the edge of the receptor to minimize tissue superimposition from the arm and shoulder over the image field.

7) Clear any folds from the inframammary area.

8) Select the appropriate AEC cell position.

9) Ask the patient to stop breathing. Complete the exposure and release the compression immediately.

HELPFUL HINTS

a) The most common error experienced with this view occurs when the patient leans to the side, to comfortably align her sternum with the edge of the image receptor; when this occurs, in effect a 90 degree lateromedial projection will be obtained. The patient must remain upright for a true SIO view to be imaged.

b) A true SIO view, performed with the patient remaining straight, rather than leaning over against the bucky, provides an orthogonal view to the axillary tail projection.

 Many abnormalities occur in the axillary tail. A complete study must demonstrate this area on at least one projection.

c. Axillary Tail View

(AT View, Axillary view, previously the Cleopatra View)

 The glandular tissue in the axillary tail area.

This view is used to isolate the tail of the breast from the remaining breast tissue.

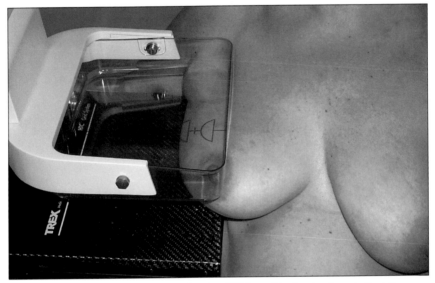

Figure 4.170 A patient positioned for the AT View (Projection); note that the beam is directed in an AP projection (rather than a lateral or oblique projection) to the axillary tail of the breast.

PROCEDURE

1) Rotate the C-arm approximately 25 - 30 degrees, to allow the glandular tissue in the tail of the breast to rest comfortably on the surface of the bucky.

2) Place the correct film marker on the axillary side of the image receptor.

3) Rest the patient's hand on the handlebar; her elbow should be bent behind the receptor to keep the axilla loose and relaxed.

4) The technologist should be standing on the patient's opposite side, as she would be when positioning the MLO view. With the patient's thorax *facing* the technologist, rest the patient's lateral ribs against the edge of the bucky.

5) Gently pull the tail area of the breast away from the chest wall and support it against the receptor; advance the compression down to secure the tissue in this position. *Compression will be applied anterior to posterior rather than medial to lateral*; this is often done improperly.

6) Select the appropriate AEC cell position.

7) Ask the patient to stop breathing. Complete the exposure and remove the compression immediately.

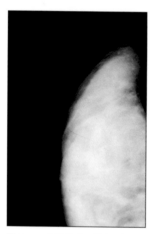

Figure 4.171 A clinical image of the AT view; the tail area of the breast is imaged without superimposition from adjacent breast tissue.

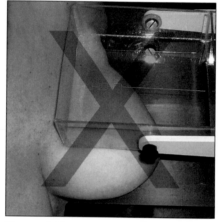

Figure 4.172 Incorrect patient positioning for the AT view; the patient's breast is imaged in a lateral projection, which will superimpose medial and central tissue over the axillary tail. Compare this with the correct positioning in Figure 4.170.

HELPFUL HINTS

a) *Do not rotate the patient's thorax toward the receptor*, similar to her position for the MLO view. This position would include the remainder of the breast on the receptor as well; central and medial tissue would then be superimposed over the axillary tail.

b) Only the tissue in the tail area should be under the compression paddle, in an anteroposterior (AP) projection.

c) When there is an abundance of tissue in the superior lateral area of the breast, it is often difficult to image the posterior border of the glandular tissue with an XCCL view. The AT view will provide an alternate projection of this area.

d) This view does not provide an orthogonal view to the CC or the Lateral view; therefore, it cannot be used to determine lesion orientation relative to the nipple.

e) Try to include enough tissue to cover the AEC device and allow you to use an automatic exposure technique. Otherwise, a manual exposure technique will have to be selected.

f) This projection is frequently confused with an axillary view, which is simply a high MLO projection that is used to image deep superior tissue and nodes in the axilla area. A brief description of this position can be found under *Helpful Hints n* for the MLO View.

d. Tangential View

(TAN View)

Any peripheral area of the breast. Masses and glandular abnormalities must be palpable; dermal calcifications may also be the focus of tangential views.

This view is utilized when a palpable peripheral lesion is projected over glandular tissue on the standard mammography images. Tangential views project these lesions into the subcutaneous fatty tissue, allowing them to be evaluated free of superimposed structures. As well, positioning these structures in the subcutaneous adipose tissue enhances radiographic contrast which also facilitates their evaluation.

Tangential views are also the projection of choice to confirm the dermal location of calcifications.

Any area of the breast can be examined tangentially. *Landmarks* are needed to indicate the orientation of the area radiographically. The nipple is used as a landmark as well as a *lead BB* marker attached to the skin surface to mark the location of the lesion.

With tangential views, lesions can be evaluated without superimposition from surrounding breast tissue. Also, projecting the area of concern into subcutaneous adipose tissue will enhance radiographic contrast for the images.

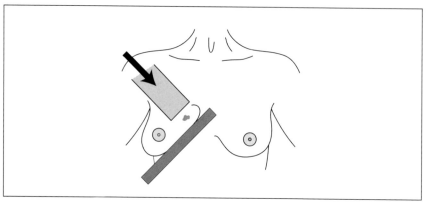

Figure 4.173 The TAN View (Projection).

i. Procedure for Masses

1) Tape a lead BB marker on the surface of the breast to mark the location of the lesion.

2) *Draw an imaginary line from the BB to the nipple.* Rotate the C-arm to position the bucky parallel to this line. (Helpful Hints *a.*)

3) Place the correct film marker on the axillary side of the image receptor.

4) Palpate the lesion and attempt to roll and manipulate the adjacent tissue to bring the area of interest as close as possible to the subcutaneous tissue and away from glandular structures.

5) Hold this position firmly in place until the compression paddle has secured the tissue against the image receptor.

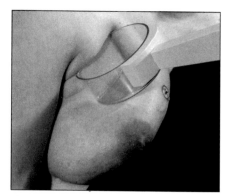

Figure 4.174 A patient positioned for a tangential view.

6) Attempt to include the nipple for orientation purposes. In a large breast, or one with remote lesions, this will not be possible. The lead BB marker will be the only landmark imaged.

7) Include sufficient tissue under the compression paddle to cover the photocell. Otherwise, a manual exposure technique will need to be selected.

8) Ask the patient to stop breathing. Complete the exposure and release the compression immediately.

ii. Procedure for Dermal Calcifications

1) Determine in which quadrant the calcifications are located.

2) Choose the appropriate view that will position the open alpha-numeric biopsy paddle closest to the area of concern (use the localization breast map in Figure 4.185). Place the correct marker on the axillary side of the image receptor.

3) Compress the breast in the selected projection, with the open window of the biopsy paddle positioned directly over the general area where you expect to visualize the calcifications.

4) Expose the film; do not release the compression. Process this image.

5) Examine the image to locate the microcalcifications, and note their location using the alpha-numeric coordinates on the biopsy paddle (e.g. B - 4).

6) Using the coordinates marking the location of the calcifications, place a BB marker on the patient's skin.

7) Release the compression. Replace the biopsy paddle with a standard or a spot compression paddle.

8) Draw an imaginary line from the BB to the nipple; turn the bucky, or the breast, or the patient so that this *line* will be parallel to the receptor for the next image. Place the appropriate marker on the axillary side of the image receptor.

9) Compress the breast tissue, making sure the shadow of the BB marker is projected tangentially onto the surface of the image receptor.

10) Include sufficient tissue under the compression paddle to cover the photocell. Otherwise, a manual exposure technique will need to be selected.

11) Ask the patient to stop breathing. Complete the exposure and release the compression immediately. The calcifications should be visualized beneath the BB marker, along the skin line if they are truly located in the patient's skin.

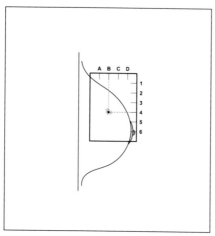

Figure 4.175 The location of suspected dermal calcifications is determined with the alphanumeric compression paddle.

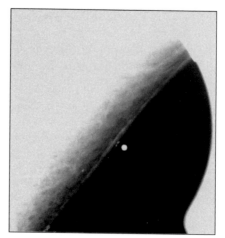

Figure 4.176 A clinical image confirming the dermal location of calcifications.

HELPFUL HINTS

a) *The appropriate C-arm angle is determined by the location of the lesion*; use Breast Localization map, Figure 4.185.

b) It is ideal to visualize the nipple, the lesion and the BB marker on the image. With a large breast and a remote area of interest, this may not be possible; only the BB marker and the lesion may be visualized.

c) Magnification is frequently utilized and is very complimentary for tangential views.

d) Deep lesions cannot be visualized with this technique. It is only appropriate for peripheral breast tissue.

e) Always attempt to include enough breast tissue under the compression paddle to cover the AEC cell and allow you to use a phototimed exposure technique. Otherwise, a manual exposure technique must be selected.

3. Lateral Views

(90 Degree Lateral, True Lateral, Orthogonal Lateral)

 All of the breast tissue; the axillary tail and the deep posterior breast tissue may not be demonstrated as completely as they would be on the MLO projection (where breast mobility and compression are maximized).

There are two variations of lateral (orthogonal) views:
- Lateromedial View
- Mediolateral View

Lateral projections are the view of choice for demonstrating milk of calcium cysts. Air and fluid levels are best imaged with a horizontal beam. Accurate lesion localization and triangulation for interventional procedures also require a lateral image. Finally, the lateral projection presents an alternate view of the glandular tissue and may clarify structures that were superimposed on the oblique projection.

Although geometric consideration may influence the choice of beam direction for a lateral view, the Lateromedial projection is by far the most popular choice (see Breast Mapping section, page 116). When taking scout images prior to an interventional procedure, the lesion should be imaged with the same projection that will be utilized for the examination. This means the lesion will be located away from the image receptor, close to the compression paddle. This will simulate the breast position for the interventional procedure, when the shortest needle path to the lesion will be utilized. *The nipple should always be imaged in profile with lateral views.* These views are used to localize abnormalities. Measurements are frequently made from the images; therefore, it is important to accurately visualize the nipple position.

a. Lateromedial View (LM View)

PROCEDURE

1) Rotate the C-arm 90 degrees so that the beam is projected horizontally to enter the lateral surface of the breast.

2) Place the correct film marker on the axillary side of the image receptor.

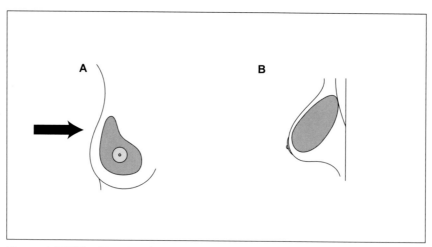

Figure 4.177 The LM View (Projection)

3) Rest the patient's sternum against the edge of the bucky so that the medial surface of the breast is in contact with the image receptor; the top of the film should be located at the level of the sternal notch.

4) Have the patient extend her head forward and rest her chin along the top of the image receptor. This will help to relax the shoulder area.

5) Raise the arm of the side you are imaging and rest the patient's hand on the handlebar. Bend the elbow to keep the pectoral muscle loose and relaxed; this will facilitate inclusion of the axillary tail and the deep posterior breast tissue on the image.

6) Lean the patient slightly back from the receptor to facilitate access to the medial tissue as you proceed.

7) Place your hand flat against the patient's ribs directly under the breast being examined and slide it upward, elevating the breast to position the parenchyma perpendicular to the chest wall. Grasp the breast from below in a similar fashion to that utilized for the MLO view, with your thumb in front and your fingers along the medial tissue. Instruct the patient to relax her shoulder and chest muscles and gently pull as much tissue as possible forward onto the receptor. Offset the edge of the image receptor slightly toward the opposite breast as the sternum contacts the bucky; this will ensure that all the medial tissue will be included in front of the receptor.

8) Carefully guide the compression paddle past the latissimus dorsi muscle, adjusting the position of the arm if necessary.

9) Just before the compression paddle contacts the lateral breast, rotate the patient medially to bring
   more lateral tissue forward onto
   the receptor; the breast should
   be lateral with the nipple in profile. The compression paddle
   should secure the breast in this
   position to ensure that as much
   lateral tissue as possible has
   been included.

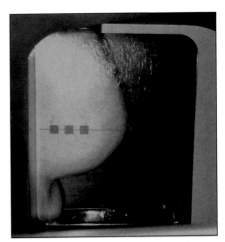

Figure 4.178 A patient positioned for a LM view.

10) Complete the compression, en-
    suring that the breast is sup-
    ported up-and-out, away from
    the chest wall and not allowed to
    droop. The nipple should be in
    profile. Always include tissue in
    the inframammary area. Clear
    any folds in this area.

11) Select the appropriate AEC cell position.

12) Ask the patient to stop breathing. Complete the exposure and release
    the compression immediately.

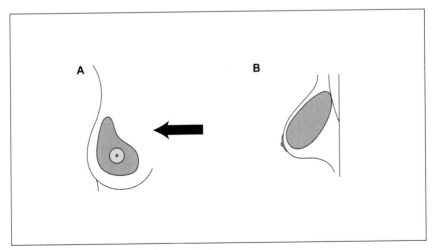

Figure 4.179 The ML View (Projection).

b. Mediolateral View (ML View)

PROCEDURE

1) Rotate the C-arm 90 degrees so that the x-ray beam will enter the medial side of the breast, projecting the image onto the film which is adjacent to the lateral aspect of the breast.

2) Place the correct film marker on the axillary side of the image receptor.

3) Have the patient face the mammography unit as with a CC view and bend the arm of the side you are imaging at a 90 degree angle, resting it along the top of the receptor.

4) Rotate the patient somewhat laterally to help bring medial tissue forward, and bend her hips back somewhat to bring the axilla forward and the abdomen slightly away from the film.

5) Place your hand flat against the patient's ribs directly under the breast being examined and slide it upward, elevating the breast to position the PNL perpendicular to the chest wall. Grasp the breast from below in a similar fashion to that utilized for the MLO view, with your thumb in front and your fingers along the lateral tissue. Instruct the patient to relax her shoulder and chest muscles and gently pull as much tissue as possible forward onto the receptor.

6) The breast should be lateral with the nipple in profile.

7) Have the patient hold the opposite breast out of the way while the compression paddle eases past the sternum. Roll the patent laterally, to include as much medial tissue as possible on the image.

8) Gently pull the breast away from the chest wall and support it up-and-out, to prevent drooping until the compression paddle secures the breast in this position. The compression should now be complete.

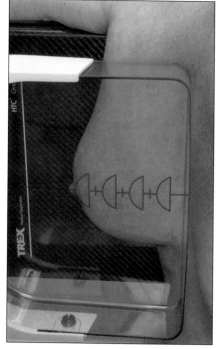

Figure 4.180 A patient positioned for a ML view.

9) Always include tissue in the inframammary area. Clear any folds in this area.

10) Ensure that the patient continues to keep the opposite breast back and out of the image field.

11) Select the appropriate AEC cell position.

12) Ask the patient to stop breathing. Complete the exposure and release the compression immediately.

HELPFUL HINTS

a) Both lateral projections are used to provide an orthogonal view to the CC projection for accurate lesion localization prior to a needle localization procedure. The location of the lesion will determine which approach will be utilized; the lesion should be placed as close as possible to the compression paddle for interventional procedures.

b) It is essential that the nipple is imaged in profile because it will be utilized as a landmark to measure and calculate lesion location for localization or for surgical purposes.

c) Lead nipple markers are frequently used to clearly indicate the nipple location on lateral projections.

d) The lateromedial projection is sometimes used with very slim patients to pull more pectoralis muscle into the image field. It is also helpful to keep protruding abdomens back and to minimize tissue superimposition in the inframammary area with obese patients.

e) The correctly positioned lateral projection will image a smaller wedge of pectoral muscle than would normally be imaged on the MLO projection. With very dense breasts, the posterior margin of the glandular tissue may not be demonstrated as well as on the MLO projection.

f) A lateral projection can be used to image posterior inferior breast tissue in the inframammary area when this has not been adequately visualized on the standard MLO view or when folds or wrinkles limit tissue evaluation in this area (Figure 4.138).

g) Generally, less tissue will be visualized on a lateral projection compared to a MLO projection. This is because compression will not be applied parallel to the pectoral muscle fibers, and therefore the muscle will resist the action of the compression paddle. As a result, it will be difficult to accomplish the same degree of tissue compression and there may be incomplete anterior displacement of the breast away from the chest wall.

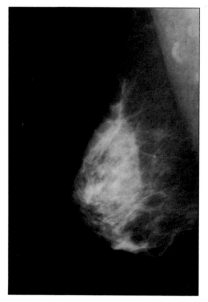

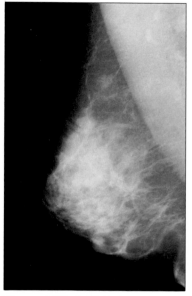

Figure 4.181 A clinical image of a LM view.

Figure 4.182 A MLO view of the same patient in Figure 4.181.

h) The horizontal beam in a lateral projection is advantageous to demonstrate fluid levels in cysts and abscesses.

c. Spot Compression Views

i. Contact Spot Compression Views

(Contact spots, Regular Spots)

 FOCUS
Any area in the breast that may require further clarification, primarily because of overlapping structures.

A spot compression view can be performed with any positioning approach. Focal spot compression helps to define structural margins by minimizing local tissue superimposition. These views are useful to clarify specific areas in the breast through improved tissue detail. In order to accomplish this goal, several important principles must be employed. These are:

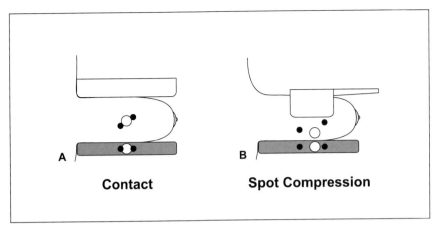

A   B

Contact   **Spot Compression**

Figure 4.183 Spot Compression Views.

a) Spot compression films are performed with bucky technique, using the large focal spot (identical parameters to standard mammography imaging).

b) A small compression paddle, designed to apply *focal compression* should be used. The field size should include tissue beyond the area of interest; the entire film is frequently exposed.

c) The area of concern can be imaged with either lateral projection. Positioning the abnormality close to the receptor will maximize geometric sharpness; positioning it away from the receptor will provide a minimal degree of magnification (which may be advantageous) on the image. This decision will be made by the individual radiologist.

d) *Taut compression is even more important with spot views* because optomizing the information on these images is critical and has serious implications for the patient. High quality spot compression views may be directly responsible for eliminating the suspicion of malignancy. The patient's anxiety will be immediately alleviated, needless surgery will be avoided, and the patient

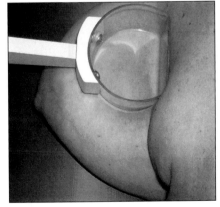

Figure 4.184 Spot compression views, performed with a small compression paddle, provide improved focal compression in a specific area.

will be spared future mammography complications due to residual scar tissue.

PROCEDURE

1) The area in question is usually indicated by the radiologist on the routine mammography images.

2) The location of the lesion will determine which views will be utilized. Generally two views are obtained, one in the CC projection and one in the lateral or the MLO projection; other projections are utilized according to the individual situation.

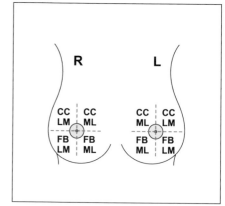

Figure 4.185 Breast localization Map, to select appropriate views for spot images.

3) Place the correct film marker on the axillary side of the image receptor.

4) Center the area in question beneath the spot compression device. Use a compression paddle appropriate for the area in question; a variety of sizes and configurations are available from equipment manufacturers.

5) Select the appropriate AEC cell position. Ask the patient to stop breathing. Complete the exposure and release the compression immediately.

HELPFUL HINTS

a) As with standard mammography, the axillary side of the film must be labeled with radiopaque markers that indicate laterality and projection. This is especially important when the image does not include breast landmarks that can orient the interpreter to the location of the coned area in the breast.

b) To maintain a similar relationship to the standard mammography views (again for orientation purposes), similar breast positioning should be utilized for spot views whenever possible. However, imaging the lesion is always the primary goal and any position that may accomplish this should be employed in the event that an unusual lesion location may require *creative* positioning.

c) AEC cell position is critical with spot compression views, particularly when the density of the abnormality is significantly different from the surrounding breast tissue. *The cell position must coincide with the*

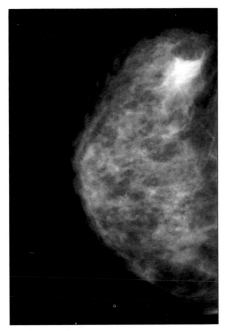

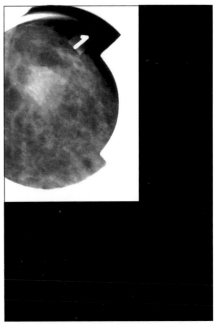

Figure 4.186 An irregular mass is seen in the lateral part of this CC view.

Figure 4.187 Spot compression views were performed to provide detailed information about the characteristics of this area.

abnormality in order to achieve the optimal exposure technique for this tissue.

d) *Contact* or *Regular* spots are generally used to spread out and clarify superimposed tissue. In these situations, the magnification technique is not necessary.

 Taut compression is even more important with spot views *because optomizing the information on these images is critical and has serious implications for the patient. High quality spot compression views may be directly responsible for eliminating the suspicion of malignancy. The patient's anxiety will be immediately alleviated, needless surgery will be avoided, and the patient will be spared future mammography complications due to residual scar tissue.*

ii. Magnification Spot Compression Views
(*Mag* Spots, Magnified Spots)

 FOcus   Any area in the breast that may require further clarification.

Magnification spot compression views are particularly useful to clarify the structural characteristics of microcalcifications and to better delineate the borders of irregular masses.

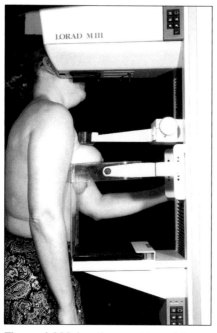

Figure 4.188 A patient positioned for a magnification spot view.

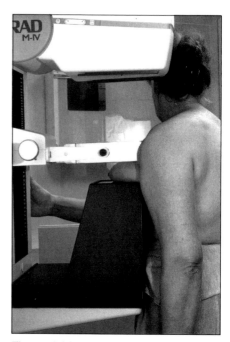

Figure 4.189 An alternate equipment set-up for magnification spot views.

PROCEDURE

1) The procedure is identical to that outlined for Coned-Down Compression Spot Views with one exception. Magnification studies are performed non-bucky and the small focal spot is used routinely.

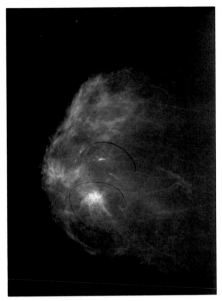

Figure 4.190 A CC view demonstrating a suspicious area of calcifications.

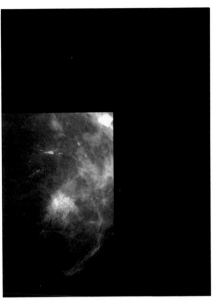

Figure 4.191 Magnification spot views of the suspicious area in Figure 4.190 provide detailed information about the characteristics of this area.

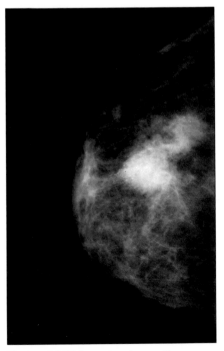

Figure 4.192 An extensive malignancy was noted on this patient's examination.

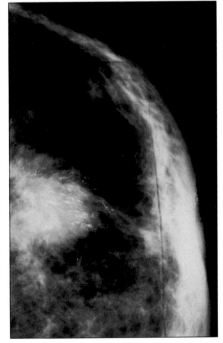

Figure 4.193 Magnification spot views provided improved detail about characteristics of the microcalcifications in this lesion.

HELPFUL HINTS

a) With magnification studies, *the use of the small focal spot is critical* to maximize geometric sharpness and resolution. *A bucky (grid) should never be used*; scatter from the breast dissipates in the air gap before it reaches the film below.

b) Motion is the most common problem encountered with magnification spot films. The time factor is considerably longer than that used for standard mammography images because the mA capacity of the small focal spot is much lower than that of the large focal spot. In order to overcome these inherent difficulties, there are five factors that are critical for successful magnification imaging:

1. Use a slightly higher kVp than that used for standard mammography imaging - 27 or 28 kVp is a good range for magnification views of the average breast. This will shorten the exposure time.

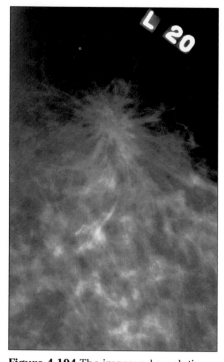

Figure 4.194 The improved resolution of magnification imaging helped to define the characteristics of this spiculated lesion.

2. Use as much compression as the patient can tolerate. This will also shorten the exposure time correspondingly, because there will be less tissue to penetrate.

3. Prepare the patient for the longer exposure time so that she is not surprised. She will otherwise expect a very short exposure time, similar to her standard mammography examination. Explain that this is a special imaging technique and she will need to stop breathing and hold perfectly still for a much longer time.

4. Always ensure the patient is steady for these images; make sure her position is as comfortable as possible, separate her feet for better balance, and have her hold the handlebars with both hands if possible.

5. Give the patient plenty of time to stop breathing before the exposure. In fact, as you position her, it is a very good idea to ask her to breathe in slowly and then breathe out slowly several times before positioning is complete. The last time you ask her to do this, finish by saying *Now just stop breathing and hold very still.* Give her a few seconds to finish breathing before you expose the film.

c) Refer to page 236 for Helpful Hint items *a*, *b*, and *c* which also apply to magnification spot views.

C. POSITIONING CHALLENGES

1. Nipple Profile Problems

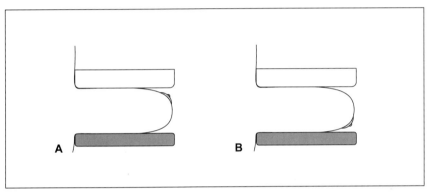

Figure 4.195 With an off-centered nipple location, it is difficult to project the nipple in profile and include all of the breast tissue on the same image.

In the majority of mammography examinations, the nipple will be imaged in profile without difficulty. This is both desirable and important because the nipple is the only natural breast landmark from which measurements can be made to indicate precise lesion location in the breast. However, when performing mammography examinations, the technologist should NEVER sacrifice tissue coverage to obtain a profile projection of the nipple on her standard views. *In general, a mammogram is considered acceptable* (without requiring additional views) *as long as the nipple is projected in profile on one of the two routine images.*

Occasionally, with an off-centered nipple location or when surgery has distorted the breast tissue, difficulty arises in obtaining a profile projection of the nipple area on the standard mammography images. Often the discrepancy is minimal, and simply manipulating the skin may bring the nipple into profile without tissue loss. When this is not possible, an additional anterior view should be obtained to demonstrate the nipple and retroareolar structures in a profile projection. Occasionally, the retroareolar tissue may be so dense that the loss of profile is not radiographically apparent. Should this be the case, mark the film *nipple not in profile* for follow-up comparison purposes. A radiopaque BB marker is very helpful to provide a definitive indication of nipple location, particularly when it will be imaged over glandular breast tissue rather than in profile.

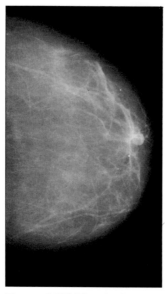

Figure 4.196 The nipple was not projected in profile on this clinical image.

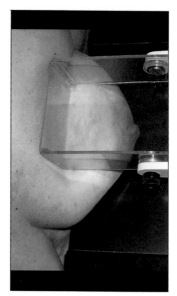

Figure 4.197 An anterior compression view can clarify the retroareolar tissue in these situations.

A nipple that is not imaged in a profile presentation can produce a deceiving appearance on the mammogram and it may be mistaken for a mass, especially when the retroareolar structures are dense or nodular. Alternately, it may obscure an underlying mass. For these reasons, it is advisable to clearly mark the film as *nipple not in profile* or *nipple out of profile*. This should alleviate misinterpretation and facilitate comparison for follow-up examinations. A lead BB marker to indicate nipple location is very helpful in these situations.

2. Flaccid, Pancake Breasts

Flaccid breasts that are composed of little more than loose skin are extremely difficult to image free of wrinkles and skin folds, particularly in the axillary area. The technologist must be very conscious of this and she must make every effort to smooth the inferior tissue as well as the superior tissue as she positions the breast on the image receptor. The greatest challenge in positioning these breasts comes during the process of breast compression. If the technologist uses her hands to position the breast tissue, as she does with other patients, the compression paddle will encounter her hands long before it is close to the breast tissue. A rubber spatula may be helpful to *hold* the tissue in position until the compression paddle is close enough to secure the patient's breast in the desired position.

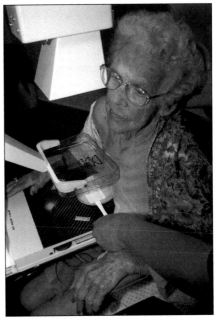

Figure 4.198 A rubber spatula is useful to hold a thin, flaccid breast in position until the compression paddle has secured its position.

3. Large Breasts

Fortunately, modern mammography equipment provides technologists with two sizes of image receptor in order that small, average, and large sized breasts can all be imaged adequately and efficiently. Always select the appropriate size of image receptor in order that all the breast tissue can be included on each mammography view. When compression is applied, breast tissue spreads out; therefore the breast that just fits on the image receptor as positioning begins, may require a larger film size once compression has been applied. With larger breasts, the smaller receptor may be adequate for the CC view, but the larger size is often required for the MLO view to provide coverage from the axilla to the inframammary area. Receptor size must always be selected on the basis of facilitating optimum breast positioning; convenience or esthetics in mounting images of similar size on view boxes is a poor excuse to sacrifice image quality.

Occasionally we encounter breasts so large that they must be imaged in overlapping sections. This process is difficult for the technologist, the patient, and the radiologist who must piece a view box full of breast sections together in a jig-saw fashion. Often, routine positioning protocols are difficult to follow. The standard position of the technologist at the patient's side may not always work when positioning large breasts. The volume of breast tissue may be difficult to control and position adequately with only one hand. As positioning begins, the technologist may need to stand behind the patient and use both hands to lift the breast and generally center it on the image receptor. At this point the technologist can usually resume her normal side position to complete the positioning process.

Keeping in mind the basic principle of demonstrating ALL the breast tissue, the technologist must *proceed in a systematic fashion to cover the entire breast in overlapping sections*. Because some of the images may not include natural landmarks (skin edges, nipple, etc.), it is extremely important to *maintain the correct axillary placement of markers* to assist in correctly *piecing* the examination together. Also, a metal BB or other similar skin marker can be attached to the breast tissue in a central area to provide a landmark to confirm the overlapping of tissue on multiple breast images. Always clearly indicate on the patient's history sheet that the metal BB marker has been placed on the patient's breast *only* for orientation purposes to assist with piecing the numerous mammography images together during interpretation.

The specific breast shape will determine the pattern of coverage. Tailor the examination to the individual patient's presentation.

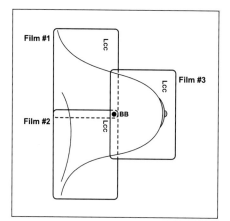

Figure 4.199 A metal BB marker is used to confirm overlapping views on this CC view that must be imaged in 3 individual sections.

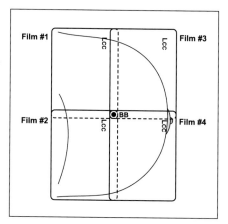

Figure 4.200 This breast shape must be imaged in 4 sections for the CC view; again, a metal BB marker is used to confirm overlapping tissue on these views.

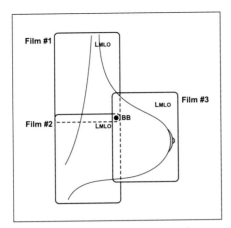

Figure 4.201 A metal BB marker is used to confirm overlapping views on this MLO view that must be imaged in 3 individual sections.

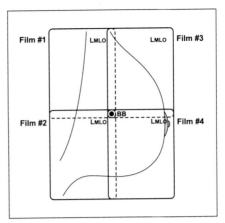

Figure 4.202 This breast shape must be imaged in 4 sections for the MLO view; again, a metal BB marker is used to confirm overlapping tissue on these views.

NOTE: When planning an examination that will be performed in multiple pieces or sections it is important to note that two independent methods exist to accomplish this task.

TRADITIONAL IMAGING: Uses the standard protocol of imaging for all individual images in an examination that is performed in multiple sections. This means that if a MLO projection must be imaged in pieces, all of the individual images will be performed with the standard MLO positioning technique.

ALTERNATE IMAGING: Points out that the primary function of the MLO view is to demonstrate tissue in the U.O.Q. Once this goal has been accomplished, additional views for the remaining breast tissue will not benefit from an oblique projection. In fact, this school of thought proposes that the anterior and inferior breast tissue are best imaged with a 90 degree approach. In the event that a lesion is detected and must be localized for a surgeon, the lateral projection required to pinpoint the true orthogonal location of the abnormality will already be performed and available for the radiologist. This means that if a MLO projection must be imaged in pieces, the image that includes the U.O.Q. will be performed with the standard MLO protocol. However, any additional images of the remaining breast tissue will be performed with a 90 degree lateral projection.

It is important for the reader to consider both of these protocols and determine which may be most appropriate for their individual practice.

The following descriptions have been presented with the alternate imaging protocol.

1) THE WIDE BREAST (from side to side):

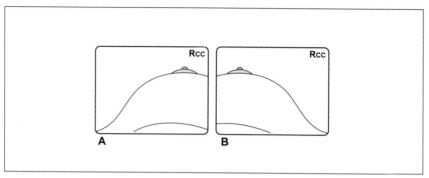

Figure 4.203 For CC views of a wide breast, two images must be taken; the first will focus on lateral tissue and the second on medial tissue. The nipple will provide a common point of overlap in the center of these two images.

- CC VIEWS: This breast shape should be imaged from side to side in two sections: one should focus on lateral, axillary tissue, to include the nipple medially; the second image should focus on medial tissue and include the nipple laterally (Figure 4.203).

- MLO VIEWS: A breast that is wide from side to side (a broad thorax) presents specific imaging difficulties in the MLO projection, especially when the breast is also large. In particularly difficult cases, two views may be necessary: one for the posterior and axillary tissue (the anterior breast will not be well compressed; it may also be overexposed due to the thickness of the posterior tissue) and one for the anterior breast (with this tissue compressed optimally, the technique will also be improved). The anterior film should be imaged with a 90 degree C-arm orientation.

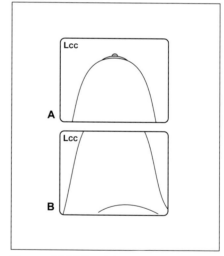

Figure 4.204 For CC views of a long breast, 2 images must be taken; the first will focus on posterior tissue and the second on anterior tissue.

2) THE LONG BREAST (from front to back):

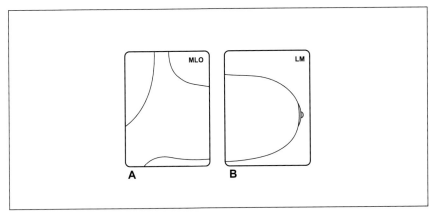

Figure 4.205 For MLO views of a long breast, two images are required; one will image posterior tissue and the other will image the anterior breast.

- CC VIEWS: If the breast will fit from side to side on a 24 x 30 cm film, complete the examination with two images: one image should include the posterior tissue and as far anterior as the film covers; the second image will include the nipple and as far back as the film covers. These two images will overlap in the central breast area (Figure 4.204).

- MLO VIEWS: If the breast will fit from top to bottom on a 24 x 30 cm film, complete the examination with two images: one image is for the posterior tissue, with standard MLO positioning, taking care to include from the axillary tissue above to the inframammary area below; the second image should include the anterior tissue and as far back as the film covers using a 90 degree lateromedial projection (Figure 4.205).

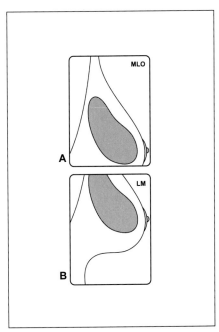

Figure 4.206 The breast that is long at its chest wall dimension will require a superior and an inferior image to completely visualize the tissue in the MLO projection.

3) The Long Breast (from top to bottom):

- MLO VIEWS: This breast shape will not fit from top to bottom on a 24 x 30 film and therefore it must be examined with a superior and an inferior image. The superior MLO image should be positioned high in the axilla to cover the U.O.Q. and the deep axillary tissue. The inferior tissue should be imaged with a lateral projection and should include from the inframammary fold to as far up as the film dimension will cover (Figure 4.206).

4. Small Breasts

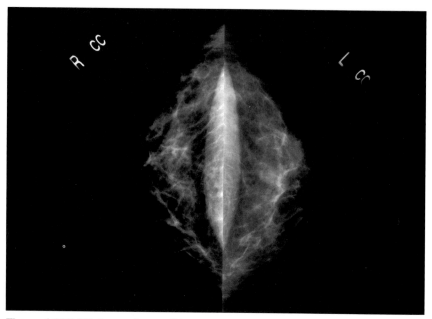

Figure 4.207 CC views of a small-breasted patient.

Although this is not always the case, small breasted women are frequently also very slim. They may find mammography positioning uncomfortable due to a deficiency of fatty tissue which can act as a cushion and provide padding along their ribs and thorax. These patients often present with solid, fibrous breasts that are firmly attached to the chest wall, exhibiting no pendulous tendencies. These breasts may be difficult to ease forward onto the image receptor, despite every conceivable effort. Concurrent with this presentation is difficulty in demonstrating tissue in the inframammary area.

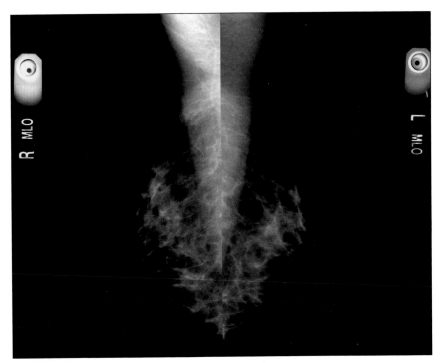

Figure 4.208 MLO views of a small-breasted patient.

Occasionally, the musculature of emaciated, nutritionally deficient, or extremely ill patients has atrophied and visualizing the usual generous amount of pectoralis muscle on the MLO view may be very difficult.

When imaging small breasts, there are two factors that cannot be compromised. First, *the technologist MUST achieve relaxation in the patient's shoulder and pectoral area*. This is essential in order to ease the breast tissue forward onto the image receptor. Encourage the patient to slouch. Have her roll her shoulders forward, drawing her shoulders together as much as possible. This will help the breast tissue to fall forward and away from the chest wall. Without changing her shoulder position, encourage her to relax her shoulder and chest muscles; this will allow you to manipulate and position the loose breast tissue. Second, *the technologist must maintain a very firm hold on the tissue, keeping it against the receptor until the compression paddle has secured its position.* Releasing the breast too early will allow tissue to *slip back* against the chest wall. This presents a positioning dilemma. If the technologist uses her hands to position the breast tissue, as with other patients, the compression paddle will encounter her hands long before it is close to the breast tissue. A rubber spatula may be helpful to *hold* the tissue in position until the compression paddle is close enough to secure the patient's breast. Careful attention to these two factors will result in a successful examination for the majority of small breasted patients.

When the technologist experiences difficulty performing a routine CC projection on an extremely small breast, the FB view will provide an excellent alternative that is often very successful in capturing more tissue close to the chest wall.

Also, the LMO projection can be very helpful in demonstrating more of the pectoralis muscle when this is difficult to accomplish with standard MLO positioning. If the patient relaxes her shoulder muscles and the compression paddle is positioned directly adjacent to the ribs with the corner into the axilla, it will lift the flaccid pectoralis muscle, bringing more of this tissue up to meet the image receptor above. If the LMO view is difficult to accomplish for any reason, a 90 degree lateromedial projection may be helpful to improve visualization of the pectoral muscle.

5. Augmented Breasts

Mammography examinations of augmented breasts can be difficult and *the presence of breast implants interferes with ideal evaluation of the breast tissue*. Augmented breasts have been imaged for years using standard mammography positioning with limited compression. A manual technique is required because the presence of the implant precludes the use of a phototimed exposure technique. Visualization of breast tissue is compromised due to the physical presence of the implant; it is very difficult to provide complete global coverage of the natural breast tissue that is located around the perimeter of the implant. Additional mammography projections (90 degree lateral views, SIO views) can provide multiple tangential views of the natural breast tissue surrounding the implant; however, detailed tissue visualization remains sub-optimal due to inadequate compression.

A modified positioning technique called implant displacement (ID) has been developed to improve visualization of the natural breast tissue in patients with breast implants. This technique involves additional mammography views with manual displacement of the implant position. The patient is often encouraged to participate in this specialized technique because she is most familiar with the way her implants move and the degree of mobility that they exhibit. Most patients are very receptive to a protocol that will provide a more complete evaluation of their implant and natural breast tissue. The implant displacement technique consists of two additional views of each breast with the implant displaced posteriorly allowing normal, taut compression to be applied to the anterior breast tissue. With practice, the technologist will become quite comfortable with this positioning technique. A phototimed exposure technique can be used when the volume of compressed tissue covers the photocell.

Breast implants which have been surgically placed behind the pectoral muscle (*subpectoral*) are very easy to image using the implant displacement technique and the resulting mammography examination is of excellent quality. Implants that have been surgically placed between the pectoral muscle and the breast tissue (*intramammary or retromammary*) may be very difficult to maneuver for a number of reasons. Under these circumstances, the resulting mammography examination is frequently suboptimal.

There are situations when the implant displacement technique will not be successful. These include:

1) Implants that are firmly encapsulated and exhibit minimal mobility

2) Patients who have minimal natural breast tissue surrounding the implant

3) Post mastectomy implants that are only surrounded by a thin layer of skin

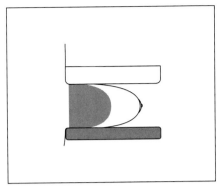

Figure 4.209 Images are first taken to include the breast implant; manual technique and limited compression is used.

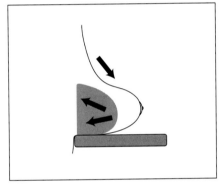

Figure 4.210 The implants are then gently displaced back as the anterior tissue is brought forward and compressed.

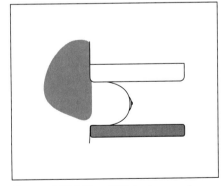

Figure 4.211 The AEC device can be used to phototime the ID views; taut compression can be used on these images because the implant has been excluded from the compressed tissue.

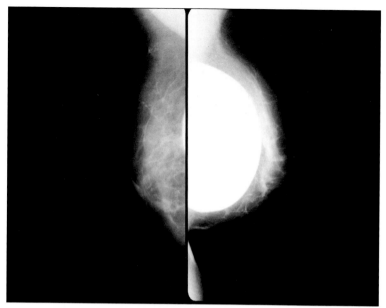

Figure 4.212 Retromammary implants may move well for ID views, provided they have not become encapsulated.

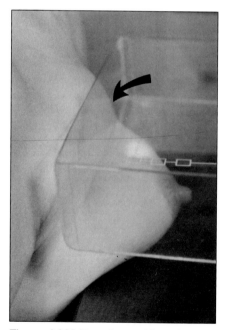

Figure 4.213 Note the position of the implant, behind the compression paddle for the ID views.

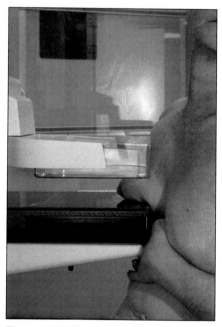

Figure 4.214 The patient may feel more stable for ID views if she uses her hand to fill the space between the bucky and her ribs for these images.

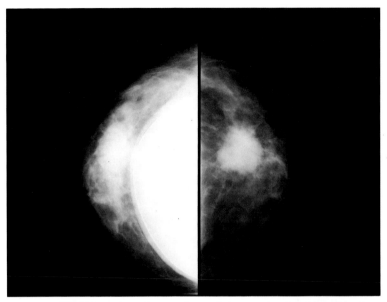

Figure 4.215 This patient detected a nodule near her implant. Her physician believed she was feeling the filling stem of her implant. Mammography revealed a large carcinoma in this woman's breast.

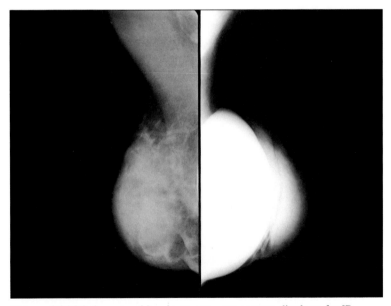

Figure 4.216 Subpectoral Implants are very easy to displace for ID views; these examinations are very successful and provide thorough tissue coverage.

a. Positioning Protocol - Mobile Implants:

1. Routine CC and MLO Views (to include implant, limited compression, manual technique)

2. Implant Displaced CC and MLO Views (without implant, taut compression, phototimed technique)

The complete examination for a patient with mobile breast implants consists of eight rather than four exposures. The examination begins with the standard mammography views (CC and MLO); the implant is included in these images. Manual technique and limited compression are required. These images visualize the deep breast tissue, close to the chest wall. Implant displacement views follow. Phototimed exposure technique and normal, taut compression provides improved visualization and enhanced image detail of the anterior breast tissue.

b. Positioning Protocol - Encapsulated Implants:

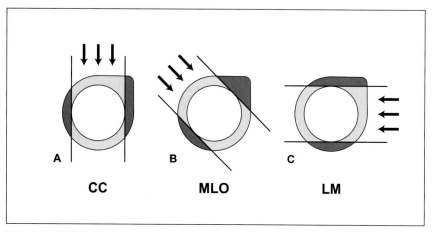

Figure 4.217 Multiple views of the encapsulated implant provide global coverage of the surrounding breast tissue.

1. Routine CC and MLO Views (to include implant, limited compression, manual technique)

2. 90 degree LM View (to include implant, limited compression, manual technique) for more complete global coverage of natural breast tissue

The complete examination for a patient with encapsulated breast implants or for a patient with minimal natural tissue consists of six rather than four

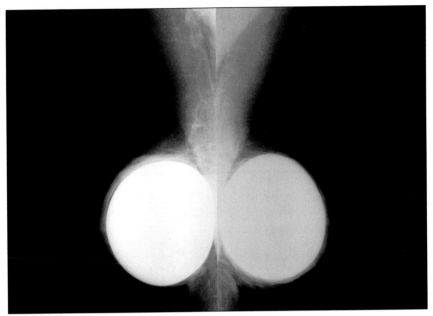

Figure 4.218 These encapsulated implants were unable to be displaced; therefore, CC, MLO, and LM views were performed to provide more thorough global coverage.

exposures. The examination begins with the standard mammography views (CC and MLO); the implant is included in these images. Manual technique and limited compression are required. These images visualize the deep breast tissue, close to the chest wall. A third, 90 degree LM projection is then performed to provide more complete global coverage of the natural breast tissue around the perimeter of the implant.

 A modified positioning technique called implant displacement (ID) has been developed to improve visualization of the natural breast tissue in patients with breast implants. This technique involves additional mammography views with manual displacement of the implant position.

Breast implants which have been surgically placed behind the pectoral muscle (subpectoral) are very easy to image using the implant displacement technique and the resulting mammography examination is of excellent quality.

c. Implant Displacement Views

(Push-Back Views, Modified Views, previously the Eklund Technique)

 Implant displacement views are designed to image the breast tissue anterior to breast implants. Posterior breast tissue will be imaged on the standard views that include the implant in the image.

i. Implant Displacement - Craniocaudal View (I.D.)

PROCEDURE

1) It is advisable to take a few moments to explain this procedure very thoroughly to the patient, indicating that the additional views taken will provide a much more complete examination. This is important in order to obtain her cooperation for the examination and to build her confidence in your technical expertise.

2) Place the correct film marker on the axillary side of the image receptor.

3) Adjust the height of the image receptor slightly higher than that used for the images that included the breast implant.

4) Encouraging the patient to relax her shoulder and chest muscles, grasp her breast near the chest wall with both hands and, feeling for the implant, work forward, *gently pulling as much tissue as possible over the implant anteriorly, easing the implant posteriorly as you proceed.*

5) Once the breast tissue has been brought forward, hold it firmly and lean the patient forward so that the implant is located at the edge of the image receptor and the anterior displaced breast tissue is resting flat on its surface.

6) *Gradually apply compression*, easing the compression paddle past the anterior implant surface to meet the breast tissue resting on the image receptor. Have the patient lean against the compression paddle slightly to keep the implant back and to keep as much breast tissue forward as possible. Rest the patient's opposite hand on the handlebar to stabilize her position. Apply normal, taut compression.

7) Use a phototimed exposure technique for the implant displaced images. When there is not enough compressed tissue to cover the photocell, a manual exposure technique will need to be selected.

ii. Implant Displacement - Mediolateral Oblique View (I.D.)
PROCEDURE

1) Rotate the C-arm to the appropriate angulation for the individual patient, according to her body habitus.

2) Place the correct film marker on the axillary side of the image receptor.

3) The patient should be standing slightly back from the image receptor. Bend the patient's elbow and rest her hand on the handlebar; ensure that she remains very loose and relaxed in the shoulder area.

4) Grasp the breast near the chest wall with both hands and, feeling for the implant, work forward, *gently pulling as much tissue as possible over the implant anteriorly, easing the implant posteriorly as you proceed.* Always begin pulling superior and axillary tissue forward first, then work downward with implant displaced views for the MLO projection. Beginning the displacement process with the inferior tissue may lodge the implant solidly in the U.O.Q. making it very difficult to image the patient's natural breast tissue in this area.

5) Firmly hold the tissue anterior to the implant; lean the patient forward slightly until the implant is at the edge of the image receptor and the anterior displaced tissue is resting flat on its surface.

6) *Gradually apply compression,* gently guiding the compression paddle along the anterior implant surface to meet the breast tissue resting on the receptor. Ease the shoulder and axillary tissue forward to include as much of the axilla as possible before the final, taut compression is applied.

7) Use a phototimed exposure technique for the implant displaced views. When there is not enough compressed tissue to cover the photocell, a manual exposure technique will need to be selected.

HELPFUL HINTS

a) If you have difficulty palpating the implant in the breast, have the patient bend forward; with the breast pendant, it may be easier to detect the margins of the implant. Pull the breast tissue forward and hold it firmly before the patient stands and approaches the mammography unit.

b) The displaced breast tissue must be firmly secured on the surface of the image receptor before compression is applied. This is easily done using your index and middle fingers, spreading and securing the tissue between them, rather than having them tightly grouped in the central

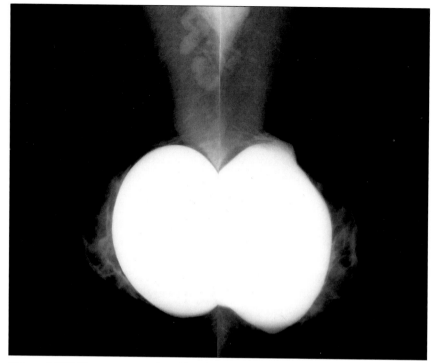

Figure 4.219 These encapsulated implants are demonstrating signs of rupture and leakage.

retroareolar area. This will provide better tissue control and will be more comfortable for the patient.

c) If the patient appears unsteady for the implant displacement views, place her hand against her ribs beneath the breast to act as a stopper, filling the space between her thorax and the image receptor and providing stability as she leans against the receptor. When the space is larger than the width of her hand, the patient can make a fist and place it against her ribs in the same fashion.

d) Magnification views are very successful with the implant displaced technique. Interventional procedures such as needle aspirations, needle biopsies and wire localizations may also be performed with implant displacement.

e) Tangential views should be utilized (as with standard mammography) whenever a palpable mass is obscured by superimposed tissue on the routine projections.

If the patient appears unsteady for the implant displacement views, place her hand against her ribs beneath the breast to act as a stopper, filling the space between her thorax and the image receptor and providing stability as she leans against the receptor. When the space is larger than the width of her hand, the patient can make a fist and place it against her ribs in the same fashion.

f) If the technologist is unsure that the modified technique will be successful when a patient has minimal natural breast tissue, she should initially perform only one displaced projection and process this image. If the patient has a clinical symptom, choose the view that has the greatest potential for demonstrating the abnormality for the radiologist. Evaluate the additional information gained by this image; a decision can then be made to abandon the process or to continue with the remaining implant displaced images.

g) Use caution when attempting an implant displaced view on patients with encapsulated implants or on patients with very little natural breast tissue surrounding the implant. This may cause the patient a great deal of discomfort and often will yield very little useful information on the examination.

h) Patients with subpectoral implants may experience discomfort when the pectoral muscle is compressed. They should be informed and prepared for this possibility before the examination begins.

i) Some patients are very helpful in manipulating their implants and moving them into the most posterior location for the displacement views. Always encourage the patient to participate in the examination if she is willing and comfortable doing so.

j) It is important to note that many women are very protective of their implants and they may be very anxious or even skeptical of the implant displacement process. Always explain the technique and the benefit they will gain in order to gain their cooperation and their trust before you begin.

k) Mammography examinations of implant patients are often asymmetric. One breast may be severely encapsulated and exhibit minimal displacement characteristics. The opposite side may be soft and mobile and easily displaced for the imaging study.

6. Deformities Of The Sternum

a. Pectus Excavatum (Depressed Sternum, Sunken Chest)

Pectus excavatum is a condition characterized by a *depressed sternum*. The primary concern with mammography examinations on patients with this anomaly relates to adequate coverage of the medial breast tissue that extends along the ribs as they curve inward, toward the sternum.

Occasionally, when the anterior ribs are bowed very acutely, a routine CC view will not be able to visualize a satisfactory amount of breast tissue on either side of the nipple. In these circumstances, the most thorough coverage can be achieved with two overlapping CC views, one exaggerated medially (to include tissue adjacent to the medial ribs and sternum, over to the nipple area) and one exaggerated laterally (to include tissue adjacent to the lateral ribs, over to the nipple area). Both of these images should include the nipple. Maintain the standard axillary placement of markers to provide the appropriate orientation of the images for the interpreting physician.

The standard MLO view will image the majority of the breast tissue. A LMO view (reverse oblique) will demonstrate deep medial tissue more clearly than the standard MLO view when there is extreme curvature of the thorax. Alternately, a 90 degree lateromedial projection may be used.

b. Pectus Carinatum (Pigeon Chest, Barrel Chest)

Pectus carinatum is a condition characterized by a *protruding sternum*, creating a very rounded, barrel-like thorax. The severity of the rib curvature will dictate the imaging deficiencies and the number of images that will be required to provide thorough breast tissue coverage.

The CC view will frequently need to be imaged in two overlapping views, one exaggerated medially (to include tissue adjacent to the medial ribs and sternum, over to the nipple area) and one exaggerated laterally (to include tissue adjacent to the lateral ribs over to the nipple area). Both of these images should include the nipple and they should be labeled in the standard manner in order to provide appropriate orientation of the images. When the curvature of the rib cage is minimal, a standard CC view may provide adequate tissue coverage.

The MLO view may also need to be imaged in two individual projections. A standard MLO view will image the lateral tissue well and a LMO view (reverse oblique) or a 90 degree lateromedial view can be used to image the medial tissue. When the curvature of the rib cage is minimal, the standard MLO will provide adequate tissue coverage.

7. Deformities Of The Spine

a. Kyphosis

Kyphotic patients present with a *C-shaped, anterior-to-posterior curvature of the spine*. The degree of this curvature varies, and as it becomes more pronounced, positioning this patient for standard mammography projections becomes progressively more difficult. These patients are physically unable to *straighten up* and stand erect with their shoulders back. The problems they present for mammography examinations relate to the superimposition of their shoulders, neck, and upper thorax over the breast area. Also, if the patient is of small stature, the compression paddle may be physically too wide to fit into the constricted area between her shoulder and lower ribs for the MLO view.

Kyphotic patients present with a **C-shaped, anterior-to-posterior curvature of the spine.** *The degree of this curvature varies, and as it becomes more pronounced, positioning this patient for standard mammography projections becomes progressively more difficult.*

Patients with severe kyphosis are very difficult to image mammographically. These patients are also frequently frail and the positions they must assume make them unsteady. Mammography positioning is often very uncomfortable for them and they may find it difficult to remain still during the x-ray exposure.

For the CC view, have the patient hold onto the handlebars with both hands. Encourage her to slowly inch forward and walk under the image receptor to bring her breasts closer to the receptor surface at the same time that her shoulders tip back, out of the path of the compression paddle. If this is too difficult, have her sit in a chair and slip the chair under the image receptor until her shoulders will clear the edge of the compression paddle above. Alternately, rotate the C-arm 180 degrees and perform a From Below (reverse CC) view. This is an excellent option. The image receptor will be in contact with the superior tissue and the compression paddle will contact the inferior breast surface.

The standard MLO projection may be possible to perform if the curvature of the spine is not excessive. With pronounced kyphosis, a narrower compression paddle may be much more successful at fitting into the limited chest wall space from the axilla down to the IMF. Often the compression paddle is not able to clear the neck and shoulder area, or, when it does, these structures immediately roll forward, overshadowing the breast tissue below. When this is the case, a LMO (reverse oblique) view will be much more successful to avoid the neck and shoulder problems and image the breast free of superimposition from adjacent body parts.

b. Scoliosis

Scoliosis is a condition characterized by *lateral curvature of the spine*. This condition exists in a wide range of severity from being so minor that one would barely perceive an abnormality to being so pronounced that the patient's thorax is markedly twisted and deformed. The challenge is to image the breast tissue as it follows the abnormal contour of the rib cage. According to the severity of this abnormality with an individual patient, mammography examinations of patients with spinal scoliosis may follow a completely normal protocol or they may require significant alteration. The one outstanding characteristic of mammography examinations when modification is required is that the images are almost always asymmetric; this presents a challenge to the interpreting radiologist because the symmetrical comparison of images from one side to the other is not possible. Depending on the direction and the severity of the spinal curvature, the individual breasts may exhibit very different characteristics regarding their physical relationship to the rib cage and chest wall. Therefore, one breast may be imaged with near-normal conditions and the mammography images may be very normal in appearance. On the other hand, the opposite breast may require a number of additional views to completely image the breast tissue and the mammography images will be obviously abnormal in appearance.

Imaging studies of scoliosis patients often follow a similar protocol to that outlined with pectus excavatum and pectus carinatum because both of these conditions relate to imaging breast tissue as it follows the deformed and abnormal contour of the rib cage. The best advice one can offer is to remain focused on imaging all of the breast tissue. When the standard protocol of symmetrical imaging for both of the breasts is not possible, manage each breast individually in the best manner possible, given the existing physical limitations. Always maintain the axillary placement of markers indicating view and laterality to facilitate correct orientation of the images for interpretation purposes. Finally, as with any mammography study when the examination must be *pieced* together in a jig-saw fashion, always remember to include overlapping tissue; a BB skin marker may be used on the patient's skin to facilitate the confirmation of overlapping breast tissue on the mammogram. This should be noted on the patient's requisition to avoid misinterpreting the BB marker to indicate the location of a palpable mass.

8. Difficult to Position Patients

The most important factor to keep in mind when positioning difficult patients is that they are, without question, difficult. An attempt to obtain the best possible images on these patients must always be made. However, the technologist and radiologist must realize that, with these patients, it is often difficult to produce films that meet the criteria of the images that we regularly obtain with *average / normal* patients. Perfect films are often difficult to obtain, even with the most *perfect* patients. Formidable body shapes and sizes test our skills even further. Not only does this present a positioning challenge for the technologist, it also creates an overlying sense of frustration. The patient often shares this frustration, along with an acute sense of embarrassment, as she acknowledges the difficulty that her body size and /or shape has presented for this examination. The resulting mindset of both the patient and technologist can be counterproductive to achieving high quality mammography images.

Rather than focusing on what can't be done, it is far easier and more productive to focus on what can be done. An example of this would be to consider the kyphotic patient. Many times it is virtually impossible to perform an adequate MLO on such a patient because the neck and opposite shoulder may impede the proper movement of the compression paddle over the thorax. *Pulling* these body parts back and out of the way may result in the loss of medial tissue on the breast that is being imaged. A *normal* MLO cannot be done, yet many technologists proceed with the standard protocol, repeating film after film in an attempt to image all the breast tissue using this standard projection.

In general, if the positioning does not improve after two or three attempts, it most likely cannot improve. When this occurs, an alternate projection that can *work around* the physical restrictions should be performed. *Your first choice should always be the single projection that can adequately substitute for the routine view which cannot be performed.* If the patient's limitations are such that one image will not include all the required tissue, *the next best choice would be a number of projections that together will provide complete tissue coverage.* Under difficult circumstances such as this, the fate of the examination has little to do with the skill of the mammography technologist. Even the most experienced technologist will encounter real limitations directly related to the patient's body structure and other physical conditions.

Unfortunately, when these challenging circumstances occur, both the patient and technologist experience a heightened level of tension and frustration each time another attempt is made to improve the previous image. This situation can quickly escalate into a negative experience for both parties. Rather than continue to be frustrated by the inability to perform a proper *standard* view, the technologist should *consider what options are available* to produce the best possible images given the circumstances she is faced with. *A positive, constructive approach is important* to maintain the trust and cooperation of the patient.

To remain focused on what can be done, one should look for another view or approach that would demonstrate the same anatomic information as the standard view that cannot be performed. For example, it is apparent that the LMO view is the direct reverse of the MLO view; the bucky and the compression paddle simply change positions and the direction of the x-ray beam is reversed as it traverses the breast tissue. Technically, these views should demonstrate the same anatomic information. When you are performing the LMO on a kyphotic patient, the compression paddle will encounter the tissue of the lower, outer quadrant first, thereby avoiding the neck and shoulder area. This is often a very successful alternative for this patient presentation.

An important point to keep in mind when performing these non-standard views is that often, despite our best efforts, the amount of breast tissue that is demonstrated may not be consistent with what we are accustomed to seeing on our standard images. This is primarily due to the difficult physical limitations of the patient, combined with the awkwardness of the positioning technique and the inexperience of the technologist in performing these unfamiliar positioning maneuvers. During the course of a normal working day, a mammographer performs many of the standard projections. Naturally, she is well versed in these techniques and is comfortable and competent with every step in this process. Even in the busiest of practices, mammographers seldom have occasion to practice non-standard positioning techniques, and therefore, their expertise and comfort level have not had the opportunity to develop. Also, many technologists find their body mechanics much more difficult when performing these projections; they may need to assume a very uncomfortable and awkward position for an extended time as they work with the patient. They often need to work under the mammography unit or at least below the level of the patient's breast.

 Your first choice should always be the single projection that can adequately substitute for the routine view which cannot be performed.

While it is natural for the technologist to focus on the frustrations and difficulties of the situation at hand, she must maintain an awareness of the patient's perspective. There is a large psychological component that accompanies the physical limitations of these situations. On the psychological side, a basic but easily forgotten fact is that these patients are also people - with the same feelings, fears, worries, and needs that we all have. They should be treated with the same respect and courtesy that every other patient receives. Speak directly to them rather than communicating through a companion. Always explain the procedure and inquire about their capabilities in assisting with the positioning procedure rather than focusing completely on their limitations. Physically challenged patients frequently live with a great deal of discomfort and compromise on a daily basis. They have limited agility and their muscles and tendons may be very rigid. A very simple maneuver, such as raising an arm, turning their head, or bending forward may be very difficult to accomplish. In general, many of these patients find mammography examinations very challenging and uncomfortable. Their patience may deteriorate as the examination proceeds. All of these factors contribute to the fact that, although alternate views provide an excellent alternative for the difficult-to-position patient, they seldom yield optimal results. Document on the requisition, when adequate tissue coverage has not been achieved in these situations.

In general, the alternate views that are useful in positioning the difficult patient are as follows:

LMO View - This view should be performed when it is not possible to achieve standard MLO positioning. This should be easy to determine. Anytime that it is difficult to apply compression to the medial breast tissue, as would normally be the case with a standard MLO, the LMO view should be substituted. Examples of patients that may benefit from the LMO projection are those with the following conditions:

- Kyphosis
- Pectus excavatum (depressed sternum)
- Pectus carinatum (prominent, protruding sternum / pigeon chest)
- Frozen shoulder
- Recent open heart surgery
- Hickman catheter/other miscellaneous catheters
- Prominent pacemaker
- Protruding, distended abdomen
- Well developed pectoral muscles

FB View - This view should be utilized whenever it is difficult to perform the standard CC view. Its use would apply to many of the same patients that would benefit from the LMO positioning, as described above. Along with this basic alternative position, a FB exaggerated CC view and a FB cleavage view can also be performed when clinical presentations warrant information specific to these areas.

LM View - There are occasions when it may be difficult to perform the LMO view as the most logical substitution for the standard MLO view. The patient may have an extremely limited range of motion. She may be confined to a wheelchair in which the arms are not removable. In these circumstances, after considering the overall limitations, the technologist should then proceed with the *next best* option, which would be the 90 degree LM view. This is the best alternative to the MLO on patients that have the greatest physical limitations.

a. Patients in Wheelchairs

When performing mammography examinations on patients seated in a wheelchair, two important factors must be considered. First is the general mobility of the patient herself. Second, the ability to remove the side arms of the wheelchair will have a major impact on the success of the examination.

Begin by assessing the patient and any limiting conditions that will impact her positioning for the mammography examination. Many patients that arrive in a wheelchair are able to stand unassisted for a limited period of time. It is critical that the condition of the patient must be verified and carefully considered before asking her to stand. Her safety is the primary consideration and it must not be compromised. As well, it is important to determine if the patient may be disoriented or confused before you begin the examination. Some questions that you may want to ask before standing a wheelchair patient are:

- Can you stand alone for several minutes, unassisted?

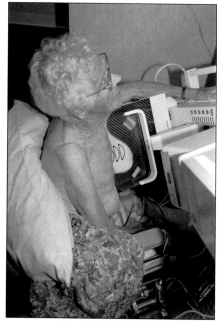

Figure 4.220 Occasionally, a patient must be done in a wheelchair. Placing a pillow behind her back will help to keep her leaning forward, into the mammography unit.

- Can you step minimally from side to side or raise one arm at a time without losing your balance?
- Do you often walk around your room (or home) unassisted?
- Do you dress yourself? This task generally encompasses a similar degree of agility and range of motion that would be required to perform a standing mammogram.

If there is any hesitation on the part of the patient or if you have any doubt about her stability, do not stand the patient for the mammogram. Leave her seated for the examination. If it is at all possible, enlisting the assistance of another technologist will facilitate the speed and safety of performing a mammography examination on a patient seated in a wheelchair. Always engage the wheelchair brakes once the chair is in place as you begin to position the patient. The patient will be most stable when her hips are situated at the very back of the chair. The two most critical factors that will facilitate positioning with a seated patient are keeping the patient's back as straight as possible and keeping her thorax leaning slightly forward.

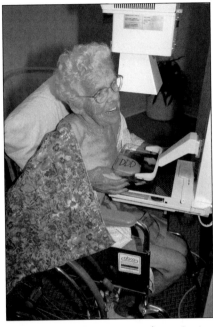

Figure 4.221 The two most important factors to keep in mind when performing mammography on a patient in a wheelchair is to keep her back as straight as possible and to keep her leaning forward from the waist.

If the arms of the wheelchair can be removed, proceed to perform a standard CC and MLO of each breast, removing only one of the arms at a time to allow the patient to use the remaining arm for support and security as you position her for the examination. Pillows can be used to support the patient as you lean her forward in the chair. If the patient has a protruding abdomen, leaning her forward into the image receptor will often help to keep the abdomen pushed back somewhat. A straight back, as opposed to a slumped posture will also be very helpful in minimizing interference from the abdomen below as well as from the shoulders above.

If the patient is kyphotic, lean her back in her chair just enough to *counteract* the kyphosis by moving the clavicle and shoulder out from under the path of the compression paddle. The position is similar to that used when performing a lordotic chest x-ray.

If the arms of the wheelchair cannot be removed, the next best option would be to transfer the patient to a mammography positioning chair (available from many equipment manufacturers) or to another chair that has adjustable or removable arms and wheels that can lock. You will require the assistance of several individuals to safely transfer the patient and someone may be required to remain near the patient, providing support and stability as the examination proceeds. If a companion has accompanied the patient, this person may be willing to fulfill this function, provided the companion is female and not pregnant. Always discuss this with the patient to be sure that she will also be comfortable with this arrangement. Every effort should be made to encourage this assistant to step behind the radiation shield after the pa-

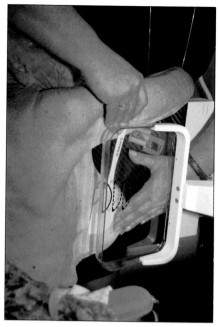

Figure 4.222 When the arms of the wheelchair cannot be removed to manipulate the C-arm into an angled position, a LM view is usually the next best choice for a second view of the breast.

tient's position has been secured for the x-ray exposure. If the patient needs to be held, a protective lead apron must be provided for the assistant; *the staff of the imaging department should not hold patients for x-ray examinations.* Should the option of transferring the patient to a suitable chair not be possible, the mammography examination should be performed to include a CC and LM projection. The wheelchair arms will interfere with the position of the image receptor and compression paddle for the MLO or LMO views, respectively. The LM projection would also be a good alternative for a patient with limited range of motion (frozen or fractured shoulder), kyphosis, or deformities of the sternum.

Always *exercise caution* when you determine that a patient is, in fact, able to stand and you elect to perform a standing mammogram. Deactivate the automatic compression release function on the mammography unit. This allows you to stand next to the patient and provide her with support as the compression is released. This will also minimize the chance that the patient may be startled and perhaps lean back, losing her balance, when the compression paddle releases her breast after the x-ray exposure. You may want to warn the patient that the compression will not be released until you return to her side after each exposure.

Also, you must be aware that a patient who is elderly, very ill, or on medication may not be able to provide an accurate and reliable assessment of her ability to stand and tolerate the mammography examination. The technologist must always use her best judgment despite information the patient might willingly offer. Chances must never be taken; *the patient's safety is always the first priority.*

b. Patients on Stretchers (Gurneys or Carts)

While mammography examinations performed on stretcher patients are very time consuming and often awkward, they are not, in fact, technically difficult. Some patients are able to sit with their legs over the side of the stretcher. If this is the case, a standard CC and MLO can be done with the patient leaning slightly forward into the mammography unit. It is very important to lock the stretcher brakes to stabilize the patient after she has been moved into position against the mammography unit. You may also choose to transfer the patient to a chair if she exhibits this degree of mobility.

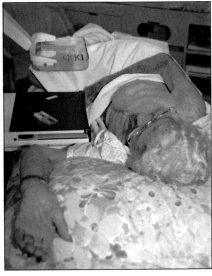

When a patient cannot sit, the recumbent examination should proceed to include a LM and a FB projection.

The LM projection will be substituted for the standard MLO projection.

Figure 4.223 The patient on a stretcher should lie on the side opposite to the side being imaged to begin positioning.

The patient should be rolled onto the side opposite to the side being imaged. For example, if the left breast is being imaged, the patient should be lying on her right side. Support her head with a pillow that has been doubled over to provide extra height. Both of her arms should be brought forward, bending her elbows and resting her hands above her head. Her knees should be bent for balance; a pillow placed between her knees may make her more comfortable, enabling the patient to remain in this position for a longer time.

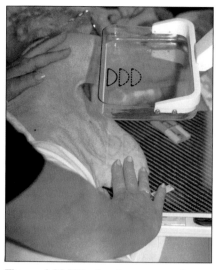 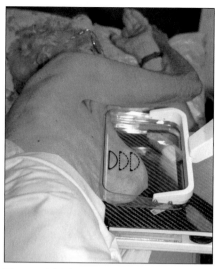

Figure 4.224 The bucky supports the breast medially; the patient leans forward onto the bucky to include lateral tissue on the image.

Figure 4.225 The breast is compressed in the LM projection; the forward position of her arm will help to keep lateral and axillary tissue on the bucky.

With the C-arm in the *normal* CC position (beam perpendicular to the floor), the image receptor will be parallel to the stretcher. Adjust the height of the receptor so that it can be positioned between the breasts, lifting the breast laterally and supporting it with the medial tissue on the receptor and the nipple in profile. Lock the stretcher brakes. Rotate the patient slightly forward to include as much lateral tissue as possible. With her elbow bent, place her hand at shoulder level on the handlebar; this will keep the pectoralis muscle relaxed. Compression is applied to the lateral breast tissue, gently retracting the latissimus dorsi muscle back to allow the corner of the compression paddle to pass by the shoulder and compress the axillary tissue. At this point the patient's arm can be raised up and over the edge of the image receptor to prevent it from overshadowing the image field. The side rail behind the patient should always be raised to provide additional security for the patient should she feel unstable or lose her balance.

The FB projection should be substituted for the standard CC projection.

With the patient in the same position as for the LM projection, the C-arm should be rotated 90 degrees, so that the tube head is toward the patient's feet and the receptor is toward the patient's head. The beam will project parallel to the stretcher and the floor.

Elevate the breast in the same manner you normally would when positioning the CC view, and adjust the height of the bucky so that the breast is centered with the superior tissue resting on the receptor surface. Supporting the breast in this manner, apply compression to secure the breast position. The purpose for substituting the FB projection for the standard CC projection with a stretcher patient relates to the size of the x-ray tube head and to the SID (source-to-image-receptor-distance). With the patient lying on her side, the large tube head will be near her abdomen and knees. There is much greater flexibility in moving these body parts out of the way of the equipment as opposed to attempting to move the patient's head and neck away from the equipment.

Again, it is important to remember that often these positioning alternatives may facilitate the examination under difficult conditions, but their use does not guarantee optimal imaging of the entire breast. While the results may be a compromised examination when compared with a *normal* mammogram, it may, nevertheless, be the best that can be achieved under the circumstances and a preferable alternative compared to postponing or canceling the examination entirely. *It is extremely important to record the patient's limitations for the radiologist's information and review when he interprets the examination. It is also recommended that this information be maintained as part of the patient's permanent medical record.*

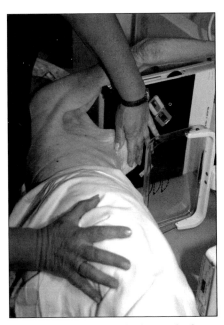

Figure 4.226 Elevate the breast in the same manner as you would for a CC view; adjust the height of the bucky so that the breast will be centered for this image.

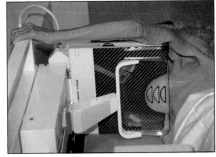

Figure 4.227 The FB view is substituted for the CC view to provide more comfortable patient positioning (the large tube head will be located near the patient's knees rather than close to her head).

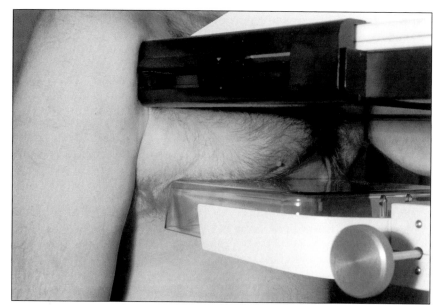

Figure 4.228 A well developed pectoral muscle may limit compression in the CC projection with a male patient. The FB view is an excellent substitute in these situations.

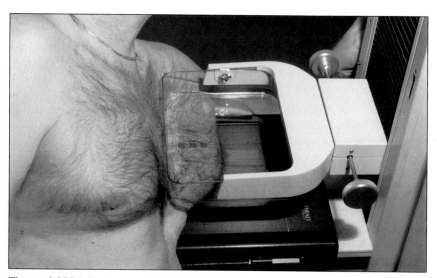

Figure 4.229 It is no more difficult to image a male breast than it is to examine the breast of a small woman.

9. Male Mammography

With few exceptions, the male breast is basically a dormant structure, with a similar anatomical makeup to that of a pre-adolescent female. It consists primarily of fatty tissue with a small, rudimentary nipple and minimal duct formation in the retroareolar area. The hormonal sensitivity of these ductal structures predisposes them to stimulation during adolescence, much the same as with females. This may result in minimal subareolar tissue proliferation which is often clinically asymmetric. The prolonged use of some medications may also stimulate breast changes in men. Although any female breast condition can occur in males, the most common disorder that is clinically encountered is gynecomastia. This transient condition may be unilateral or bilateral and is characterized by an increase in the fibroglandular tissue in the retroareolar area. Male breast cancer is rare; it accounts for only 1-2% of all breast cancers.

Male mammography is only pursued when a clinical abnormality has been detected; it is never used on a routine basis to diagnose or screen for breast cancer. It is most important for the mammography technologist to conduct herself in a professional, competent manner when performing male mammog-

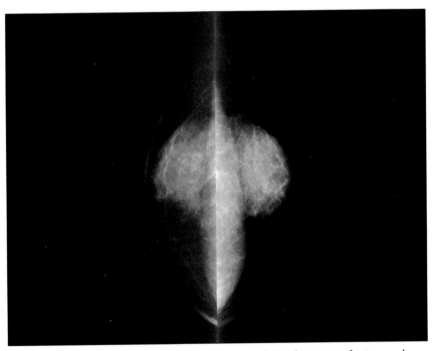

Figure 4.230 CC views of a male patient; bilateral development of retroareolar glandular tissue is evident.

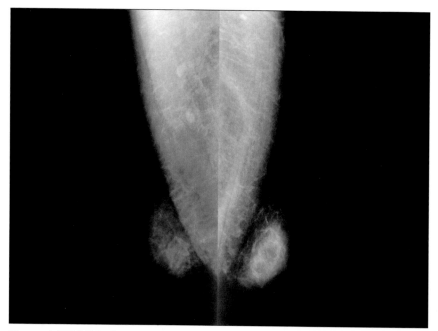

Figure 4.231 MLO views of a male patient; note the prominent pectoralis muscle.

raphy examinations. Many men are extremely self-conscious and embarrassed in this situation; a compassionate and understanding technologist can facilitate the examination and make the situation as comfortable as possible for her patient.

The basic mammography examination is identical for both male and female patients: bilateral CC and MLO views. It is no more difficult to position and image a male breast than it is to examine the breast of a small female. Breast compression with male patients may be more difficult when the pectoral muscle is highly developed and rigid. Should this situation create positioning difficulties, a FB (From Below) view can be used as an alternate CC projection and a LMO view can be performed rather than the standard MLO view. This may also be necessary should an abundance of hair on the chest result in slipping of the breast tissue from beneath the compression paddle. The tissue will be held much more securely when the compression paddle encounters skin directly. Again, the FB and the LMO view will effectively accomplish this objective.

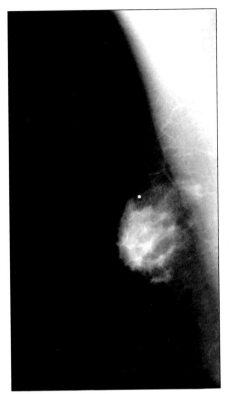

Figure 4.232 This male patient had developed a significant component of glandular tissue in his right breast.

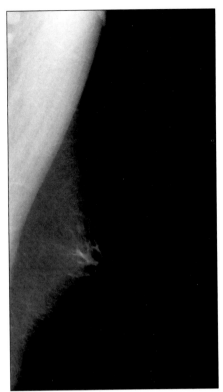

Figure 4.233 Minimal ductal formation was noted in the retroareolar area on this mammography examination of a male patient.

Additional views, magnification spot films, tangential projections, etc. may be required and are very successfully performed on the male patient.

D. TRIANGULATION

There are times when an area of concern is imaged on only one of the two standard mammography images (CC and MLO). Frequently a LM view will be performed to provide additional information. If the abnormality is again seen on this projection, it then becomes important to determine the orthogonal location of this area in order to perform spot compression images and perhaps an interventional procedure. By analyzing the location of the abnormality on the two images where it has been visualized, the general area where it will be located on the *other* standard mammography image can be accurately deter-

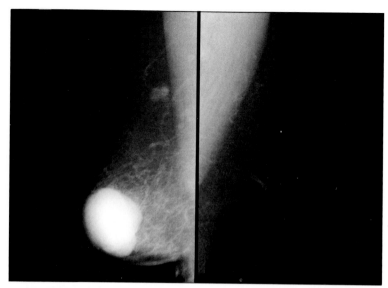

Figure 4.234 This 70 year old male patient presented with a large carcinoma of the right breast. His mother and sister both died of breast cancer; one brother died of lung cancer and another of leukemia.

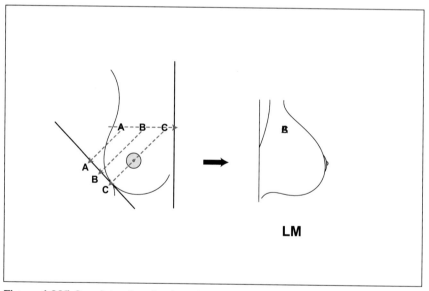

Figure 4.235 On a lateral projection, these three lesions (located in the superior part of this breast) will be superimposed. Compare this appearance to that in Figure 4.236 to develop an appreciation of the principles of lesion location that is used for triangulation.

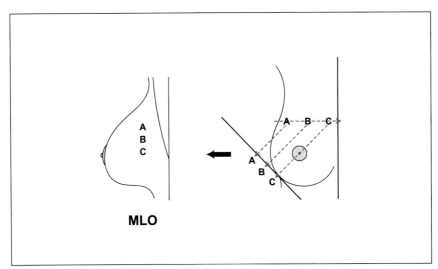

Figure 4.236 These same lesions will be imaged in completely separate locations on an MLO projection.

mined. This information will direct the technologist to select the most appropriate supplementary views to demonstrate the abnormality.

Triangulation is a process of determining in which area of the breast a lesion will be located based on its known position on two other mammography images.

Using the triangulation diagram in Figure 4.237 as a reference, follow along with the following discussion. *A lesion that moves DOWN on a lateral view,* compared to its location on the MLO view - *will be located in the LATERAL part of the CC projection.* Perform an XCCL view to *find* the abnormality in the CC projection.

A lesion that moves UP on a lateral view, compared to its location on the MLO view - *will be located in the MEDIAL part of the CC projection.* Perform a CV view to *find* the abnormality in the CC projection.

Occasionally, an abundance of glandular tissue may *hide* an abnormality on the MLO projection. By following the lines in the Triangulation diagram in Figure 4.72, you will be able to determine the general area where the abnormality is located on the MLO view. Coned compression spot views can then be performed to demonstrate the abnormality for the radiologist.

Note: Refer to additional information on Triangulation on page 118.

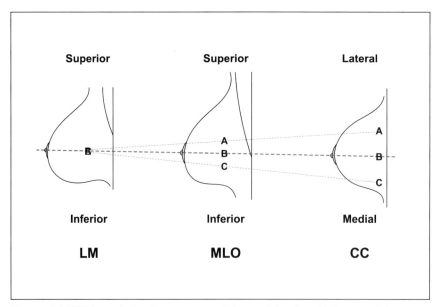

Figure 4.237 Triangulation is a process of determining in which area of the breast a lesion will be located based on its known position on two other mammography images.

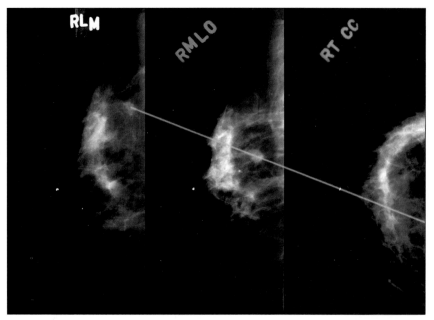

Figure 4.238 The location of this mass in the CC view was discovered by triangulation, using the LM and MLO projections that had visualized this abnormality.

E. SPECIMEN RADIOGRAPHY

In many cases a biopsy specimen must be imaged to provide confirmation that the abnormality in question has indeed been surgically removed. This is particularly important when the abnormality is characterized only by suspicious microcalcifications. If the lesion is not in the biopsy specimen, the surgeon then has the opportunity to obtain another tissue sample while the patient is still in the operating room. Also, when the lesion is located close to the edge of the biopsy specimen, additional tissue along the edge in question should be excised to obtain clear margins of disease and therby improve the patient's prognosis. The edges of the biopsy specimen can be marked with sutures, wires, etc. to facilitate correct orientation in the event that additional tissue must be excised. Alternately, the surface of the specimen may be coated with multiple colored inks to identify orientation to breast tissue.

Specimen radiography can be performed with a dedicated mammography unit (using the small focal spot and magnification), with a digital spot receptor, or with a stand-alone specimen radiography unit.

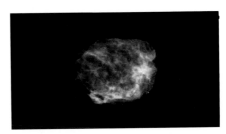

It is important to be aware that the radiographic appearance of an abnormality on the specimen image may be very deceiving. The absence of superimposition from skin and from surrounding tissue, particularly if it was fibrous or dense in nature, may result in a very different appearance from that observed on the

Figure 4.239 When clear margins have not been obtained with the first biopsy specimen, the surgeon must excise more tissue along the border where the lesion has been visualized on the specimen image.

original mammogram. Most often, however, specific lesion features or characteristic microcalcifications will clearly identify the abnormality within the biopsy specimen. Because the image quality of the specimen radiograph is far superior to presurgical full-breast and coned compression images, important information regarding the true nature and extent of the breast abnormality, including mutiple areas of involvement, can be determined from these images. *This information is critical in planning appropriate treatment protocols.* For this reason, the entire specimen, including all tissue borders, must be radiographed. Because the magnification technique is recommended, this may require multiple images with large tissue specimens.

Although frequently difficult to perform, orthogonal views of a biopsy specimen are both desirable and valuable. When an abnormality is not clearly identified in a specimen, an orthogonal image, or an image with an alternate orientation of the tissue sample, may be very helpful in confirming specific lesion characteristics. Also, a single specimen image can demonstrate clear lesion margins in only two dimensions; an orthogonal image may present an entirely different perspective. Specimens that are large and firm will be easily imaged in multiple planes.

The specimen radiograph can also be used to direct pathological studies to the specific abnormality within a biopsy sample. After reviewing the specimen image, the radiologist can insert a needle into the tissue, adjacent to the lesion; this will act as a marker, directing the pathologist to the exact location of the abnormality. This will facilitate direct histologic correlation with radiographically identified abnormalities; multiple lesions or multiple areas of involvement will require this correlation. Marking the abnormality is also important when the specimen is large in relation to the abnormality and when the localizing wire marker is distant from the target lesion. The entire specimen should be examined for pathology, however, to detect additional, unsuspected areas of involvement that would indicate multifocal disease. This information is extremely important in planning an appropriate treatment protocol for the patient.

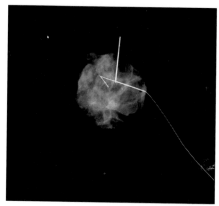

Figure 4.240 A needle can be inserted into the specimen to mark the exact location of the lesion for the pathologist.

It is also desirable to image the localizing wire marker in the specimen tissue. Besides correlation that the marked lesion was indeed excised, it also confirms that the intact localizing wire has been removed (Figure 4.240).

Specimen radiography, then, serves a number of functions:

1. Confirms lesion excision

2. Identifies the size and characteristics of the lesion

3. Identifies (unsuspected) multifocal disease

4. Assists in evaluating margins of disease

5. Directs pathology evaluation to the lesion

6. Confirms complete removal of localizing marker

When biopsy specimens are prepared for pathologic evaluation, they are processed in a number of chemical solutions and then embedded in paraffin blocks. These blocks are sliced into a number of sections; several thin slices are then taken from each section and examined for disease. Occasionally, when the pathology report does not identify the disease that was expected, based on the specimen radiograph, additional tissue samples must be obtained from the paraffin blocks. Imaging the individual blocks can help to identify the appropriate section to examine further. Calcifications require special consideration when there is a discrepancy in correlation. When the specimen radiograph clearly demonstrates microcalcifications and they are not apparent pathologically, a number of options must be considered. First, the pathology specimens should be examined with polarized light. One specific kind of calcium (calcium oxalate) is visible radiographically but not microscopically; its presence in tissue samples can be easily identified with a polarized light source. Alternately, the possibility exists that the calcium may have been inadvertently *washed out* of the specimen during the process of preparing the tissue samples in the lab. They also may have been shattered or dislodged as the blocks were sliced into individual sections. Always indicate that a specimen contains calcium when it is sent to pathology; this will help alleviate these oversights in processing the specimen tissue.

The following protocol will produce specimen images of very high quality:
- Use the small focal spot size for optimum definition.
- Use the lowest possible kVp setting for optimum contrast; dose is not a consideration with specimen radiography.
- Use magnification technique for improved resolution.
- Use a high definition (detail) screen for improved resolution; again, dose is not a consideration.

Many abnormalities have been identified better with ultrasound than with mammography on the pre-biopsy work-up. Specimen imaging of these abnormalities can also be performed with ultrasound. Gel can be applied to the tissue bag containing the surgical specimen; alternately, a stand-off pad may be used. Lesion location in the specimen can be marked in the same manner that was described in the above discussion.

HELPFUL HINTS

a) *Gently compress a surgical biopsy specimen*, particularly with large tissue samples. The benefits of compression are identical to those obtained with standard mammography images. If the facility uses biopsy specimen containers, compression of the tissue sample will not be possible. Tissue specimens from a LCNB (large core needle biopsy) are small and much more fragile; they should not be compressed.

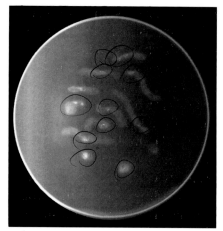

Figure 4.241 Core specimens can be collected in a small dish during the biopsy procedure. They should be imaged to document the presence of microcalcifications.

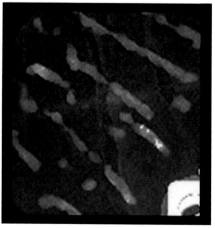

Figure 4.242 Core specimens can also be collected on a telfa pad for imaging.

b) The specimen is usually transported to the x-ray department in a small plastic bag. When this is not the case, place a piece of x-ray film on both sides of the biopsy specimen before compressing the tissue. This will minimize clean-up and keep the mammography equipment and accessories more sanitary.

c) With abnormalities characterized by suspicious microcalcifications, it is important to image the core tissue samples from a LCNB (large core needle biopsy) to document the presence of microcalcifications in the specimens. Try to minimize the overlapping of the core samples on the image.

d) To achieve a higher degree of magnification (particularly desirable with core biopsy specimens), use the following protocol rather than imaging the specimen(s) on the magnification platform from the equipment manufacturer: Remove the face shield. Turn one of the standard compression paddles upside down in the paddle housing and raise the compression carriage to its highest position. Place the specimen(s) on the compression paddle, which should now be located very close to the tube head. Place the cassette on the receptor platform or on top of the bucky. Use the imaging parameters previously outlined.

e) The images of core biopsy specimens will be most clear when there is minimal fluid surrounding the cores. At the same time, the cores must not be allowed to become dry with exposure to air during the biopsy procedure or while they are being imaged after the procedure. They should be lightly sprinkled with saline to keep them moist but not excessively wet. They can be covered with plastic wrap to retain their moisture if there will be any delay in imaging. After they have been radiographed, they should be placed in a preservative (formalin) immediately.

f) With a surgical biopsy specimen, if there is sufficient tissue to cover the AEC device, a phototimed exposure technique can be used. With small surgical specimens and with core biopsy specimens, a manual exposure technique will need to be selected.

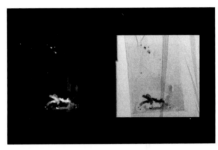

Figure 4.243 The core specimens may be imaged digitally after the biopsy procedure. This will also document that microcalcifications have been removed.

g) It is also important to image any additional tissue samples that are excised when this is deemed necessary on the basis of the initial specimen image. Subsequent samples should be labelled or coded appropriately.

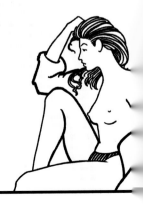

CHAPTER 5:
FILM CRITIQUE

CHAPTER 5:
FILM CRITIQUE

A. INTRODUCTION

A thorough evaluation of mammography images requires the careful examination of a number of relevant factors. These factors can be broadly classified into two groups: those that relate to the content of the image itself and those that are independent of the image content. Factors which are not related to the image content are film identification and the general aesthetic presentation of the film. Factors associated with the image content include breast positioning and compression, exposure factors, image quality features, and the presence of artifacts. The latter two factors (image quality and artifacts) require individual focus; they are described in the following two chapters.

B. FILM PRESENTATION

1. Film Identification

A mammography image is an important medical document that contains valuable clinical information. Clear, standard film labeling is important to establish accurate and consistent communication between colleagues and professionals in related fields. Labeling also facilitates proper interpretation of the examination and minimizes confusion and the possibility for errors in diagnosis.

A mammography image is an important medical document that contains valuable clinical information.

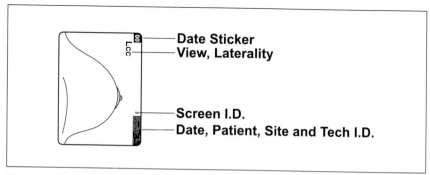

Figure 5.1 Mammography accreditation programs have established clear guidelines for the identification of mammography images.

The Canadian Association of Radiologists (CAR) and the American College of Radiology (ACR) mammography accreditation programs have established clear guidelines for the identification of mammography images.

All mammography images *must* be *permanently* identified with the following information:

Facility name and location (city, state/province, zip/area code), patient name (first and last), patient identification number (medical record number, social security number, or date of birth if others are not available), examination date, radiopaque markers indicating laterality (R, L) and projection (CC, MLO), technologist identification, cassette/screen identification, and the mammography unit number (if multiple units are at site).

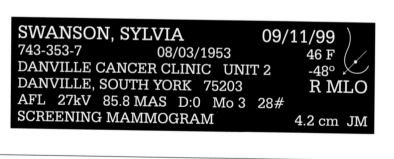

Figure 5.2 An example of the technical information that is imprinted on each mammography image with a patient identification system that is connected to the mammography unit.

Also *recommended* are a separate date sticker and a read-out of the technical factors. Labeling codes that indicate laterality and projection have been outlined in the discussion on mammography positioning techniques in Chapter 4. Refer to Figures 5.1 and 5.2 for examples of image identification for mammography images.

2. Aesthetic Presentation

The technologist should attempt to have her images symmetrically centered on the film for a pleasing artistic appearance. This is important because the films will be mounted side by side on viewboxes and compared as mirror images during the interpretation process.

Radiopaque markers indicating both view and laterality should be placed on the axillary side of the image and somewhat away from the image itself (closer to the film edge) so as not to distract the radiologist during his or her examination of the films. The markers should be clearly visible but not overpowering or distracting. They should use the standard labeling codes that have been outlined by the national mammography accreditation programs.

Finally, for all full-breast images, the collimation of the mammography unit should be adjusted to expose the entire film area. Images with an exposed, black background are much easier for the radiologist to examine and interpret with the greatest degree of accuracy. For compression spot views, consideration should also be given to exposing the entire film, or, at the very least, for extending the field beyond the physical dimension of the spot compression paddle. Minimizing extraneous bright light from the illuminators will dramatically increase the visual acuity and perception of the interpreter's eye. The same effect can be achieved with collimated images if masking is used to cover the clear, unexposed areas on clinical images. Unfortunately, masking is cumbersome and awkward. This practice would be impractical for high volume viewing situations such as those encountered with screening programs.

 Radiopaque markers indicating both view and laterality should be placed on the axillary side of the image and somewhat away from the image itself (closer to the film edge) so as not to distract the radiologist during his or her examination of the films.

If the clinical area of concern has not been imaged on the standard views, the technologist should proceed to obtain an image of this area, especially with an unusual lesion presentation.

C. IMAGE CONTENT

The technologist should regularly assess her films for both content and radiographic technique. In most situations, the technologist will have the opportunity to observe her films before the radiologist reviews them. She possesses the distinct advantage of having first-hand knowledge regarding the patient's physical condition and body habitus as well as detailed information about her clinical concerns. Only she will be able to appreciate the reasons for less-than-optimal images due, perhaps, to an uncooperative or a less-than-ideal patient. Also, if the clinical area of concern has not been imaged on the standard views, the technologist should proceed to obtain an image of this area, especially with an unusual lesion presentation.

1. Patient Positioning

Two sizes of image receptor are available for mammography: 18 x 24 cm and 24 x 30 cm. It is important that the appropriate size of film be utilized for each examination. Consideration of the breast size and contour will direct the appropriate selection. The breast tissue should not *flow* over the edges of the film; the receptor should be large enough to accommodate *all* of the breast tissue for each view. The exception to this would, of course, be the very large breast that must be imaged in overlapping sections because the large receptor is not able to image one view in its entirety. On the other hand, although patient positioning would not be jeopardized in any way, using a large receptor for the craniocaudal projection of a small breast would result in a waste of film area and an unusual visual presentation. However, using a large film for the mediolateral oblique projection of a small breast will seriously compromise patient positioning. One of two possibilities will occur. First, in order to center the breast on the film, the patient's shoulder will not be positioned correctly with the latissimus dorsi muscle behind the corner of the bucky. While this position will accommodate appropriate AEC selection, it will result in an unacceptable image because, with the latissimus muscle also positioned on the receptor, the pectoralis muscle and axilla will not be lying flat on the bucky and therefore they will not be well compressed. Also, under these circumstances, breast compression is frequently very uncomfortable for the patient. Alternately, should the correct shoulder position be selected, the centrally located AEC device would be positioned over inferior breast tissue, which is typically fatty. The AEC will be unable to select an optical film density that will adequately demonstrate the central, glandular breast tissue; this exposure will be light and will need to be repeated. Also, with this receptor position, the inferior corner of the bucky will poke into the ribs and abdomen of the patient, creating unnecessary discomfort and encouraging her to lean away from the receptor.

Evaluation of clinical images may proceed in the following manner:

a. The Mediolateral Oblique (MLO) Projection / View

When properly performed, this projection demonstrates more breast tissue than any other single view. Refer to Section III of Chapter 4 for a detailed discussion of patient positioning for the MLO view. The following criteria are typical of a good mediolateral oblique image:

1. A generous amount of pectoralis muscle (A) is seen as an inverted triangle with a wide margin at the axilla and the apex directed inferiorly; the inferior margin should reach the level of the nipple or slightly lower; a convex contour indicates a flaccid muscle. The latissimus dorsi muscle should not be included on the film. The pectoralis muscle shadow should be radioluscent.

2. The breast is supported; the parenchymal pattern should be perpendicular to the chest wall.

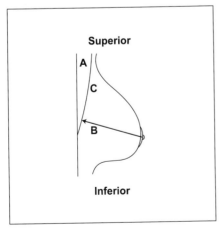

Figure 5.3 Evaluation criteria for a good MLO view.

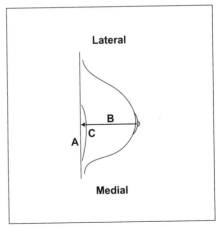

Figure 5.4 Evaluation criteria for a good CC view.

Minimizing extraneous bright light from the illuminators will dramatically increase the visual acuity and perception of the interpreter's eye.

3. The breast parenchyma is well separated, indicating good compression.

4. The breast parenchyma is well penetrated, indicating correct exposure technique.

5. A layer of retromammary fat (C) is seen behind the parenchyma.

6. The inframammary fold is clear (free of superimposed tissue).

7. The nipple is in profile for most examinations.

8. There are no folds or wrinkles in the tissue.

Note: The depth of tissue demonstrated on the MLO view is calculated in a plane perpendicular to the pectoralis muscle, measured posteriorly from the nipple to either the pectoralis muscle or the edge of the film, whichever comes first. This is called the Posterior Nipple Line (PNL); see (B) in figure 5.3.

b. The Craniocaudal (CC) Projection / View

The craniocaudal projection is designed to include all of the medial breast tissue because this area has the greatest risk of being excluded from the mediolateral oblique view. Refer to Section III of Chapter 4 for a detailed discussion of patient positioning for the CC view. The following criteria are typical of a good craniocaudal image:

1. All the medial tissue is visualized.

2. The depth of tissue (B) measured with the Posterior Nipple Line (PNL) is within 1.0 cm of the PNL measurement from the MLO view. The PNL on the CC view is measured posteriorly from the nipple to the edge of the film.

3. As much lateral tissue as possible is demonstrated.

4. A layer of retromammary fat (C) is seen behind the parenchyma.

5. The breast is centered on the film.

6. Pectoralis muscle (A) is seen on approximately 30 % of craniocaudal images.

7. The nipple is in profile for most examinations; it should be centrally located — without medial or lateral deviation.

8. There are no folds or wrinkles in the tissue.

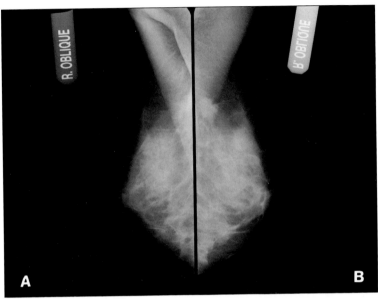

Figure 5.5 These images illustrate the importance of good patient positioning. A lesion is clearly demonstrated in the axilla of examination B. In retrospect, the lesion was present on the previous examination (A), but was difficult to appreciate due to tissue folds that were superimposed over this area of the breast.

2. Breast Compression

As has been stated previously, the value of compression cannot be overestimated.

After positioning, breast compression is the most critical component of mammography imaging.

The amount of compression applied will, of course, vary with the individual patient's tolerance and with the degree of compressibility of the tissue itself. Dense, fibrous breasts resist compression; these breasts also tend to be more sensitive, making patient compliance more difficult. Some patients will voice their objections too soon and others not soon enough. While the technologist must encourage her patients to comply with compression, she must also assess each individual situation and stop when the appropriate level of taut breast compression has been achieved. The skill of the technologist has a significant impact on the cooperation and compliance of the patient in achieving taut breast compression. Refer to Section II of Chapter 4 for more information on the specific benefits of breast compression.

3. Exposure Factors

The general principles for exposure technique are as follows:

1. Use sufficient kVp to penetrate the breast tissue. The optimal kVp for breast imaging using a grid (bucky) ranges from 25-28-30 kVp. With exceptionally dense breasts or perhaps with breasts that have been treated with radiotherapy, more than 30 kVp may occasionally be required. Modern mammography equipment also utilizes an alternate filter or focal spot material (Rhodium, Tungsten) when the required penetration reaches these higher levels. Small changes in kVp can result in marked changes in the tube output and in the overall film density.

2. The AEC will select the appropriate mAs to provide adequate film density. Long exposures times (over 2.0 seconds) are generally avoided in order to minimize problems with patient motion and reciprocity failure. All mammography units have a maximum allowable mAs based on specific features of the tube design; the heat loading capacity of the target material is the primary limiting factor.

3. The significant contribution of taut compression in reducing the required exposure while promoting the best possible imaging conditions must always be emphasized.

Ultimately, exposure factors are chosen to demonstrate the breast parenchyma. It is breast density, not size, that dictates the x-ray exposure. Although it plays a lesser role, breast thickness is also a contributing factor. This is

The amount of compression applied will, of course, vary with the individual patient's tolerance and with the degree of compressibility of the tissue itself.

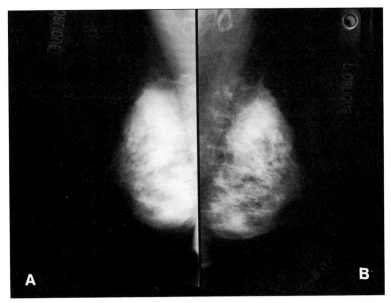

Figure 5.6 Note the benefits of properly performed breast compression with image B, where the patient is relaxed, allowing more tissue to be brought forward onto the receptor. Also, with improved tissue separation, far more information is demonstrated in the anterior glandular area of this mammogram.

apparent from our appreciation of how compression contributes to lower exposures (patient dose), primarily due to thickness reduction.

It is important to appreciate that, in the majority of examinations, a properly exposed mammogram will NOT demonstrate the skin and subcutaneous tissue on the viewbox. A bright light or *spot* viewer will facilitate assessment of these areas.

With fatty, atrophic breasts, the optical density that will optimally image this breast tissue happens to coincide with a density that may also enable the subcutaneous structures to be seen relatively well. However, this will not be a common occurrence, given the average patient age and breast tissue characteristics that typifies mammography investigations. With an average breast (50% fibrous and 50% fatty tissue) and especially with a dense breast, the exposure required to penetrate the breast parenchyma will naturally result in overexposure of the skin and subcutaneous tissue. This is normal and to be expected. It is the breast parenchyma that is at risk for the development of breast cancer and therefore it is this tissue that must be the focus of the mammography examination. Again, a bright light or a *spot* viewer will facilitate the examination of the skin and subcutaneous areas on the mammogram.

It is the breast parenchyma that is at risk for the development of breast cancer and therefore it is this tissue that must be the focus of the mammography examination.

The exposure level, or the optical density, of each image is selected with an Automatic Exposure Control (AEC) device. The optical density of the AEC system is programmed when the mammography equipment is installed; it is based on the processing parameters, the screen-film combination, and the individual preference of the radiologist. A variety of density settings or levels are operator-selectable; they typically allow density changes in plus or minus 10-20% increments. With an Auto-Time mode, the AEC will select the exposure mAs to produce the desired film density based on a given selected kVp. Current AEC systems now also select the appropriate kVp for each image (Auto kV mode), within a limited optimal range. Equipment that offers an alternate filter or anode selection for the dense breast may also have an Auto Filter mode; with this option, the AEC will select the most appropriate anode and / or filter for each exposure, along with the appropriate kVp and mAs. For each of these programs, the technical factors must be clearly displayed after each exposure for documentation purposes. AEC devices are invaluable in producing consistent optical film density and thereby minimizing repeat exposures. The technologist must, however, position the AEC device correctly for each image; the *selection* of the x-ray exposure can only be based on the tissue the AEC *sees* during the exposure. The correct AEC position is based on the location of the tissue we wish to image (the breast parenchyma). On a typical mammogram, retromammary fat will be imaged in the posterior breast area; this is not a good location for the AEC device. As breast tissue matures, fatty tissue begins to replace the fibrous components. Experience tells us that this process occurs in an orderly manner, from the posterior tissue forward; the prominent glandular tissue in the U.O.Q. remains the longest and, in the final atrophic state, retroareolar ductal structures remain as the only glandular component in a totally fatty replaced breast. Based on this information and because the AEC device moves forward in the central film plane, the best AEC location will be

AEC devices are invaluable in producing consistent optical film density and thereby minimizing repeat exposures.

toward the nipple area. For optimal film density, keep the AEC device positioned forward, toward the nipple area, making sure that it is completely covered by well-compressed breast tissue.

D. FILM INTERPRETATION

- For radiologic interpretation, the mammography images should be viewed on high intensity mammography illuminators.
- Mount the films with the axillas up, side by side (CC and MLO views together, respectively) in order to facilitate symmetrical comparison.

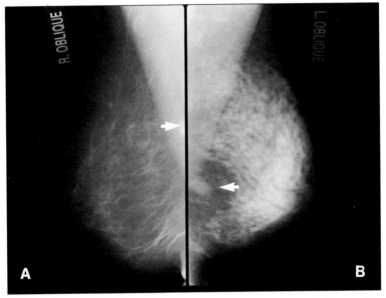

Figure 5.7 In both of the above cases, it is apparent that careless positioning techniques could have easily resulted in the lesion being excluded from the image. The importance and focus of the skill of the mammographer in positioning the patient cannot be overstated.

- Bring the side shutters to the edge of the films if you are using dedicated mammography viewers, or, if you are using standard viewboxes, utilize masking to eliminate all unnecessary illuminator light. Ensure that ambient room light is at an appropriate low level. A bright light spot viewer should be available for examining areas of high density (skin and subcutaneous tissue). Illuminator characteristics are discussed in detail in Chapter 8.

- Using the magnifying glass (usually 2X magnification), begin examining the images in the axilla area and proceed downward, comparing symmetry. Normal lymph nodes vary in size and frequently contain a peripheral notch or a central umbilication. Their size is not a good indication of malignant change. Very large nodes may be infiltrated with fat; this is a normal finding. Diseased nodes will appear increased in density (regardless of their size), with an irregular shape or with spiculated margins; they may contain microcalcifications.
- The upper outer quadrant, adjacent to the pectoralis muscle shadow, is a particularly vulnerable area for breast disease; examine this area carefully for asymmetric tissue.
- Continue the inspection down to the inframammary area, to examine the extreme inferior breast tissue.
- Next, examine the nipples and retroareolar structures for symmetry; this is the second most common location of breast abnormalities.
- Finally, scan over the interior breast tissue, noting glandular contour and density, and watch for any disruptions in the tissue balance or pattern. Coopers ligaments are responsible for the characteristic concave, scalloped appearance of the glandular tissue on a mammogram. Straight lines and bulging convex borders should raise suspicion in the absence of trauma and surgery.
- Fatty replacement begins in the posterior tissue and proceeds forward, with the retroareolar area remaining dense and glandular until complete tissue atrophy has occurred. The medial component of the breast on the CC view is typically fatty replaced; glandular tissue remains in the axillary tail area, often extending to the edge of the film.
- The interface between the posterior fatty tissue and the anterior glandular components must be carefully examined; this is again a particularly vulnerable area for breast disease.
- Additional views may be required to characterize masses, areas of asymmetry, architectural distortion, or microcalcifications. Compression spot views are useful to spread out clusters of tissue and minimize superimposition. Magnified compression spot films are essential to evaluate microcalcifications and to delineate the borders of irregular masses.
- The nipple, skin, and subcutaneous structures may be evaluated with a bright light spot viewer.

The current examination should always be compared to previous studies, when they are available. It is best to begin the comparison with the earliest previous examination of comparable image quality. Subtle changes will not be apparent when comparing short interval examinations; a longer time frame

MAMMOGRAPHY IMAGE EVALUATION

_____ Date

_____ Signature

Patient Name: _____ ID #: _____ Technologist: _____

Image Content

☺ ☹

Position

_____ All tissue imaged	_____ Inframammary area	_____ Droop
_____ Axilla	_____ Retroareolar area	_____ Symmetry
_____ Posterior tissue	_____ Folds / wrinkles	_____

☺ ☹

Identification

_____ Present	_____ Legible
_____ Location	_____ Correct

Image Quality

☺ ☹

Compression

_____ Parenchyma separated	_____ Uniform density
_____ Tissue perpendicular - chest wall	_____ Motion

☺ ☹

Density

_____ Underexposed	_____ Parenchyma penetrated
_____ Overexposed	_____ Fatty tissue overexposed

☺ ☹

Contrast

_____ Poor	_____ Excessive

☺ ☹

Detail

_____ Structural Clarity	_____ Mottle excessive

☺ ☹

Artifacts

_____ Dust, lint	_____ Screen Contact
_____ Processing	_____ Handling
_____ Equipment	_____ Miscellaneous

Additonal Comments

Figure 5.8 A suggested format for mammography image evaluation.

between studies will often improve the perception of small or subtle tissue changes. Additional, more recent studies can also be utilized for comparison with an earlier study, if necessary after this initial overview.

The radiologist can complete a detailed technical critique of the examination; a suggested format is presented in Figure 5.8. This is very useful to establish consistent communication between the radiologist and the technologist, especially if they do not have the opportunity for direct communication, as is the case in many facilities. This practice will also provide valuable feedback for the ongoing improvement of mammography examinations.

E. CONCLUSION

The routine evaluation of clinical images for both content and quality should be an ongoing process that is incorporated into the routine protocol for every imaging facility. Only through a dedicated continuous focus on the quality of the examinations that are produced every day will the opportunity for improvement and growth become a reality. This process will naturally position these facilities on a completely different level of performance compared to the average site which chooses not to devote the time and energy to this important focus.

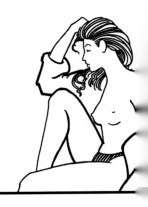

CHAPTER 6:
IMAGE QUALITY

CHAPTER 6:
IMAGE QUALITY

A. INTRODUCTION

Image quality is a global term that encompasses all the variables that can have an effect on the final radiographic image. A wide variety of factors contributes to the characteristics of the final image: mammography equipment features, adequate breast compression, film and screen characteristics, cassette design features, film handling techniques, radiographic exposure techniques, darkroom conditions, the processing environment, viewing conditions, as well as the patient's body habitus, cooperation for the examination, and the composition of her breast tissue, and, finally, the technologist's positioning skills. These factors challenge us daily. We are fortunate to be able to exercise direct control over many of these variables; the others we must simply strive to optimize. The final image represents the combination of choices and tradeoffs that we select between these components.

Mammography poses a unique imaging challenge. It commands high spatial resolution to identify microcalcifications, as well as high contrast resolution to identify masses surrounded by tissue of similar density.

Maintaining high image quality requires a skilled, knowledgable, dedicated technologist and a stringent quality control program.

A single quotable standard does not exist for image quality; it will vary with different breast types and with individual preferences. Frequently, mammography image quality is described by three distinct factors: radiographic contrast, radiographic blurring (or sharpness), and radiographic mottle (or noise).

FACTORS AFFECTING IMAGE QUALITY
RADIOGRAPHIC SHARPNESS

RADIOGRAPHIC CONTRAST	RADIOGRAPHIC BLURRING (Unsharpness)

Subject Contrast
 	
• Absorption Differences in Breast
    • Thickness
    • Density
    • Atomic Number
    • Breast Size
    • Contrast Material
 	
• Radiation Quality
    • Target Material
    • Kilovoltage
    • Filtration
 	
• Scatter Radiation
    • Kilovoltage
    • Beam Collimation
    • Compression
    • Grid
    • Air-Gap
 	
Receptor Contrast
 	
• Film Type
 	
• Processing
    • Chemistry
    • Temperature
    • Time
    • Agitation
 	
• Optical Density
 	
• Fog
    • Safelight
    • Light Leaks
    • Chemical
    • Storage
	Motion Blurring
	
	• Breast Immobilization (Compression)
	• Exposure Time
	• Patient Preparation
	
	Geometric Blurring
	
	• Focal Spot Size
	• Focal Spot - Object Distance
	• Object - Image Receptor Distance
	
	Receptor Blurring
	
	• Screen Factors
	    • Phosphor Thickness
	    • Phosphor Particle Size
	    • Light Absorbing Dyes and Pigments
	
	• Film Factors
	    • Crossover
	    • Halation
	    • Film - Screen Contact

Figure 6.1 Factors affecting radiographic sharpness

FACTORS AFFECTING IMAGE QUALITY
RADIOGRAPHIC NOISE

RADIOGRAPHIC MOTTLE	RADIOGRAPHIC ARTIFACTS
Receptor Graininess	**Handling**
• Films	• Crimp Marks
	• Fingerprints
Quantum Mottle	• Scratches
	• Static
• Film Speed	
• Film Contrast	**Fog**
• Screen Conversion	
Efficiency	• Exposure
• Screen Absorption	• Safelight
• Light Diffusion	
• Radiation Quality	**Equipment**
• Radiation Quantity	
	• Grid Lines
Structure Mottle	• Holder Assembly
	• Filtration
• Screens	• Collimation
	Processing
	• Streaks
	• Spots
	• Scratches
	Screen - Film
VIEWING CONDITIONS	• Dirt
	• Stains
	• Light Leaks
	• Screen Contact
• Bulb Wattage	**Patient**
• Viewbox Light Color	
• Viewbox Cleanliness	• Motion
• Ambient Lighting	• Foreign Objects
	• Body Parts

Figure 6.2 Factors affecting radiographic noise

Mammography image quality is described by three distinct factors: radiographic contrast, radiographic blurring (or sharpness), and radiographic mottle (or noise).

B. RADIOGRAPHIC CONTRAST

The detection of subtle architectural structures is highly dependent on radiographic contrast. Detail only becomes visible through differences in optical density, or, in other words, through contrast. Radiographic contrast represents the combined effect of subject contrast and receptor contrast.

1. Subject Contrast

Subject contrast can be described as the varying x-ray pattern that exits the breast (given a uniform x-ray exposure) due to the differential absorption and scattering that occurs as radiation traverses the breast tissue. The individual factors that contribute to subject contrast are breast thickness, density (mass per unit volume), tissue atomic number, and, to some degree, breast size. Subject contrast is the one factor that we cannot control or alter to suit our imaging needs. Breast compression, once again, plays a major part in reducing tissue thickness and separating structures to facilitate differential absorption. Although kVp is the most critical exposure factor affecting contrast, the quality of the x-ray beam is also affected by other inherent tube features. The kVp should be kept relatively low, consistent with adequate breast penetration. Finally, the very nature of the interaction between radiation and tissue requires attention to measures that will control scatter. The two major factors that affect the amount of scatter generated during an exposure are kVp selection (just enough to penetrate the tissue) and breast compression (to reduce tissue thickness). Secondary control is then accomplished with grids and the air gap technique; these measures serve to *clean up* the scatter that has been generated during the x-ray exposure.

Mammography poses a unique imaging challenge. It commands high spatial resolution to identify microcalcifications, as well as high contrast resolution to identify masses surrounded by tissue of similar density.

2. Receptor Contrast

Receptor contrast determines how the varying x-ray pattern exiting the breast will be recorded as varying optical densities on the film. It is highly dependent on the inherent characteristics of the film and screen products that the site has selected. The best indicator of receptor contrast is average gradient. A host of film products are available for mammography applications; each requires individual characteristic processing conditions which, in turn, will determine the optical density, average gradient, and D-max achievable for that specific product. The critical role of processing parameters has been described in Chapter 2.

3. Optical Density

Concurrent with the considerations of subject and receptor contrast is another factor: the exposure level or radiographic optical density of the mammography image. For optimal breast imaging, an appropriate optical film density must be selected that will maximize the imaging capabilities of the screen-film combination. This, in turn, will ensure that subtle density differences between the glandular tissue components will be visually appeciated.

The contrast of the screen-film system will be optimized with a high quality x-ray beam, taut breast compression, a grid receptor, and a properly exposed and optimally developed high-contrast film. Refer to the troubleshooting guides in Chapter 10 for helpful solutions to image contrast problems.

C. RADIOGRAPHIC BLURRING

Ironically, radiographic sharpness is frequently described in terms of its opposite entity — radiographic blurring. The degree of sharpness that an image displays is closely related to the radiographic resolution of the image. Resolution can be defined as the ability to identify two closely spaced objects as being separate. Should any factor degrade our ability to perceive distinct margins between structures, these separations will quickly become fuzzy and blurred,

 The two major factors that affect the amount of scatter generated during an exposure are kVp selection (just enough to penetrate the tissue) and breast compression (to reduce tissue thickness).

Ironically, radiographic sharpness is frequently described in terms of its opposite entity — radiographic blurring.

and our perception of fine detail will diminish rapidly. Considering the low inherent contrast of breast tissue and pathology, maximizing resolution (sharpness) and minimizing blurring (unsharpness) becomes a critical focus; mammographers must be able to identify structures that are as small as 0.1 to 0.2 mm in size.

Resolution is frequently described in terms of modulation transfer function (MTF). Modulation transfer function is defined as the ratio of output information to input information (in other words, how much information is lost in the process of recording an image); it is expressed as a function of spatial frequency (line pairs per millimeter). Each component in the imaging system can be assigned an individual MTF value; their combined values will indicate the limit of the spatial resolution for the system. Metal bar test objects with various arrangements of lead strips provide a simple method of evaluating spatial resolution. Typical values for mammographic screen-film combinations are 15-21 line pairs per mm (lp / mm).

Radiographic blurring (unsharpness) can be categorized into motion blurring, geometric blurring, and receptor blurring.

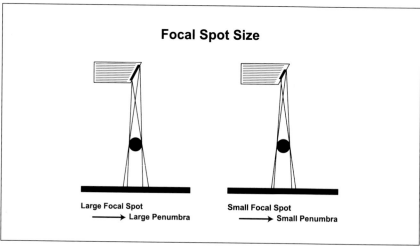

Figure 6.3 The effect of focal spot size

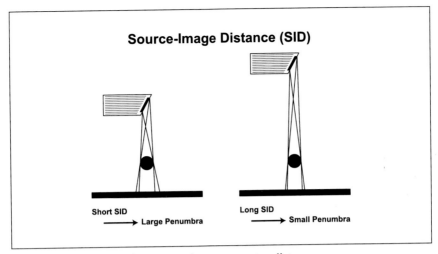

Source-Image Distance (SID)

Short SID
→ Large Penumbra

Long SID
→ Small Penumbra

Figure 6.4 The effect of source-to-image receptor distance

1. Motion Blurring

Motion blur can frequently be resolved with careful patient preparation and with taut breast compression. Should this not be effective, the effects of motion can be minimized with a shorter exposure time or with a faster screen-film combination.

2. Geometric Blurring

Geometric unsharpness is equipment related; it is determined by three factors: focal spot size, focal spot-object distance, and object-receptor distance. These factors are determined by the basic design of the mammographic equipment. The critical impact of these factors emphasizes the tremendous importance of equipment selection for mammography.

The size of the focal spot will control the effect of penumbra. Penumbra can be defined as the blurred margin that is imaged at the edge of an object. The smaller the focal spot size, the more that penumbra will be minimized and the clearer our images will be.

Modulation transfer function (MTF) is defined as the ratio of output information to input information (in other words, how much information is lost in the process of recording an image).

Chapter 6

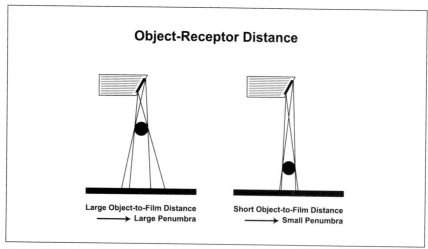

Figure 6.5 The effect of object-receptor distance

The last two factors are collectively encompassed by the focal-film distance (FFD) or the source-to-image receptor distance (SID) of our mammographic equipment. A longer SID will minimize penumbra; however, an excessively long SID should be avoided because of the accompanying need for higher mA values, which will result in increased tube loading. The one factor that we can control to some degree is the object-receptor distance. Again, taut compression is extremely important and the position of the receptor relative to the area of interest (lesion) is a distinct consideration for specialized views with diagnostic work-up examinations.

3. Receptor Blurring

The receptor factors noted in the image quality charts at the beginning of this chapter are basically controlled by the characteristic features of the screen-film system that has been selected. With this in place, our participation is limited to ensuring that adequate screen-film contact is maintained on a regular basis.

 Radiographic mottle can be defined as random undesirable variations in optical density on a radiograph that has received a uniform x-ray exposure.

Quantum mottle is the major contributing factor to the appearance of radiographic mottle. It is related to the random distribution of x-ray quanta in the x-ray beam.

D. RADIOGRAPHIC MOTTLE

Radiographic mottle can be defined as random undesirable variations in optical density on a radiograph that has received a uniform x-ray exposure. The following factors contribute to radiographic mottle.

1. Receptor Graininess

Film granularity, which becomes increasingly pronounced with the larger grain size that accompanies high-speed film, contributes significantly to radiographic mottle.

2. Quantum Mottle

Quantum mottle is the major contributing factor to the appearance of radiographic mottle. It is related to the random distribution of x-ray quanta in the x-ray beam.

High speed imaging systems (requiring less radiation exposure due to faster screen and film speeds) generate images with increased noise, which translates to reduced sharpness or resolution. Noise limits our ability to detect and to characterize small structures on a radiographic image.

To describe the concept of quantum mottle, an analogy can be drawn between the appearance of quantum mottle on an x-ray film and rain falling on a sidewalk. Droplets of rain (x-ray 'bundles' or quanta) begin to fall on the sidewalk. With a light shower (small x-ray exposure), we will see a very 'speckled' appearance on the sidewalk (grainy, mottled image). A heavier shower (increased exposure) will 'fill in' many of the dry areas on the sidewalk and the individual raindrops will begin to blend together (smooth out the speckles on the x-ray). As more rain falls (increased exposure), the additional raindrops (x-ray quanta) fill in the dry areas on the sidewalk (more information on the film) and it begins to take on a uniform, wet appearance (x-ray film is 'filled' with information; there are no 'empty holes' in the image, as there were earlier). Fast imaging systems that require small x-ray exposures (light rainfalls) will produce mottled, grainy (speckled) images. The more exposure (mAs) the x-ray receives (heavier rainfall) the more information will be captured by the film and the smoother and more uniform the image will appear.

3. Structure Mottle

Screen structure mottle arises from non-uniformity of the phosphor layer of the intensifying screen; this is a minor consideration with radiographic mottle.

4. Film Artifacts

The concept of radiographic noise also incorporates the artifacts that appear on our images. Artifacts can be defined as unwanted densities that are visible on the image. Artifacts can be related to equipment features, patient factors, positioning, film handling, and darkroom difficulties. They degrade image quality and, even more critically, they can mimic microcalcificatiions on the examination.

To appreciate the image clarity that exists on our films, the images must be viewed under optimal conditions that would include dedicated, high intensity mammography illuminators, adequate masking features, and the appropriate low level of ambient light in the viewing room.

E. CONCLUSION

The visualization of fine detail on mammographic images is a complex process that incorporates a number of factors. Contrast, sharpness, and noise are major factors; however, viewing conditions make significant contributions as well. Coupled with all these factors is the subjective evaluation of the individual observer who is operating on the basis of his or her personal perception and criteria of the image evaluation process.

Today, we have a wide variety of choices in x-ray equipment, image receptors, and processing conditions. The selection of our unique imaging *package* will be directed by our individual perception of the ideal compromise between image quality and patient dose. This selection will then dictate the limits of the achievable contrast and sharpness resolution that we can expect on our images. Our goal should be to optimize all the factors that affect image quality, consistent with our prescribed expectations for image quality and patient dose.

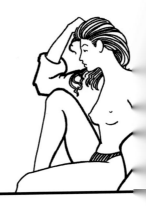

CHAPTER 7:
ARTIFACTS

CHAPTER 7: ARTIFACTS

A. INTRODUCTION

Artifacts are defined as unwanted defects or irregularities on processed films. Mammography film demonstrates increased susceptibility to artifacts of many types for two reasons. First, the film is coated on one side only; we are unable to take advantage of the masking effects that would be furnished by a second emulsion layer. Second, the emulsion layer is by nature somewhat thicker than that of double emulsion films. This thick emulsion becomes very soft during film processing, thereby increasing the likelihood of processor related artifacts.

Determining the source of a particular artifact is necessary before the problem can be corrected. The fact that many artifacts are intermittent or, worse, very random, only complicates and delays the problem solving process. Artifacts are particularly worrisome because they have the ability to both mask and mimic breast disease. In fact, this author often cites a *Murphy's Law* pertaining to artifacts: they occur on the most difficult patients, or they occur in the primary area of interest. A fine-tuned quality control program is essential to minimize their occurrence.

Artifacts are defined as unwanted defects or irregularities on processed films.

Mammography film demonstrates increased susceptibility to artifacts of many types for two reasons. First, the film is coated on one side only; we are unable to take advantage of the masking effects that would be furnished by a second emulsion layer. Second, the emulsion layer is by nature somewhat thicker than that of double emulsion films.

B. SOURCES OF ARTIFACTS

1. Processing Environment

The processor is the source of many film artifacts. The mechanical components must be maintained on a regular basis to keep the processor in optimum working condition. Unfortunately, thorough processor service is sometimes performed only after problems surface. In many ways, processors are like automobiles. When routine maintenance is done and parts are replaced as they show signs of wear, the processor will perform as expected, with optimum results for a long time. When good preventative maintenance is not carried out on a regular basis, the processor will perform in a less than optimal manner and it may have a shorter life span.

The chemicals used for processing are equally important to the production of quality films. Again, the processor service provider is key to consistency. The chemicals must be properly mixed, properly replenished and stored, and maintained with an acceptable degree of freshness. Exhausted chemicals may cause a number of problems, including artifacts and poorly processed films.

Proper film washing and drying is also critical. Of particular importance in mammography is fixer retention. Mammography films must be kept for longer periods of time than other radiographic examinations, and the thicker single emulsion tends to retain fixer more readily. For these reasons, an appropriate

The fact that many artifacts are intermittent or, worse, very random, only complicates and delays the problem solving process.

balance of processor service and budgetary considerations must be maintained. If the processor is serviced less frequently in order to save money, the facility will soon find that the economy is short-lived as films are repeated and quality diminishes.

There are excellent comprehensive books and publications that focus exclusively on processing (see appendix), so our intention here is to cover common issues that occur with mammography so that the technologist can use this chapter as a checklist to eliminate artifacts when they occur.

For specific descriptions and examples, see *Processor Related Artifacts*.

 Of particular importance in mammography is fixer retention. Mammography films must be kept for longer periods of time than other radiographic examinations, and the thicker single emulsion tends to retain fixer more readily.

2. Darkroom Environment

One of the most frequently overlooked sources of airborne artifacts such as dust, dirt, and lint is the darkroom. It is often helpful to use an ultraviolet (black) light to identify sources of dust; this light should be used with appropriate safety precautions to protect the eyes, face, and skin. While not all dust or dirt particles are demonstrated by ultraviolet light, the great majority will be visualized with this tool. Remember to use the black light again following corrective measures to verify their effectiveness and to confirm that improved working conditions have been restored.

Other areas of concern in the darkroom include:

- *Humidity.* Relative humidity should be maintained between 30 and 50 percent.
- *Cassette storage.* Mammography cassettes should not be stored or placed on the floor. Passboxes may have dirt or other particles that can be deposited in cassettes during film loading.
- *Air quality.* Incoming air should be properly filtered to eliminate airborne particles. Be sure to replace air filters regularly.
- *Ventilation.* Proper ventilation is important for air quality. Make certain that air vents are cleaned frequently.

- *Storage.* Wherever possible, storage of items in the darkroom should be avoided, especially on open shelving. Cabinets help contain any airborne particles. Personal items such as sweaters, purses, and packages contribute to the circulation of dust. Clutter should be kept to a minimum.
- *Cleanliness.* The need for darkroom cleanliness cannot be overstated. The darkroom must be cleaned daily, prior to processing images.
- *Darkroom design.* Older or poorly designed darkrooms may have inherent features that contribute to airborne particles, such as suspended ceilings, which are known to be sources of dust and dirt. Chronic dust problems should be investigated.
- *Safelights.* Make certain that safelight filters are correct for the type of film used. Older filters can become cracked and faulty over time. Bulb wattage must be appropriate; if the wattage is too high, safelight fog may result. There must also be enough distance between the safelight and any surface such as the processor feed tray and countertops where exposed film may lie, waiting to be processed.

For specific examples and descriptions, see *Darkroom Related Artifacts*.

 It is often helpful to use an ultraviolet (black) light to identify sources of dust.

3. Film Handling

Film handling accounts for many artifacts seen on mammography film. Fortunately, film handling artifacts can easily be eliminated by careful attention to the manner in which the films are loaded into the cassettes and then processed. The most common types of handling artifacts are crimp marks due to bending the film, fingerprints, scratches, and static due to improper clothing or lack of humidity in the darkroom. Handling artifacts that are minus density (white) result from improper film handling prior to exposure. Handling artifacts that have plus density (black) result from improper film handling after exposure. The exception to this rule pertains to tabular-grain or cubic-grain films, which may have plus density artifacts prior to or after exposure.

For specific descriptions and examples, see *Handling Related Artifacts*.

Film handling artifacts can easily be eliminated by careful attention to the manner in which the films are loaded into the cassettes and then processed.

4. Image Receptor

The image receptors used for screen-film mammography are very sensitive and are easily damaged. Intensifying screens must be cleaned regularly and properly to prevent dust and other foreign materials from being imaged on the film. As mentioned previously, the darkroom environment is critical. Cleaning screens with frequency will not be effective if the darkroom is not properly designed and maintained. The screen manufacturer must approve any cleaning solutions that are used for intensifying screens. The use of other solutions and devices may void the manufacturer's warranty. Also, the phosphor layer of the intensifying screen has a protective layer that must be protected. Excessive force during cleaning can wear the surface and make the screen susceptible to stains and rapid aging, which will result in a reduction in screen speed and image quality. See the additional comments on image receptors (screen-film contact, screen identification, etc.) in Chapter 3, Quality Control.

For specific descriptions and examples, see *Image Receptor Related Artifacts*.

5. Film Fog

Fog from any source results in undesirable film density. This in turn results in a decrease in film contrast and an increase in film density. The darkroom integrity should be routinely verified by performing a darkroom fog test with the mammography phantom (see *Imaging the Mammography Phantom* and *Darkroom Fog Test* in separate chapters); this will help to prevent film fog. Film storage conditions are also important; temperature and humidity must be controlled and maintained within acceptable limits (see *Darkroom Environment*). In addition, care should be taken to avoid unintentional exposure by

Intensifying screens must be cleaned regularly and properly to prevent dust and other foreign materials from being imaged on the film.

Fog from any source results in undesirable film density. This in turn results in a decrease in film contrast and an increase in film density.

opening the film bin in white light, improperly loading the film into the cassette, or leaving cassettes where they can be exposed to scatter radiation. Over-development fog or chemical fog due to overactive chemicals should also be avoided.

For specific descriptions and examples, see *Fog Related Artifacts.*

6. Equipment

The mammography unit can also be the source of artifacts. Failure of the grid to move appropriately and grid flaws or defects may create an objectionable appearance on the image. Faulty grid function can cause this problem. The use of higher kVp may result in an exposure time that is too short to accomplish correct grid motion, while exposure times that are too long can result in exposures continuing after grid motion has stopped. For this reason, it is important to know the limitations of each mammography unit with regard to exposure times. The carbon fiber surface on the bucky can deteriorate and result in unwanted artifacts. The compression device, film holder, collimators, and tube filtration may also contribute to film defects. Routine equipment maintenance will minimize potential problems.

In addition, it is recommended that a phantom image be used for *acceptance testing* of any new device or equipment that will be used for patient imaging. Detailed information regarding imaging of the phantom is provided in Chapter 3, Quality Control. Unsuspected items such as the paint used to mark AEC positions on the compression paddle can sometimes result in shadows or artifacts. These unwanted densities are often more readily seen on the phantom image than on clinical images. Most equipment related artifacts can be reproduced in the same location using a number of different cassettes.

For specific descriptions and examples, see *Equipment Related Artifacts.*

7. Patient

The patient also serves as a potential source for artifacts that are frequently noted on clinical images. If the patient is wearing deodorant or other body powders, creams, or oils, these substances may be imaged on the clinical films. Large earrings, necklaces, and other similar articles are often removed prior to beginning the examination to avoid their accidental inclusion on the clinical images. Hair is often imaged over the medial half of the CC view, particularly when it has been sprayed or coated with hair products. Also, chins, ears, glasses, etc. are frequently imaged if the patient turns her head toward the breast being imaged before the exposure has been made. Finally, other body parts may be imaged if the patient inadvertently moves prior to the x-ray exposure.

For specific descriptions and examples, see *Patient Related Artifacts*.

C. ARTIFACT ANALYSIS

Identifying the probable source of an artifact is the first important step towards solving the problem. Isolating the processor as the probable source is relatively easy, and should be done first.

Using the phantom or an acrylic sheet, make two exposures. Run one film through the processor lengthwise, and one through the processor crosswise.

If the artifact is equipment related, the artifact will run across the long axis or the short axis of both films. If the artifact is processor related, the artifact changes direction according to the way it was processed, i.e., the artifact will be either perpendicular to the direction of film feed, or it will be parallel to the direction of film feed, on both films.

Thus, when the films are hung on the viewbox side by side, the artifacts run in opposite directions if the processor was the culprit. Attention can then be focused on the processor, and the charts below can be used to determine the specific source within the processor. In addition, it helps to then focus on

Identifying the probable source of an artifact is the first important step towards solving the problem.

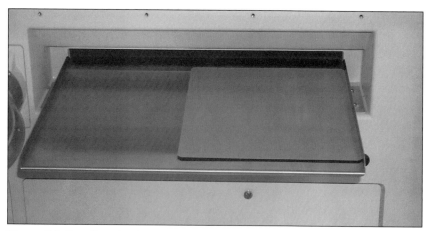

Figure 7.1 One film should be run through the processor lengthwise.

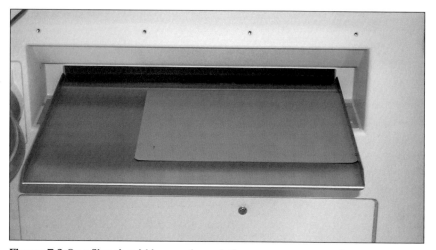

Figure 7.2 One film should be run through the processor crosswise.

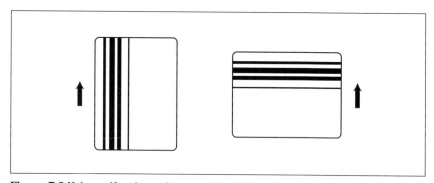

Figure 7.3 If the artifact is equipment related, its orientation will remain the same, no matter which direction the film has been processed. Its appearance will be similar on two films that have been fed into the processor in different directions.

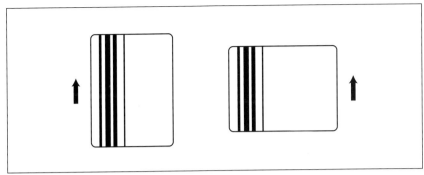

Figure 7.4 If the artifact is processor related, its orientation will change according to the direction of feed into the film processor. Its appearance will be different on two films that have been fed into the processor in different directions.

several additional questions. Is the artifact demonstrated in both transmitted and reflected light? If this is so, the source can be anywhere in the processor. Does the artifact demonstrate equally well when the film is fed emulsion side up and emulsion side down?

Artifacts that are demonstrated on emulsion side up processed films may be caused by the inside rollers of the racks and/or by the crossover rollers. Artifacts that are demonstrated on emulsion side down processed films may be caused by the outside rollers of the racks and/or by the turnaround rollers.

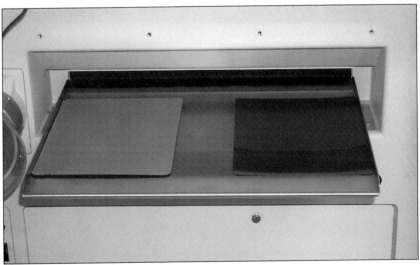

Figure 7.5 Determine if the artifact changes in appearance depending on whether the film is oriented emulsion up (left side) or down (right side) in the film processor.

It is also important to identify the leading edge of the film. Once films have dropped into the film bin it may be difficult to remember or identify which edge is which. Making a small pencil mark to identify the top right-hand corner of the film before you feed it into the processor will eliminate this confusion.

Of course, once the leading edge of the film is identified, the trailing edge is easily recognized. This also identifies the top surface of the film versus the bottom surface, and which side of the processor feed tray was used. Additional identification, such as emulsion side up or down, can also be done with a pencil prior to processing (Figure 7.7).

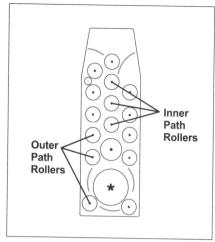

Figure 7.6 Artifacts that are demonstrated when the emulsion is oriented up may be caused by the inside rollers of the main racks or by the crossover rollers. Artifacts that are demonstrated when the emulsion is oriented down may be caused by the outside rollers of the main racks or by the turnaround assembly rollers.

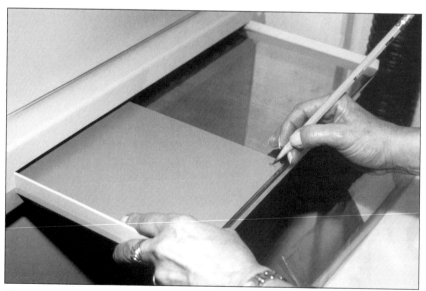

Figure 7.7 Identify the direction of film travel before you feed the film into the processor.

1. Processor Related Artifacts

Artifacts may be either plus density (dark) or minus density (white). Processor artifacts may occur parallel to the direction of film travel, perpendicular to the direction of film travel, or randomly. Once you have determined density and direction, the following descriptions can be visually compared.

Previous editions of this book may have included other artifacts that are no longer current, or have been renamed. The following classifications are the most current as of this publication.

Guide Shoe Marks: ▬▬▬▬▬▬▬▬▬▬▬▬▬▬▬▬▬▬▬▬▬▬▬▬▬▬

Direction: Parallel to film travel.   *Density:* May be either plus or minus.
Description: Guide shoe marks are small, evenly spaced marks that most often occur on the leading edge or trailing edge of the film, but may occur anywhere.

Causes:
- Plus density marks are made by guide shoes in the developer tank.
- Minus density marks with no surface damage are made by guide shoes in the fixer tank or fix-to-wash crossover. Marks that show surface damage can occur anywhere in the processor.
- Marks on the top surface of the film originate in the crossover assemblies. Marks on the bottom surface of the film originate in the turnaround assemblies.
- Chemical deposits on guide shoes can result in guide shoe marks.

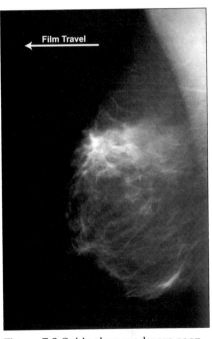

Figure 7.8 Guide shoe marks are seen along the chest wall edge of this image.

Solutions:
- Examine guide shoes and replace any that are bent or damaged.
- Remove dried chemicals from guide shoes.
- Make certain crossover assemblies and racks are positioned squarely in the processor and that they are always handled carefully.
- Mammography film should be processed lengthwise. The image should not be on the leading edge of the film.

Delay Streaks:

Direction: Parallel to film travel.   *Density:* Plus.

Description: Delay streaks are ill-defined randomly spaced narrow bands of varying widths. They occur on the first film processed after the processor has been on standby or inactive for a time.

Causes:
- Oxidized developer buildup on the developer to fix crossover assembly or on the re-wet roller.
- Poor ventilation of the processor.
- Low level of developer in tank.
- Re-wet roller not functioning properly.
- Evaporation covers on tanks not installed.

Solutions:
- Process clearing film if the processor has been on standby for over 30 minutes.
- Ensure proper processor ventilation.
- Keep rollers clean.
- Maintain proper level of developer.
- Install evaporation covers.

Entrance Roller Marks:

Direction: Parallel to film travel.

Density: Plus.

Description: Entrance roller marks are plus-density bands about 1/8 inch wide.

Causes:
- Moisture on entrance rollers.
- Pressure on film by entrance rollers.
- Trailing edge of film exposed to light.

Solutions:
- Dry entrance rollers thoroughly after cleaning. Avoid immersing during cleaning.
- Wait for rollers to be completely dry before processing films.
- Follow manufacturer's directions for maintaining entrance rollers. Make sure the assembly is properly seated in the processor.

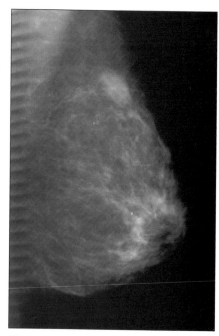

Figure 7.9 Entrance roller marks: the darkroom door was opened while the trail edge of this film was still in the entrance roller assembly.

- Wait until film is fed completely into the processor before opening darkroom door or turning on light.

Chatter:

Direction: Perpendicular to film travel.   *Density:* Plus

Description: Chatter appears as random bands of varying widths and density that occur at a consistent distance from each other. Spacing corresponds to the spacing of the sprocket or gear teeth in the developer rack.

Causes:
- Developer rack drive chain or gears too loose or too tight.
- Crossover assembly drive mechanism too loose or too tight.

Solutions:
- Adjust developer rack drive chain or gears according to manufacturer's recommendations.

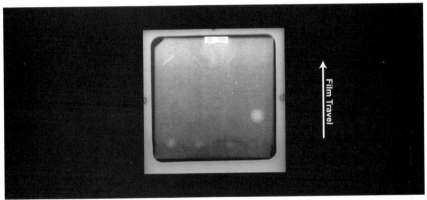

Figure 7.10 Curtain runback is noted along the chest wall edge of this phantom image.

Runback (Curtain Runback):

Direction: Perpendicular to film travel.   *Density:* Plus.

Description: Runback occurs on the trailing edge of the film and has a wavy appearance.

Causes:
- Squeegee at the exit of the developer rack is inadequate; excess developer will *run back* over the trailing edge of the film as it turns in the crossover assembly to enter the fix tank.

Solutions:
- Adjust or replace worn or damaged parts and rollers.

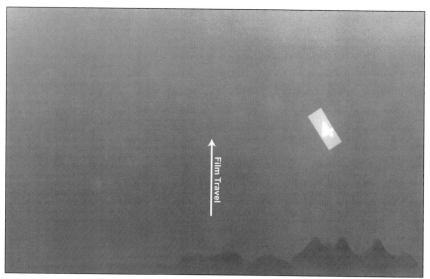

Figure 7.11 Curtain runback

Slap Lines:
Direction: Perpendicular to film travel.   *Density:* Plus.
Description: Slap lines occur as a broad band located anywhere from about 3/4 inch to 2 1/4 inches from the trailing edge of the film. The band has ill-defined edges and may be up to 1/4 inch wide.

Causes:
- Trailing edge of the film releases suddenly from the developer-to-fix crossover and slaps the top center roller of the fix roller.

Solutions:
- Ensure proper fixer replenishment rates and mix.
- Check developer exit squeegee for proper operation and uniformity.

Hesitation (Stub) Lines:
Direction: Perpendicular to film travel.   *Density:* Plus.
Description: Hesitation lines are ill-defined irregularly spaced lines that may appear on either side of the film. They may be more apparent on one side of the processor. The marks are caused by inconsistent film transport.

Causes:
- Non-uniform film speed.
- Worn chains or bearings.
- Drive chain adjusted too loose or too tight.
- Guide shoes positioned incorrectly.
- Worn or dirty rollers.

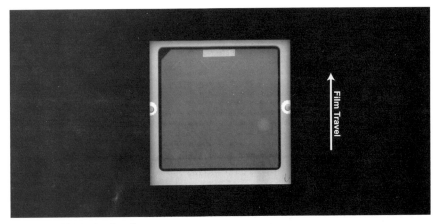

Figure 7.12 Hesitation lines

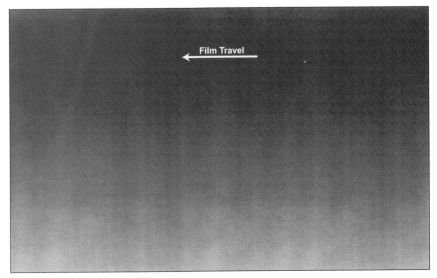

Figure 7.13 Hesitation lines

Solutions:
- Repair or replace worn rollers.
- Adjust rack chains.
- Check chemicals and replenishment.
- Clean processor.

Surface Drying Streaks and Water Spots:
Direction: Parallel to film travel.   *Density:* Plus.
Description: Narrow, wavering bands with a mottled, washed-out appearance that are randomly spaced. Seen best in reflected light.

Causes:

- Under-replenished fixer, or oxidized developer, dirty dryer or squeegee rollers, improperly seated air tubes, or excessively high dryer air temperature.

Solutions:

- Check and adjust fixer replenishment if necessary.
- Replace exhausted developer chemicals.
- Check air tubes for alignment.
- Lower dryer temperature.

Pick Off:

Direction: Random.   *Density:* Minus.

Description: Perhaps the most common processor related artifact on mammography film. Pick off occurs when the emulsion of the film is *picked off* of the film's base. The small, irregularly shaped areas appear as very bright minus-density spots in transmitted light. The edges of these areas are sharply defined. A magnifying glass should be used to differentiate pick off from shadow images caused by dust or other obstructions.

Causes:

- Dirty or worn (scratched) roller surfaces.
- Inconsistent film transport speed.
- Exhausted or improperly mixed chemicals.

Solutions:

- Ensure proper processor cleanliness and maintenance.

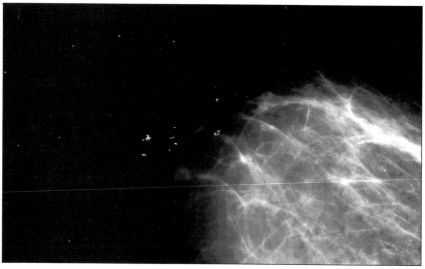

Figure 7.14 Random pick off

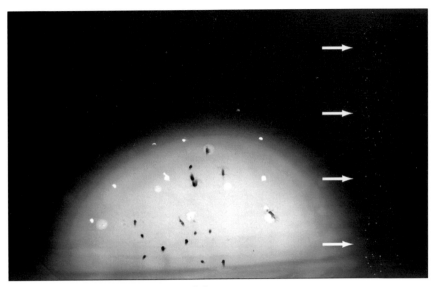

Figure 7.15 Pick off due to a roller defect

- Check film transport for uniform speed.
- Make certain replenishment rates and chemical mixing is consistent with manufacturer's recommendations.
- Be sure that shadow images resulting from dust or dirt are not mistaken for pick off. The appearance is very similar!

Wet Pressure:

Direction: Random.   *Density:* Plus.
Description: Wet pressure appears as tiny plus density areas that are often mistaken for noise or quantum mottle.

Causes:
- Excessive roller pressure applied to the film emulsion in the developer or developer-to-fix crossover assembly.
- Rough, warped or dirty rollers.

 Pick off occurs when the emulsion of the film is <u>picked off</u> of the film's base. The small, irregularly shaped areas appear as very bright minus density spots in transmitted light. The edges of these areas are sharply defined.

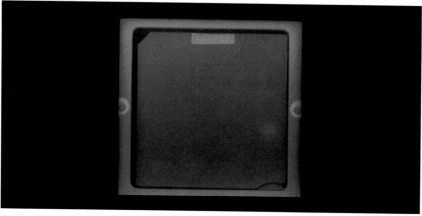

Figure 7.16 Wet pressure marks originating from the rollers in the developer tank.

- Exhausted or contaminated chemicals.
- Excessively high developer temperature.

Solutions:
- Replace chemicals if necessary.
- Check replenishment rates and developer replenishment line.
- Clean, repair, or replace rollers if worn or damaged.

Brown Films:

Description: Random, all-over discolored appearance. Odor may also be present.

Fixer retention affects film archival (keeping) quality. Mammogram record retention requires optimum archival quality, making this issue critical.

Causes:
- Incomplete, improper washing of film resulting in retained fixer in the emulsion.
- Poor quality or improperly mixed fixer.
- Improper fixer replenishment.

Solutions:
- Check fixer replenishment and mixing. Correct if necessary.
- Make certain that water and fixer temperatures are correct according to manufacturer's guidelines.
- Check water flow and wash tank levels.
- Make certain water is turned on.
- Check water filter for clogging.

Dye Stain:
Description: Lavender or pink coloration in clear areas of the film. Color varies with film type.
Causes:
- Incomplete removal of dye.
- Inadequate fixing and washing (see *Brown Films,* above).
- Transport speed through fixer too rapid.

Solutions: (see *Brown Films* above)
- Replace used chemicals with fresh chemicals.
- Make certain processing cycle is as recommended by film manufacturer.
- If fixer is recycled, check method used.

Bent Corners:
Description: Corner of film is damaged or bent.
Cause:
- Excessive recirculation of chemical solutions alters the path of the film, resulting in a bent corner.

Solution:
- Lower circulation rate of solutions.

Flame Patterns:
Description: Variations in film density, which resemble the flame of a candle. Best visualized in transmitted light.
Cause:
- Improperly seasoned chemicals.

Solution:
- Change chemicals less often as long as processor QC remains stable.

Skivings:
Description: Thin, plus density threads of emulsion that have been redeposited on the surface of the film.
Cause:
- Uneven film transport resulting in roller lifting threads of emulsion from film.

Solution:
- Perform processor maintenance as needed. Be sure to use chemicals recommended by manufacturer, and use cleanup film periodically to remove dirt and film emulsion from rollers.

NOTE: It is important that qualified personnel perform the remedial action for all processor-related artifacts. This may require involving the processor service organization or the film representative.

2. Darkroom Related Artifacts

Shadow Images: ━━━━━━━━

Description: Small minus density areas on the film surface.

Causes:

- Dust or dirt on the intensifying screen resulting in an area of non-exposure on the film. This is generally due to poor housekeeping in the darkroom or dust in the ventilation system. Screen cleanliness may also be a factor.

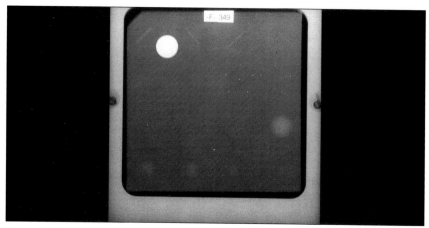

Figure 7.17 Shadow images are seen on the phantom image.

Water Marks: ━━━━━━━━

Description: Plus density wavy marks on the film surface, visible in reflected light.

Causes:

- Unprocessed film coming into contact with a wet surface. Water or liquid on the processor feed tray or film loading surface wets the emulsion, resulting in an artifact.

Static: ━━━━━━━━

Description: Plus density artifacts that may resemble smudge marks or lightning (sometimes referred to as *Christmas tree* static).

Causes:

- Low humidity. Static occurs when the air in the environment is too dry.

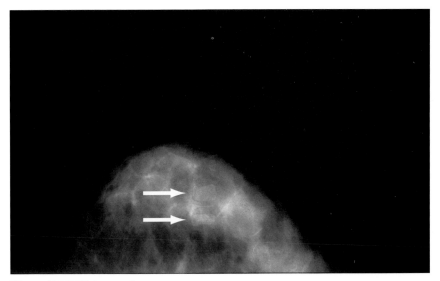

Figure 7.18 Water marks

 Static is a plus density artifact that can take on a variety of forms; it is generally due to low humidity conditions.

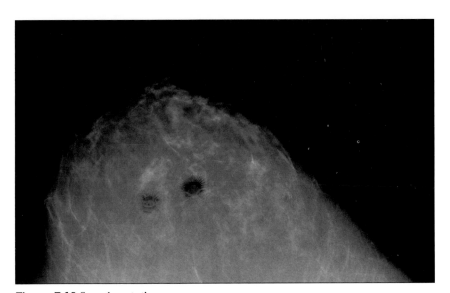

Figure 7.19 Smudge static

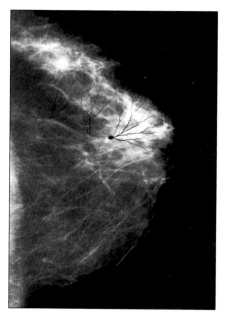

Figure 7.20 Lightning or Christmas tree static

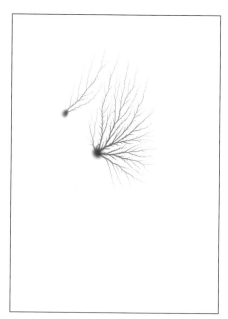

Figure 7.21 Although lightning static can be quite artistic in appearance, its effects on clinical images is very detrimental.

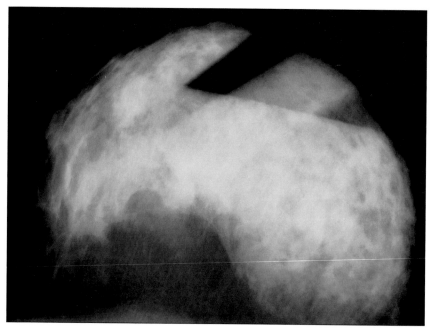

Figure 7.22 Darkroom fog

Fog: ▬▬▬▬▬▬▬▬▬▬▬▬▬▬▬▬▬▬▬▬▬▬▬▬▬▬▬▬▬▬▬▬

Description: Overall loss of contrast accompanied by an increase in image density.

Causes:
- Light leaks, damaged or aged safelight filters, improper safelight bulb wattage, safelights located too close to film loading surfaces or feed tray.

3. Film Handling Related Artifacts

Crescent Marks (Kink or Crimp Marks): ▬▬▬▬▬▬▬▬▬▬▬▬▬▬

Description: Plus or minus density marks with a curved appearance.

Causes:
- Pressure during film handling such as bending, folding, or creasing may result in a curved artifact. Minus density marks occurred prior to exposure; plus density marks occurred after exposure.

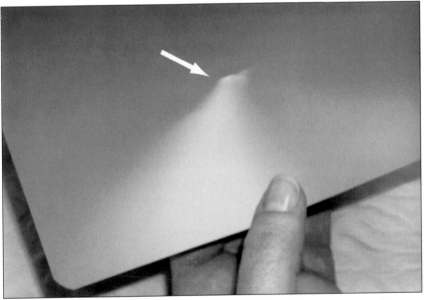

Figure 7.23 Crimping the film in this manner will result in a crescent mark on the image.

Fingerprints and Smudge Marks: ▬▬▬▬▬▬

Description: Plus or minus density image of partial or complete fingerprint.

Causes:

- Failure to handle film by the edges. Lotions and oils on the hands will increase the incidence of fingerprints on images. Minus density fingerprints occurred during film loading or handling prior to exposure. Partial minus density fingerprints may mimic calcifications and hinder film evaluation. Plus density fingerprints occurred after exposure.

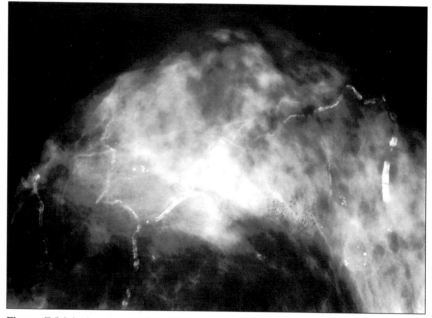

Figure 7.24 A plus density (black) fingerprint.

 The appearance of fingerprints can be controlled by handling the film by the edges. Minus density fingerprints occur prior to exposure; plus density fingerprints occur after film exposure.

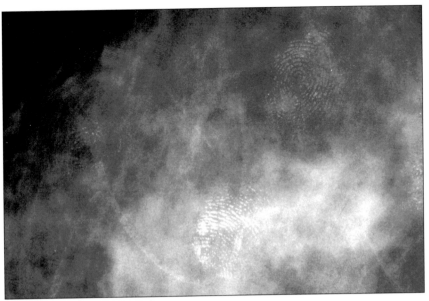
Figure 7.25 Several minus density (white) fingerprints.

Film Creases or Folds:
Description: A clearly defined line indicating a fold or crease. May be physically evident on processed film.

Causes:
- Closing cassette with film folded within the cassette or with a corner of the film sticking out of the cassette. May also result from catching film in film bin door as it is closed, resulting in damage to the emulsion. These films should be discarded rather than used for imaging.

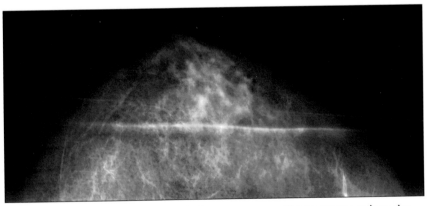
Figure 7.26 A film fold that occurs before exposure will appear as a minus density artifact.

Scratches: ■■■■■■■■■■■■■■■

Description: Minus density abrasion on the film surface.

Causes:

- Fingernails or other abrasions. Dirt may also scratch the film surface. Care must be taken not to *dig* at the film or intensifying screen when loading and unloading films into cassettes.

Pressure Marks: ■■■■■■■■■■■

Description: Plus or minus density marks on the film. May occur on single films or an entire box. If entire box is affected, the pressure marks will be repeated on multiple films and gradually decrease in appearance as you progress further into the box of film.

Causes:

- Dropping or striking a box of film. Excessive pressure on film emulsion. Marks will be minus density if film was unexposed, and plus density if film was exposed prior to damage.

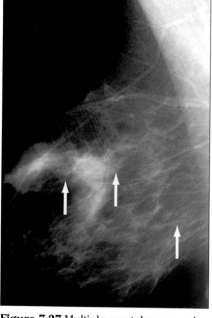

Figure 7.27 Multiple scratches are evident on this film.

4. Receptor Related Artifacts

White Specks: ■■■■■■■■■■■■■■■■■■■■■

Description: Multiple random minus density spots that occur consistently with the same cassette (Figure 7.17).

Causes:

- Poor cleaning habits or excessive abrasion of screen surface may result in permanent damage. Improper cleaning solutions can accumulate in tiny areas of the screen.

Image Blur: ■■■■■■■■■■■■■■■■■■■■■■■■

Description: An area of unsharpness resulting in a lack of detail.

Causes:

- Receptor related blur is the result of poor screen-film contact (Figures 7.28 and 9.2) or trapped air in the cassette. (Image blur can also be

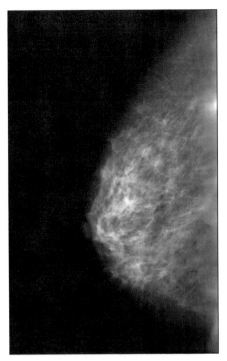

Figure 7.28 Improper film loading resulted in a blurred image along the chest wall edge.

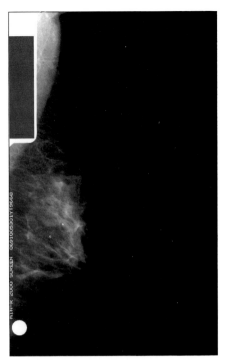

Figure 7.29 This cassette was loaded incorrectly into the bucky.

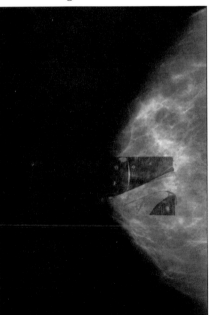

Figure 7.30 A piece of paper was found in this film cassette.

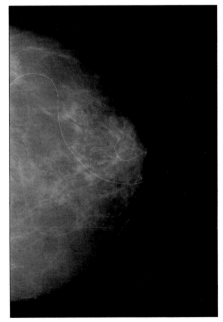

Figure 7.31 A piece of string was found in this film cassette.

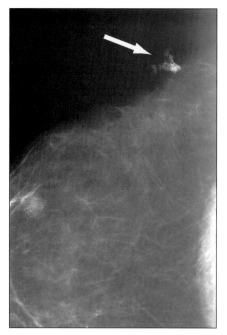 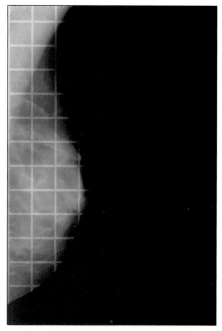

Figure 7.32 Screen damage occurred as a result of spraying canned air directly at the screen surface.

Figure 7.33 This cassette was loaded in the bucky upside down.

caused by poor compression, focal spot degradation, patient motion, or equipment motion.) Cassettes should be allowed fifteen minutes to air bleed following film loading.

5. Fog Related Artifacts

Description: Fog related artifacts are always plus density, and will result in a loss of image contrast where they occur.

Causes:
- They differ in appearance according to specific cause. For example, local areas of fog can occur around improperly closed latches (Figure 7.34), darkroom light leaks (Figure 7.22), film bin light leaks, and so forth. Generalized fog resulting from exposure to scattered radiation or improper film storage will result in an overall loss of image contrast and an increase in density. Fog can also result from over development in the processor.

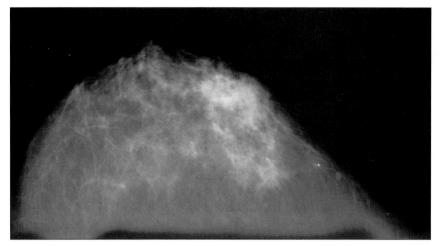

Figure 7.34 Faulty latches on this cassette resulted in film fog.

6. Equipment Related Artifacts

Once the processor and image receptor have been eliminated as possible sources of the artifact, attention can be directed towards the mammography unit.

Grid Lines: ▬▬▬▬▬▬▬▬▬▬▬▬▬▬▬▬▬▬▬▬▬▬▬
Description: Grid lines are linear striations that run parallel to the short axis of the film.

Causes: Grid lines may be the result of several possibilities, including:
- Exposure time is too short, so the grid does not have adequate time to reciprocate or move.
- Grid was flawed when manufactured, resulting in visible grid lines or uneven exposure on the image.
- Grid mechanism is not functioning properly, or is jammed.

Solutions:
- Decrease kVp, and/or increase exposure time.
- Have grid tested for uniformity, and replaced if necessary.
- Have equipment serviced; evaluate and repair grid mechanism.

Unexposed Areas on Film Perimeter: ▬▬▬▬▬▬▬▬▬▬▬▬▬
Description: Clear areas near film's edge impair viewing conditions.
Causes:
- Collimators are not properly adjusted.

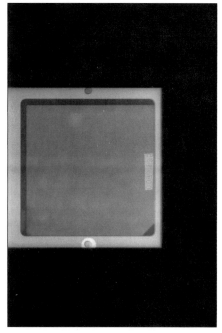

Figure 7.35 A manufacturing defect is evident on this grid.

Figure 7.36 This defect was also apparent on clinical images (note pattern).

Solution:
- Some equipment is not designed to expose all areas of the film. Under MQSA and CAR requirements this may be acceptable. However, if the equipment was designed to cover the receptor to the edges, the collimators may need to be adjusted.

Poor Compression:
Description: Inadequate image density, areas of image blur, or inconsistent compression of breast tissue.

Cause:
- It is important to rule out technical error or patient intolerance to compression. If the problem persists, it may be that the compression mechanism is not functioning properly.

Solution:
- Equipment service should evaluate the rigidity and function of the compression paddle and compression mechanism.

Inadequate Image Density:
Description: Clinical or phantom images are too light.

Causes:
- Most often technical error such as AEC position incorrect, density selection too low, inadequate compression, etc. If such variables have been ruled out, equipment calibration should be verified by equipment service.

Image Blur:
Description: Areas of image blur or poor definition.

Causes:
- Equipment causes of image blur include poor compression (see above), motion of the C-arm, and focal spot size.

Solutions:
- Equipment service or the medical physicist should evaluate focal spot size and motion of the C-arm.

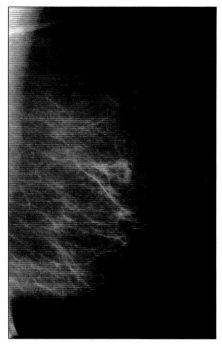

Figure 7.37 Grid lines.

Filter Artifacts:
Description: Plus or minus density shadows on the images, often better demonstrated on the phantom or a *gray sheet* using acrylic to make an exposure of about 1.00 OD.

Causes:
- Degradation of, or damage to, the moly filter.

Solution:
- Replacement of the filter.

Miscellaneous:
Other equipment related problems that may affect image quality include grid mottle, structure mottle resulting from deterioration of the grid or grid interspacing material, or the carbon fiber surface of the bucky mechanism. There may be artifacts from the compression paddle, such as the painted indicators of AEC position.

In most of these cases, evaluation by equipment service personnel is advised.

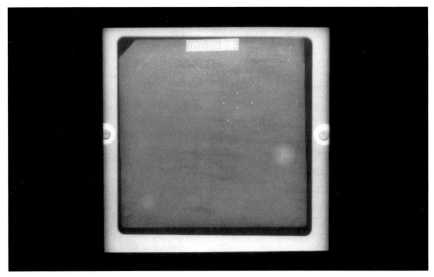

Figure 7.38 Moly filter artifact.

7. Patient Related Artifacts

Description: Foreign material, objects, or body part on clinical images.

Causes:
- Foreign material on patient's skin (powder, cream, oil), earrings, necklaces, or body parts (hair, noses, ears, fingers, etc.) that are inadvertently imaged.

Solution:
- Be sure patient removes all powder and deodorant before the examination; also all jewellery should be removed. Watch that patient's head does not lean into image field before the exposure.

D. CONCLUSION

Determining the source of artifacts that we encounter on our images requires a thorough working knowledge and understanding of the entire mammography system. Persistence and exceptional problem-solving skills are also important due to the random and intermittent patterns that are often observed. Ongoing awareness is essential. Some artifacts mimic potential pathology, such as calcifications; others obscure the proper visualization of breast tissue. The quality control program requires vigilance to ensure that artifacts occur as infrequently as possible.

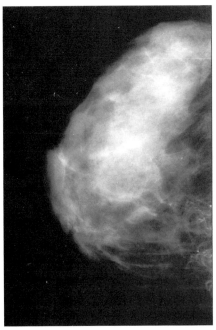

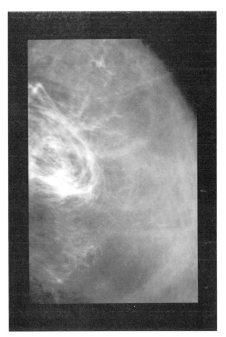

Figure 7.39 Hair is noted on the medial side of the CC image.

Figure 7.40 Again note the pronounced appearance of hair on this image.

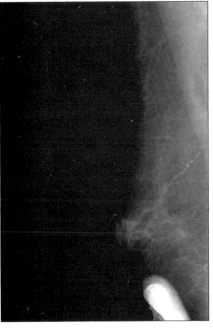

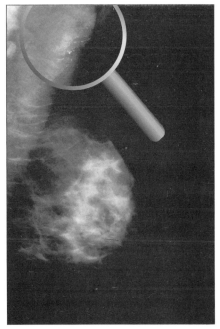

Figure 7.41 The patient's finger was imaged in the inferior part of his film.

Figure 7.42 Note the appearance of deodorant in the axilla area.

Determining the source of artifacts that we encounter on our images requires a thorough working knowledge and understanding of the entire mammography system. Persistence and exceptional problem-solving skills are also important due to the random and intermittent patterns that are often observed.

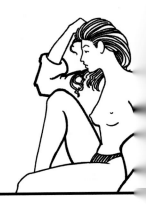

CHAPTER 8:
VIEWING CONDITIONS

CHAPTER 8:
VIEWING CONDITIONS

A. INTRODUCTION

The conditions under which mammography images are viewed have a significant influence on the interpreter's ability to perceive subtle tissue abnormalities; therefore, they have a direct impact on the accuracy of the diagnosis. Prevailing conditions such as ambient room illumination and viewbox (illuminator) luminance play important roles, although the efficiency of the observer's eyes and individual subjective factors cannot be ignored. All of these factors will influence the ease or the difficulty that will be encountered during the process of image interpretation. Unfortunately, viewing conditions in mammography departments seldom receive the care and attention that they require. Note: Throughout this text the term *viewbox* and *illuminator* are considered to be interchangeable.

B. PHOTOMETRIC MEASUREMENT

Photometry is the science of light measurement. It is a relatively complicated process that incorporates the spectral sensitivity of the human eye, specifically the sensitivity of the cones in the fovea.

With the international system of measurement (SI), units for photometric measurement are the *nit* for luminance and the *lux* for illuminance.

The amount of light emitted or scattered by a surface is known as luminance; it is measured in nit (candela per square meter). Illuminance, on the other hand, is the amount of light falling on a surface; it is measured in lux (lumen per square meter). Sufficient viewbox luminance is necessary to appreciate the diagnostic information present on properly exposed mammography images.

The conditions under which mammography images are viewed have a significant influence on the interpreter's ability to perceive subtle tissue abnormalities; therefore, they have a direct impact on the accuracy of the diagnosis.

C. VIEWBOX CHARACTERISTICS

1. Luminance Levels

On an average viewbox that is commonly found in diagnostic imaging departments (luminance of 1500 nit), the maximum optical density that can be visualized is 2.80. A bright viewbox (luminance of 3000 nit) brings the appreciable optical density up to approximately 3.10. A high intensity mammography viewbox (luminance of 7000 nit) raises this again, to the 3.40 optical density level. Mammography viewboxes will generally have luminance values of 3000 - 3500 nit. Unexposed areas on the film must be masked to exclude extraneous light that will inhibit visual perception. Although the optical density of general radiographic images does not exceed 3.50, today's mammography films frequently reach the 4.00 optical density level.

With correct luminance levels, the human eye is capable of perceiving a wide range of densities. This range diminishes rapidly when the light level is either too low or too high. Even under ideal conditions, our perception remains far from perfect. The resolving power of the human eye is always accompanied with individual shortcomings. Defects in the optical focusing system (lens) are common, as are various other forms of impaired vision and astigmatism.

Mammography images are optimally viewed with a variety of luminance levels because of the wide range of optical film densities that are represented on a typical examination. Bright-light viewers or *spot lights* are helpful in examining the darker areas of the image, particularly in the subcutaneous area.

Mammography viewboxes will generally have luminance values of 3000 - 3500 nit. Unexposed film areas must be masked to exclude extraneous light that will inhibit visual perception.

Also, many illuminators can provide overall varying luminance levels with an adjustable light switch.

2. Color Temperature

The color of the viewbox light also affects film reading conditions. Color is specified by temperature in degrees Kelvin. Low color temperatures result in a warm presentation with a color shift toward the red end of the spectrum while high color temperatures result in a cool presentation with a shift toward the blue component of the spectrum. Measurement of the color spectrum from fluorescent bulbs is particularly difficult because they produce a discontinuous spectrum. The factors that affect viewbox color temperature are type of fluorescent lamp, tint of the reflective interior component of the illuminator, and the spectral transmission properties of the viewbox covers (acrylic diffusers).

 With correct luminance levels, the human eye is capable of perceiving a wide range of densities. This range diminishes rapidly when the light level is either too low or too high.

3. Fluorescent Lamps

A variety of fluorescent lamp styles are available for viewboxes. Circular lamps are not recommended for mammography illuminators because of the light deficiency that will occur in the corner areas with this bulb (lamp) style. Many illuminators can accommodate two, three, or four individual linear fluorescent lamps. Mammographers will always prefer as many lamps as possible in order to achieve the greatest possible degree of luminance. Fluorescent bulbs diminish in brightness with age and therefore they should be replaced regularly. Refer to the quality control section of this chapter for recommended replacement criteria.

D. AMBIENT CONDITIONS

The exclusion of all sources of unnecessary extraneous light is critical in order to maximize the perception of image contrast and detail. Therefore, care should be taken to exclude light from sources such as windows, other adjacent viewboxes, overhead lights, etc. The level of ambient light in the viewing room should be no greater than the level of light that is projected through the masked

> *Mammography images are optimally viewed with a variety of luminance levels because of the wide range of optical film densities that are represented on a typical examination.*

images on the viewboxes. This will provide the best possible conditions to maximize the sensitivity of the eye for interpretation.

The ACR and the CAR MAP recommend that the ambient light level in the room where mammography examinations are interpreted should not exceed 50 lux; this is considered generally equivalent to a *moon lit night*. This light level will provide ideal conditions for visual acuity and, at the same time, allow physicians to perform their tasks without difficulty.

Proper room ventilation, temperature, and humidity will all contribute to the comfort of the interpreter. Also, a quiet, relaxed atmosphere, away from the main hub of department activity will be conducive to concentration and clear thinking; it will also minimize interruptions and distractions. The *tools* that the radiologist will need (spot viewer, magnifying glass, viewbox masking, dictaphone, paper, pens, pencils, china markers, lesion localization forms, telephone and directory of referring physicians, etc.) should be readily available.

E. IDEAL VIEWING CONDITIONS

1. Correct luminance for the film type (depends on the examination)
2. Luminance uniformity between adjacent illuminators
3. Extraneous light eliminated (masking)
4. Ambient light minimized
5. Quiet atmosphere without interruption

F. VISUAL PERCEPTION

A very important yet frequently overlooked factor is that of the visual perception and interpretation of the individual observer. The human visual system is highly complex. Photoreceptors convert light into electrical impulses that are interpreted by the brain and then presented to the conscious mind as a visual image.

This process occurs in three distinct stages: image formation on the retina, perception by the observer, and image interpretation.

The light sensitive layer that lines the posterior surface of the eye cavity is called the *retina*. Behind the retina lies a myriad of photoreceptors known as rods and cones. When exposed to visible light, these rods and cones generate nerve impulses that travel to the brain via the optic nerve fibres.

Rods are stimulated by low levels of illumination and are responsible for colorless gray tones (scoptic vision). They are highly sensitive but they cease to function in bright light conditions. They are instrumental for night vision.

Cones are the receptors that function in bright light (photoptic vision) and are responsible for color vision. A 6.0 mm focus in the centre of the retina contains a high density of cones and is called the *fovea*. This area is responsible for the best visual acuity and color vision. From this area outward, the concentration of cones diminishes and that of rods increases. Visual acuity will therefore be decreased but sensitivity at low levels of illumination will increase.

Cone response is highly dependent on prevailing light conditions; sensitivity diminishes rapidly in bright light conditions. Cone sensitivity is based on the average light intensity; therefore, an image on an unmasked viewbox diminishes optimal cone function and the image will appear overexposed and of decreased contrast. However, with appropriately masked images on bright mammography viewboxes in a room with low ambient lighting, the cones will function well to scrutinize fine detail on the images with optimal perception. The same image that previously seemed overexposed will now appear to be at a good optical density and of high image quality.

Under low light intensity conditions, rods provide coarse image resolution. High resolution will be achieved with cone vision, especially when the pupil is constricted to the point that the most densely packed central retinal area, the fovea, is being utilized.

 The level of ambient light in the viewing room should be no greater than the level of light that is projected through the masked images on the viewboxes. This will provide the best possible conditions to maximize the sensitivity of the eye for interpretation.

Again, the effects of glare and of excessive ambient light will be such that retinal signals will be suppressed and a perceived loss of contrast will result.

1. Interpretation

Image interpretation requires knowledge and expertise in a number of areas.

- An in-depth knowledge of breast anatomy and physiology is essential for the thoughtful analysis and interpretation of mammography images. A radiological appreciation of the size, shape, spatial distribution and relative attenuation properties of the breast tissue is also important.

- An understanding of both normal physiology and pathological processes is required in order to develop an appreciation for the probable etiology of abnormalities that will frequently be noted on the mammogram.

- Experience will provide a background of information that will facilitate conscious recognition of fundamental patterns that represent both normal and abnormal breast presentations.

- Clinical information relating to the patient's current symptoms and concerns is very helpful in the interpretation of the examination. It is interesting to note that a school of thought exists that believes clinical data may distract the radiologist from presenting an unbiased report. These advocates propose a brief initial examination of the films without accompanying clinical data followed by a thorough systematic search once the clinical information has been disclosed.

All images should be examined under ideal conditions that provide good visibility and comfort with minimal fatigue on the part of the interpreter.

Under low light intensity conditions, rods provide coarse image resolution. High resolution will be achieved with cone vision, especially when the pupil is constricted to the point that the most densely packed central retinal area, the fovea, is being utilized.

The concentration and focus of the observer is highly dependent on any physical discomfort that he or she may experience as a result of poor ventilation, inappropriate temperature, or excessive humidity. Also, distractions or interruptions that may occur will disrupt their concentration and train of thought; this can be particularly frustrating when thoughtfully examining multiple previous examinations with complicated clinical presentations. Individual subjective factors of fatigue, general health, and personal stress levels will also influence the perception and accuracy of the observer and, hence, the diagnostic interpretation.

G. QUALITY CONTROL

All mammography viewboxes should be checked periodically for cleanliness and for uniform light output. On a weekly basis, viewboxes should be thoroughly cleaned and any marks on their surface should be removed. At this time, a visual check of the luminance levels of all viewboxes should also be conducted.

It is important that the luminance levels of both the technologist's and the radiologist's viewboxes be similar. Otherwise, the mammography technologist may consistently accept clinical images that, to her eye, appear to be of good quality, when in fact the images may be underexposed when examined with correct light levels in the radiologist's office.

Flourescent tubes decrease in brightness with age (up to 18 % in 8 months); therefore, they should be replaced at regular intervals, usually every 18-24 months. All the tubes in an entire bank should be replaced at the same time to

Flourescent tubes decrease in brightness with age (up to 18 % in 8 months), therefore they should be replaced at regular intervals, usually every 18-24 months. All the tubes in an entire bank should be replaced at the same time to maintain uniform luminance among adjacent viewboxes.

maintain uniform luminance among adjacent viewboxes. Photometric measurement of luminance uniformity over each viewbox surface as well as uniformity with all the viewboxes in a group will ensure consistent interpretation conditions and optimal image perception.

H. PERFORMANCE CRITERIA

Suggested ACR and CAR MAP performance criteria for mammography illuminators include luminance levels of 3000 to 3500 nit, color temperature near 8400 K and ambient room illumination of 50 lux or less. In addition, masking to exclude extraneous viewbox light is highly recommended. The surface of the illuminator should provide diffused light of uniform brightness. Therefore, it is important to evaluate the uniformity of luminance across each viewbox surface as well as the consistency between adjacent viewboxes in a multiple bank presentation.

I. CONCLUSION

The film illuminator is the critical link between the high quality images that have been produced with the utmost of care and attention and the final diagnosis. The value of the illuminator is difficult to quantify. Only when viewing conditions have been maximized will the subtle density differences that may indicate early breast disease be visually appreciated during film interpretation. Without this important final process, the quality of all the other components in the system will be lost and unappreciated. The tragedy is that valuable diagnostic information will be missed and the advantage of early detection will be forfeited.

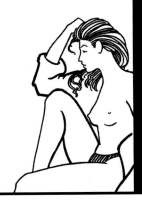

Image Problem Solving

9

CHAPTER 9:
IMAGE PROBLEM SOLVING IN MAMMOGRAPHY

CHAPTER 9:
IMAGE PROBLEM SOLVING IN MAMMOGRAPHY

A. INTRODUCTION

Analyzing the source of image problems that occur in our everyday work environment requires a skilled, analytical, and patient technologist who has developed a thorough understanding and working knowledge of mammography quality control tests and procedures. Frequently, the best means of determining the reason for the loss of image quality is a process of elimination: excluding possible factors one at a time until the most likely culprit is found. Once this task has been completed, the best resolution for the problem can be determined.

As we discussed in Chapter 3, Quality Control, single emulsion films have a higher susceptibility to any problems related to processing and handling. Since artifacts are so prevalent with single emulsion films such as those used for mammography, the most commonly occurring varieties have already been discussed in Chapter 7, Artifacts.

Analyzing the source of image problems that occur in our everyday work environment requires a skilled, analytical, and patient technologist who has developed a thorough understanding and working knowledge of mammography quality control tests and procedures.

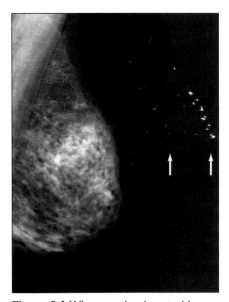

Figure 9.1 When motion is noted in the breast tissue and the identification markers are also blurred, the source of the motion can be assumed to be equipment related.

Other image quality problems include losses or increases in density or contrast, excessive image blur, and excessive noise or mottle. The factors that influence density, contrast, and blur have been discussed in Chapter 6, Image Quality.

The main difficulty you will encounter when analyzing a particular image is determining what specific cause influenced a given factor. For example, consider the possibility that image blur is encountered on a particular view. Was the blur caused by motion? If so, was the motion patient related or equipment related? Suppose the blur was not actually motion at all. It may have resulted from poor breast compression, poor screen-film contact, or entrapped air in the cassette. It is often difficult to differentiate one type of image blur from another. Only by adhering to the strictest quality control and positioning standards can one reasonably exclude some of the basic possibilities, such as poor compression, screen-film contact, or trapped air as possible causes of blur; this will help to determine that true motion was the source of blurring. If the identification markers are also blurred, the source of the motion can be assumed to be equipment related. If only the breast tissue is blurred, the source of the motion must be the patient. The most probable cause for this artifact is often determined, as noted earlier, by a process of elimination.

Similar difficulties arise when an image is too light or too dark. It is important to determine whether breast compression was adequate, and whether the AEC was positioned under the densest part of the breast or the area of interest. If

Frequently, the best means of determining the reason for the loss of image quality is a process of elimination: excluding possible factors one at a time until the most likely culprit is found.

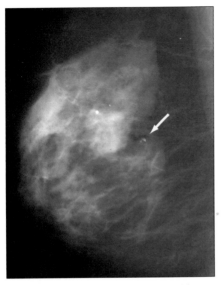

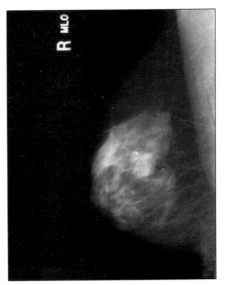

Figure 9.2 Motion was noted on this image; observe the fuzzy margins of the calcification.

Figure 9.3 An overall view of the image confirms that the *motion* is confined to one area of breast tissue (markers are clearly identified; no motion apparent along the chest wall). The source of this motion probably relates to screen-film contact.

so, perhaps a higher or lower density setting on the AEC would have produced the desired results. Was the kVp adequate for the amount and thickness of the glandular tissue for this patient? Has the equipment calibration been verified? Is processor variability a possible issue? Certainly multiple repeated films from a single processor or mammography unit would warrant further investigation. The repeat analysis is helpful in this regard. Any problem that occurs with some frequency should be investigated.

B. ANALYZING THE REPEAT ANALYSIS

The repeat analysis has always been part of every good mammography quality control program. However, under MQSA the repeat analysis has been given the importance of being specified in the legislation. There is a great deal of information available from a repeat analysis; however, many facilities fail to go beyond the basics of determining the repeat rates of the individual categories. Frequently, as long as the percentage of repeats does not exceed the maximum allowed level, no further action is taken. Under the Mammography Quality

Single emulsion films have a higher susceptibility to any problems related to processing and film handling.

Standards Reauthorization Act, corrective action is to be taken in response to increases in the percentage of repeats in any individual category.

With a comprehensive QC program it is important to look beyond the basic percentages for trends and indications of problems with positioning, technique, motion, and artifacts. For example, an increase in the percentage of repeats for light and dark films should be investigated to determine whether technical error or equipment calibration might be responsible. Once that determination has been made, corrective action can be taken to ensure that the percentages do not continue to gradually increase. For this reason, tracking repeated films as they occur, rather than waiting until the end of the analysis period, would enable the QC technologist to intervene as problems arise.

Although at least 250 patient exams are needed to obtain statistical accuracy, the repeat analysis must be performed at least quarterly under MQSA, ACR, and CAR guidelines, even if the facility does fewer exams. Some states in the U.S. require an ongoing record of repeated films.

The repeat analysis procedure can be found in the ACR Manuals for Quality Control in Mammography; it is also briefly described in Chapter 3, Quality Control.

Any corrective action should be documented. Subsequent analyses will show the success of the corrective measures. Since the repeat analysis contains images that are in some way inadequate, we shall take each of the categories and examine the possible causes of each problem.

In each circumstance, a process of elimination must be followed to determine the most likely cause of inadequate image quality. It is usually logical to

The main difficulty you will encounter when analyzing a particular image is determining what specific cause influenced a given factor.

Multiple repeated films from a single processor or mammography unit would warrant further investigation.

eliminate the processor and processing conditions first. If the problem is not with processing, the remaining variables of equipment, technical factors (kVp, mAs output, AEC selected, and proper compression), and receptor system should be evaluated.

Processing issues that result in repeated clinical images are addressed by repeat category, as are the other technical variables. Changes in processor performance that arise on the daily sensitometric strip are addressed separately. When processor variables are demonstrated on the morning QC strip, these must be addressed prior to processing clinical images so that repeated films due to processing can be avoided.

C. IMAGE PROBLEMS BY REPEAT CATEGORY (Other than processing)

1. Positioning

See Chapter 4, Positioning for Mammography.

2. Image Too Dark

Possible Causes

1. AEC density selected too high
2. KVp selected was too high
3. MAs output has increased

Suggestions

Select lighter density
Lower kVp selection
Have equipment recalibrated

 Tracking repeated films as they occur, rather than waiting until the end of the analysis period, will enable the QC technologist to intervene as problems arise.

---

3. Image Too Light

Possible Causes	*Suggestions*
1. AEC not under densest glandular tissue	Move AEC under dense tissue
2. AEC density selected too low	Select higher density setting
3. Inadequate breast compression	Increase compression as patient tolerance allows
4. KVp selected too low	Increase kVp selection
5. Film loaded upside down in cassette	Load film properly in cassette
6. Two films loaded in cassette	Make sure single film is loaded

4. Motion

Possible Causes	*Suggestions*
1. Patient motion—breathing	Patient instruction, preparation
2. Long exposure time	Reduce time; increase kVp
	Use taut compression
	Use faster receptor system
3. Other patient issues	Consider sitting patient
4. Equipment motion	Contact equipment service
5. Poor screen-film contact	Verify screen-film contact; make sure time is allowed for air bleeding from cassette after loading film

5. Other Issues

Possible Causes	*Suggestions*
1. Double exposure	Separate exposed cassettes to avoid confusion
2. Image fog	Keep unexposed cassettes away from x-ray sources
	Store film properly

It is important to note that various film products react in different, and possibly opposite ways to changes in processing conditions. For this reason, it is very difficult to establish charts or guidelines that will be universally true for all film types.

6. Grid Lines

Possible Causes	*Suggestions*
1. Grid lines due to short exposure time	Increase exposure times
2. Grid lines due to faulty grid construction	Verify proper grid construction
3. Grid mechanism jammed	Contact service representative

D. SENSITOMETRY PROBLEMS AND VARIABILITY

It is important to note that various film products react in different, and possibly opposite ways to changes in processing conditions. For this reason, it is very difficult to establish charts or guidelines that will be universally true for all film types. When you consider the number of developer types, fixer types, film processors, and processing cycles, it is easy to see how many variables there are for each situation. Also consider the number of film types and intensifying screens, and the possible combinations of these factors, and the situation gets even more complicated. The suggestions given here are meant to be a guide or roadmap to help put you on the right track. It is advisable to consult your film representative and processor service representative regarding the specific characteristics of the film and chemicals your facility uses. In addition, there are excellent books and publications that focus on film processing. Given the demanding technical requirements of mammography, it is suggested that such references be available to the quality control technologist.

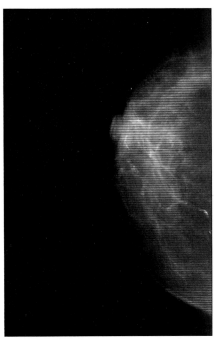

Figure 9.4 Grid lines are noted on this clinical image.

The following problems are based on daily processor QC and sensitometry results. The true speed and contrast of any film can only be determined by calculating the film's average gradient. QC strips are used for daily processor monitoring only. Day to day fluctuations are normal and are to be expected.

In the event that a problem is suspected based on the sensitometry performed on a particular day, the first step in the problem-solving process should be to repeat the sensitometry test strip, verifying that the correct film type is used, that it is inserted into the sensitometer in the correct orientation, and that the correct film feeding protocol is used to process the image. If this second sensitometry strip confirms that a proessing problem exists, you will then need to proceed to resolve the problem at hand. It is useful to recall that sudden deviations are usually the result of a mechanical breakdown (replenisher pump, developer thermostat, blocked replenishment lines) or a specific *event* (using incorrect film, mixing wrong chemicals).

1. Base + Fog Too High

Possible Causes	*Suggestions*
1. New chemicals	Inadequate starter
2. Developer over-replenishment	Reduce replenishment rate
3. High developer temperature	Reduce temperature
4. Exhausted fixer—inadequate fixing	Check fixer & replenishment rate
5. Darkroom fog	Incorrect safelight bulbs, filters
	Light leak
6. Film fog	Film fogged or outdated

2. Speed (MD) Too High
(when combined with contrast increase)

Possible Causes	*Suggestions*
1. Developer temperature too high	Reduce developer temperature
2. Developer immersion time too long	Reduce immersion time
3. Water temperature too high (resulting in increased developer temperature)	Reduce water temperature
4. Slight contamination of developer with fixer	Change developer solution

It is useful to recall that sudden deviations are usually the result of a mechanical breakdown (replenisher pump, developer thermostat, blocked replenishment lines) or a specific event (using incorrect film, mixing wrong chemicals).

3. Speed (MD) Too Low
(when combined with contrast decrease)

Possible Causes	Suggestions
1. Developer temperature too low	Increase developer temperature
2. Developer immersion time too short	Increase immersion time
3. Water temperature low, resulting in decreased developer temperature	Increase water temperature
4. Developer is under-replenished	Increase replenishment rate
5. Developer is contaminated	Change to fresh chemicals
6. Severe chemical oxidation	Change chemicals regularly
	Floating lid in replenishment tank
	Do not expose chemicals to severe temperatures, especially heat
7. Exhausted developer	Check replenishment tank & lines
8. Film is outdated	Rotate film stock to maintain current dating

E. OTHER PROCESSOR RELATED PROBLEMS

1. Wet or damp films

Possible Causes	Suggestions
1. Wash water is too warm	Lower wash water temperature
2. Fixer is exhausted or contaminated	Replace fixer solution
3. Dryer air too cold, humid, or poorly circulated	Increase dryer temperature
	Improve circulation

2. Films jammed in processor

Possible Causes	Suggestions
1. Transport system faulty	Improve film transport
2. Chemicals improperly mixed	Replace chemicals
3. Solution temperatures too high	Lower solution temperatures

3. Brittle films

Possible Causes	Suggestions
1. Excessive drying temperature	Lower dryer temperature
2. Excessive hardener in fixer	Replace with properly mixed fixer

F. CONCLUSION

Analyzing the source of imaging problems that occur in mammography requires a skilled technologist with the ability and willingness to become a detective. Since few sites have individuals dedicated specifically to image quality problem solving, the responsibility often falls on the technologist who performed the examination to make appropriate corrections. Again, one cannot over-emphasize the importance of understanding the performance criteria for the eleven quality control tests that the mammography technologist is responsible for.

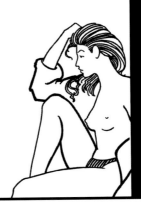

CHAPTER 10:
RADIATION EXPOSURE AND DOSE

CHAPTER 10:
RADIATION EXPOSURE AND DOSE

A. INTRODUCTION

Significant attention has been rightfully devoted to patient exposure and dose with mammography examinations. The primary reasons for this are:

- to facilitate risk evaluation to the patient; this is particularly important in screening settings where repeated examination of large numbers of asymptomatic women occurs.

- to enable professionals in the field to appropriately respond to questions and concerns from patients as well as from colleagues in the medical profession.

- to enable compliance with regulations and recommended guidelines.

- to assist with the evaluation and comparison of imaging systems.

 A frequently forgotten fact is that exposure of the general population to ionizing radiation is not restricted to doses incurred from radiologic examinations alone. There are also three naturally occurring sources of radiation that every person is exposed to on a regular basis.

The greater the amount of photoelectric absorption during an exposure, the greater will be the contrast of the resulting image.

B. SOURCES OF IONIZING RADIATION

To maintain a perspective of radiation exposure and risk, it is important to acknowledge the different sources of radiation that the population is exposed to on an ongoing basis.

A frequently forgotten fact is that exposure of the general population to ionizing radiation is not restricted to doses incurred from radiologic examinations alone. There are also three naturally occurring sources of radiation that every person is exposed to on a regular basis. Exposure to *cosmic radiation* from extraterrestrial sources is lowest at the equator and becomes higher near the earth's poles; it also increases with altitude. *Terrestrial radiation* results from radioisotope deposits in the earth; exposure to this naturally occurring source varies dramatically from one geographical location to another. It is dependent on the composition of the earth at any given location. Finally, we are regularly exposed to radiation emitted from a naturally occurring gas, *radon-222*. The atmospheric concentration of radon-222 is dependent on a number of factors, primarily the underlying earth. Although we have the option to selectively limit our radiologic exposure to radiation, no one can escape exposure to naturally occurring sources of radiation from our environment.

C. INTERACTION OF RADIATION AND TISSUE

A discussion on the subject of radiation exposure and dose from radiologic examinations should include some basics about the interaction of radiation and tissue. Two interactions occur when radiation traverses breast tissue. These processes are photoelectric absorption and compton scattering.

1. Photoelectric Absorption

Photoelectric absorption occurs when the energy of an x-ray photon is close to or slightly greater than the binding energy of an electron that the photon encounters as it traverses tissue. All of the photon's energy is used in the process of overcoming the binding energy of the electron and ejecting it from its atom. In breast tissue, this occurs at photon energies of approximately 15 to 20 keV. At this energy level, the differential absorption between fatty and fibroglandular tissue is over 40%. Increasing the photon energy from 15 to 30 keV will decrease the probability of a photoelectric absorption by a factor of 8 (probability of photoelectric absorption is proportional to the cube of the atomic number and inversely proportional to the cube of the photon energy). Hence, our goal is to keep the photon energy low, thereby enhancing the inherently low contrast of breast tissue. With photoelectric absorption, all of the energy of the incident photon is absorbed. Although this does translate to absorbed breast dose, no scatter will be produced and therefore high contrast images will result.

Photoelectric absorption is highly dependent on the atomic number of the atoms comprising the tissue being irradiated. The probability of photoelectric absorption occurring increases as the energy of the incident photon decreases and as the atomic number of the tissue increases. The greater the amount of photoelectric absorption during an exposure, the greater will be the contrast of the resulting image.

2. COMPTON SCATTERING

The other process that occurs when radiation interacts with tissue is compton scattering. This interaction occurs when the energy of the x-ray photon is considerably higher than the binding energy of the electron. After ejecting an electron from its path, the remaining photon energy is deflected or scattered within the tissue. Images with lower contrast will be produced because of the scattered radiation that is created with this interaction process. Compton scattering is dependent on density rather than atomic number. Above 20 keV, compton scattering will be the predominant interaction process. The probability of compton scattering occuring during an exposure increases as the energy of the incident photon increases.

X-ray photons below 15 keV are usually absorbed by breast tissue, contributing no useful imaging information. Therefore, for mammography examinations, where subject contrast is inherently low and must be enhanced in order to visualize minute structural details, our ideal photon energy would be between

When compton scattering occurs, images with lower contrast will be produced because of the scattered radiation that is created with this interaction process.

---

15 and 20 keV (over 20 keV scatter will reduce image contrast significantly). Molybdenum has a characteristic emission of 17 and 19 keV, making it an excellent choice of target material for mammography equipment.

As radiation interacts with the electrons in the tissue, a chain reaction is set into motion; this progresses from bond disruption to ionization (loss of the electron) to biochemical alteration to cell transformation to (finally) tissue and organ effects. The ability of radiation to produce a response in the tissue it interacts with is referred to as its relative biological effectiveness (RBE).

D. DOSE PARAMETERS

Dose is described and measured in several different ways:

> **ESE** (Entrance Skin Exposure) relates to the dose delivered to the surface of the breast (skin) where the radiation enters the breast. ESE is very easy to measure with an ionization chamber or a thermoluminescent dosimeter (TLD) placed directly under the compression paddle. However, this parameter tends to overestimate absolute risk. It does not accommodate risk variation with different beam energies and it also does not incorporate accumulated dose with multiple exposures. Therefore, its value in estimating breast dose is limited; it is seldom used in clinical practice.

> **MD** (Midline Dose) is more difficult to measure. It provides a better indication than ESE of exposure risk because it incorporates a depth measurement in the tissue. However, it also underestimates true dose risks and is therefore not frequently used to describe breast doses with mammography.

> **MGD** (Mean Glandular Dose) or **AGD** (Average Glandular Dose) cannot be measured directly, but must be calculated according to specific

 MGD appears to be the best indicator of risk today because it focuses on glandular tissue (breast cancer arises in this tissue, not fatty tissue); it reflects the amount of radiation deposited in this tissue; and it incorporates the unique exposure factors from each individual mammography image.

exposure information and calculations based on the principles of x-ray exposure. MGD appears to be the best indicator of risk today because it focuses on glandular tissue (breast cancer arises in this tissue, not fatty tissue); it reflects the amount of radiation deposited in this tissue; and it incorporates the unique exposure factors from each individual mammography image. Therefore, breast dose measurements are discussed and quoted using MGD values.

MGD is calculated using the measured ESE, the x-ray beam kVp, and the HVL for each individual exposure. The use of a grid (bucky) normally doubles the non-grid MGD value.

E. FACTORS AFFECTING DOSE

The factors that affect the radiation dose associated with screen-film mammography can be grouped into three categories: breast related factors, equipment related factors, and receptor related factors. Refer to Figure 10.1 to find a complete listing for each of these categories.

As you can see, many factors affect the radiation dose delivered during the mammography examination. The importance of maximizing each factor in order to minimize the dose delivered to the patient must be emphasised.

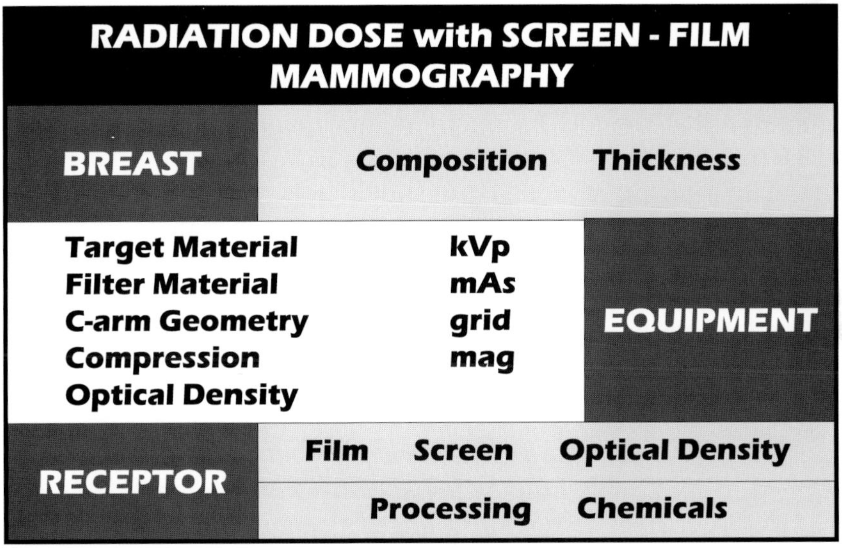

RADIATION DOSE with SCREEN - FILM MAMMOGRAPHY		
BREAST	**Composition**	**Thickness**
Target Material **Filter Material** **C-arm Geometry** **Compression** **Optical Density**	**kVp** **mAs** **grid** **mag**	**EQUIPMENT**
RECEPTOR	**Film** **Screen** **Processing**	**Optical Density** **Chemicals**

Figure 10.1 The factors affecting radiation dose with screen-film mammography.

Molybdenum has a characteristic emission of 17 and 19 keV, making it an excellent choice of target material for mammography equipment.

F. PATIENT EXPOSURE CONTROL

The cardinal principles of radiation exposure control for patients are to reduce the time of exposure, to increase the distance from the radiation source, and to use shielding when appropriate and useful (main beam within 5.0 cm of gonads). Other factors that will also contribute to reduced patient exposure are the use of filtration to remove soft rays that would be absorbed by the patient and not be used to formulate the image, the use of a faster image receptor whenever possible and avoiding repeat exposures as much as possible. The *As Low As Reasonably Achievable* (ALARA) principle should always be a guiding factor when performing patient examinations.

1. Recommended Dose Values

The definition of acceptable radiation dose is an ongoing debate; its interpretation is highly subjective. However, recommended operating parameters must be established to provide guidelines and acceptance criteria for clinical practice.

Both the CAR (Canadian Association of Radiologists) and the ACR (American College of Radiology) MAP (Mammography Accreditation Programs) have recommended that the MGD for screen-film imaging with a grid should not exceed 3.0 mGy (300 mrad) per exposure for an 'average breast' and the MGD for screen-film imaging without a grid should not exceed 1.0 mGy (100 mrad) per exposure for an 'average breast.' Pursuing further dose reduction with corresponding compromises in resolution is an individual decision. The accreditation programs have also considered including a minimum allowable dose restriction to discourage users from seriously compromising image quality in order to achieve extreme dose reduction.

The As Low As Reasonably Achievable (ALARA) principle should always be a guiding factor when performing patient examinations.

It is important to be aware that mammography image quality will be compromised if the radiation dose is too low.

G. ESTIMATED THEORETICAL RISK

To date, no woman has ever been shown to have developed breast cancer as a result of mammographic exposure, even when multiple studies at much higher doses than our current levels have been performed over an extended period of time. Excessive breast cancer rates have been noted in populations that have received extremely high doses of radiation (Japanese atomic bomb survivors, tuberculosis patients who received multiple fluoroscopic examinations, and women with postpartum mastitis who were treated with radiotherapy). Based on these high exposure levels, researchers have attempted to estimate possible risk values associated with the current low levels of radiation delivered during mammography examinations. Unfortunately, information such as this is very difficult to extract from the data and the opportunity for inappropriate estimates is both possible and likely. However, we have no experience or data with exposure levels that are more appropriate, in the lower levels that typify mammography examinations.

Interest and concern continue regarding this issue because the breast is a very radiosensitive organ and the possibility of risk is both realistic and expected.

Examination with current low dose techniques (mean breast dose of 0.17 rad for a two-view study) would carry a theoretical risk of about one excess cancer case / year / 2 million women examined. Assuming a 50 percent breast cancer mortality rate, the hypothetical risk would be one excess death / 4 million women / year; this is extremely small and can be equated with the following:

> *100 miles traveled by air*
> *15 miles traveled by car*
> *Smoking one-fourth cigarette*
> *One-third minute of mountain climbing*
> *5 minutes of being a man age 60*

Source: Feig SA: Low-dose mammography: Assessment of theoretical risk, In Feig SA, McLelland R (eds).Breast Carcinoma: Current Diagnosis and Treatment. New York, Masson Publishing USA, Inc., 1983, pp 69-76.

Glandular tissue (as opposed to adipose, skin, and areolar tissue) is the most vulnerable breast tissue for sensitivity to radiation and consequent development of breast cancer.

Since 1983, when these relative risks were quoted, we have reduced our dose for mammography significantly. Therefore, at this time, these estimations would be overstated and very high when considering current mammography exposure levels.

NCRP Report 85 describes three considerations that must be recognized when estimating potential carcinogenic risk from mammography:

- Glandular tissue (as opposed to adipose, skin, and areolar tissue) is the most vulnerable breast tissue for sensitivity to radiation and consequent development of breast cancer. Glandular tissue is understood to include acinar and ductal epithelium as well as breast stroma.

- The average rather than the maximum dose to the glandular tissue is the most useful indication of carcinogenesis. As well, an assumed linear rather than a threshold dose response relationship is utilized.

- The age group of primary interest is forty years and older. Younger women are presumed to have a limited number of diagnostic examinations. Women in the age group forty years and older will often encounter clinical breast changes requiring diagnostic examinations. Also, women in this age group are frequently eligible for participation in screening programs. Therefore, it is reasonable to assume that the breast type most commonly encountered may contain a larger proportion of adipose tissue, as is consistent with that found in older women. For this reason, breast 'models' utilized for mammography studies usually simulate a breast composed of 50% adipose and 50% glandular tissue.

Both the CAR and the ACR Mammography Accreditation Programs have recommended that the MGD for screen-film imaging with a grid should not exceed 3.0 mGy (300 mrad) per exposure for an 'average breast.'

H. BENEFIT VERSUS RISK FOR MAMMOGRAPHY

Unfortunately, breast cancer is not a disease for which we can actively pursue prevention, primarily because the exact cause of breast cancer has not been determined. We do know that almost all of our therapeutic efforts have very little effect on controlling this disease and altering mortality once the disease has invaded the lymphatic system. Only recently have we been able to detect early, noninvasive, preclinical disease and arrest its progression before it has invaded surrounding tissue. Mammography has proven to be the most reliable diagnostic modality for consistently facilitating the early detection of breast disease.

Unfortunately, mammography requires exposure to ionizing radiation. Although we have not been able to statistically prove its actual risk, we do know that the theoretical risk is low and may, in fact, be negligable when the examination is performed under ideal conditions. The fact remains that exposure to ionizing radiation does occur and the possibility for carcinogenesis does exist and must be acknowleged.

When analysing issues such as these, the benefit-risk ratio is examined and must be found to be favorable in order for a practice to be endorsed.

This puts mammography in an interesting position. The natural incidence of breast cancer clearly indicates that it is a great potential health hazard to all women. We also know that early detection is the only method of affecting mortality with this disease.

On the other hand, we do not have statistical data of the potential risk from mammography. A twenty year follow-up study of millions of exposed and unexposed women would be required to collect sufficient data to produce convincing and meaningful evidence that could answer these questions. This will never occur. Our decision must be to recognize that significant benefit can

 Unfortunately, mammography requires exposure to ionizing radiation. Although we have not been able to statistically prove its actual risk, we do know that the theoretical risk is low and may, in fact, be negligable when the examination is performed under ideal conditions.

Mammography has proven to be the most reliable diagnostic modality for consistently facilitating the early detection of breast disease.

be obtained from mammography. A theoretical risk does exist but it appears to be very low and, in fact, negligable considering the natural incidence of breast cancer as well as its insidious nature and devastating course.

Benefit-risk discussions have never been an issue with diagnostic mammography. The concern has only evolved with the introduction of screening programs that examine large numbers of asymptomatic women at regular intervals in order to detect breast cancer at an early preclinical stage of development.

For a screening examination with an average and acceptable MGD of 2.5 mGy (250 mrad) ...

> *the theoretical radiation-induced breast cancer fatalities in one million women examined with mammography is approximately 5 cases.*

This mammography radiation risk is equialent to the risk of dying as a result of an accident when traveling ...

> *5000 miles by airplane or 450 miles by car.*

In this same group of one million women, ...

> *1500 cases of breast cancer will be diagnosed in one year.*

Without the benefits of breast cancer screening, ...

> *the fatality rate from breast cancer would be about 50%.*

A breast cancer screening program would be expected to ...

> *reduce the fatality rate by 40%;*
> *this would save about 300 lives in one year.*

Analyzing these statistics, it is obvious that an extremely favorable benefit-to-risk ratio exists for mammography screening examinations.

I. RADIATION MEASUREMENT UNITS

1. Exposure

The unit of AIR KERMA (in GRAYS) has replaced the ROENTGEN (R) as the unit of exposure. The effect measured by this parameter is the ionization of air.

1 Gy	=	114.55 R	1 R = 8.73 mGy	
1 mGy	=	114.55 mR	1 mR = 8.73 µGy	

2. Absorbed Dose

The unit of GRAY (Gy) replaces the RAD (rad) as the unit of absorbed dose.

The effect measured by this parameter is the amount of energy absorbed by the subject.

1 Gy	=	100 rad	1 rad = 10 mGy	
1 mGy	=	100 mrad	1 mrad = 10 µGy	

3. Dose Equivalent

The SIEVERT (Sv) replaces the REM (rem) as the unit of dose equivalent or the effective dose. The effect measured by this parameter is the biological effect of the absorbed dose; these units are frequently quoted during discussions on radiation protection.

1 Sv	=	100 rem	1 rem = 10 mSv	
1 mSv	=	100 mrem	1 mrem = 10 µSv	

Note :   m = milli = 10^{-3} µ = micro = 10^{-6}

The natural incidence of breast cancer clearly indicates that it is a great potential health hazard to all women. We also know that early detection is the only method of affecting mortality with this disease.

J. CONCLUSION

The concern about dose relating to exposure with mammography examinations remains a very sensitive issue. The natural incidence of breast cancer compels us to pursue mammography. It would, in fact, be irresponsible to proceed otherwise in light of the fact that early detection is the single most important factor that has the ability to alter the course of breast cancer. We know that mammography saves lives. As professionals in this field, we have the ability and responsibility to perform these examinations with careful attention to minimizing patient dose, consistent with high quality imaging. Under these conditions, women can feel confident that the risk they will incur from mammography is very low; in fact, it is negligible when compared with the benefits they will receive with a quality examination that will detect breast disease at the earliest possible stage.

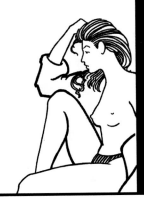

CHAPTER 11:
PREVENTING MUSCULOSKELETAL DISCOMFORT AND INJURY IN MAMMOGRAPHY

CHAPTER 11:
PREVENTING MUSCULOSKELETAL DISCOMFORT AND INJURY IN MAMMOGRAPHY

A. OBJECTIVES

The objectives of this chapter are as follows:

- Review the benefits of applying ergonomic techniques at work.
- Examine the types of discomfort experienced by mammographers.
- Review the risk factors that can contribute to specific forms of discomfort.
- Examine ergonomics techniques that can prevent specific types of discomfort.
- Review of a quick set of reminders to utilize when at work.

B. INTRODUCTION

Mammography as a career is exceptionally rewarding and satisfying; at the same time, it is also physically, psychologically, and emotionally demanding. All of these factors contribute to the overall stress that mammography technologists experience. Individually, each factor may not be considered excessive. However, together they may overwhelm the body's ability to recover and heal. The following chapter focuses on reducing the impact of the physical demands of this job on the musculoskeletal system.

The everyday tasks of a mammographer often require awkward static postures, repetitive motion, and long task duration. These factors can contribute to the development of musculoskeletal discomfort and, over time, injury. Applying

---

ergonomic techniques to mammography can help to alleviate pain and discomfort; ultimately, it has the potential to minimize injury. Ergonomics is the science that examines human performance and safety as it relates to an individual's work environment, equipment and tools, and the design of the job (Sanders and McCormick, 1993).

Common names that are used in the literature to describe musculoskeletal distress related conditions are: Cumulative Trauma Disorder (CTD), Repetitive Stress Injury (RSI), and Workplace Musculoskeletal Disorders (WMSD).

Factors that can affect your ability to use proper body mechanics or work techniques include the following:

- equipment design and set up
- design of the work task, such as pace and workload
- environmental factors, such as workplace layout and space
- patient characteristics, such as weight, height, level of stress, and level of pain or discomfort associated with the procedure
- your personal fitness, weight, general health, and body mechanics

It is important to consider all of these factors to achieve a healthy and safe workplace. Ask yourself, *which factors do I have control or influence over?* You should be able to influence some part of each of the aforementioned factors. Even minimal changes and alterations are beneficial. For example, if a patient is unfamiliar or anxious about having a mammogram, she may be quite tense, making it difficult for the technologist to position her for the examination. Describing the procedure and making the patient aware of what to expect may help to relax the individual's body posture, making it easier to position the patient and to engage her assistance as the examination proceeds.

Some factors that are extremely basic and simplistic may have a significant impact on the mammographer's ability to perform her job well and with improved comfort. An example of this would be her clothing. With tight, restrictive uniforms and lab coats, every reach, stretch and bend will be met with resistance. The technologist will be in a constant state of discomfort; over the course of a day, this can be extremely tiring. The simple measure of wearing loose, relaxed clothing that allows easy movement as the technologist positions her patient, will eliminate this source of irritation and stress.

This chapter will focus on a number of changes and options that you can incorporate into your everyday work tasks.

C. BENEFITS OF APPLYING ERGONOMICS

The process of performing mammography examinations is made up of a set of tasks that are physically demanding on the body. Specifically, the demands of the job place stress and strain on the structures of the legs and feet, the back, the shoulders and neck, and the hands and wrists. Mammography technologists frequently report musculoskeletal discomfort with years of exposure to the physical demands of their job. When these problems present, they are very real, creating a great deal of discomfort and having an impact on the individual's ability to perform their job. The good news is that musculoskeletal discomfort and injury can be prevented.

Employing ergonomic techniques in the specific areas of equipment set up, proper body mechanics, and job design can assist the mammographer to avoid musculoskeletal discomfort, or, at the very least, to minimize its effects on their health and job performance. Over the long term, practicing ergonomic principles can prevent musculoskeletal disorders such as tendonitis, carpal tunnel syndrome, back strain and sprains, and many others. The effects of these disorders are extensive, affecting the personal life and health of the technologist as well as his/her career. These disorders, if not prevented, can substantially shorten a work career in mammography. As with any profession, experience in the field of mammography is an invaluable asset. Employers do not want to lose their most valuable, experienced technologists to work related injury, particularly when the contributing factors are avoidable or at the very least, when options are available to minimize injuries.

D. MUSCULOSKELETAL DISORDERS

1. Risk Factors

The primary risk factors that contribute to musculoskeletal disorders, as reported in the literature, are grouped into the following categories: force, repetition, posture, mechanical stress, duration, vibration, and temperature.

a. Force

Forceful movements increase the stress placed on muscles, tendons, and joints. Muscle fatigue will occur at a faster pace as force increases. The degree of force required to perform a task will be affected by the weight of the object, the distribution of the load in relation to the body (stability and size of the load), the object friction or ease of handling, vibration (a vibrating hand tool will often require the individual to grip harder), and the type of grip utilized (pinch grip places much more stress on the tendons than a power grip).

There are two types of effort encountered in performing a task: dynamic and static. Dynamic effort (repetitive motion) is characterized by a prolonged period of lengthening and shortening, tension and relaxation of the muscle. Static effort (a stationary state) is characterized by a prolonged state of shortening of the muscles. This is often seen when an individual is trying to maintain a posture such as standing or forward stooping for an extended period of time. With static effort the muscle does not change length, but remains in a state of heightened tension; force is exerted over the entire duration of time. Static effort is considered significant when:

1) A high level of effort is maintained for ten seconds or more

2) A moderate effort occurs for one minute or more

3) A slight effort lasts for five minutes or more
   (Kroemer and Grandjean, 1997)

Static effort occurs when a mammographer must maintain an awkward position for an extended period of time – perhaps when bending over to position a patient in a wheelchair or when using a non-standard positioning technique with a difficult or physically challenged patient. The effect of static effort is such that, as the muscles quickly tire, they will tighten, constricting blood vessels and compressing nerves. Circulation is impeded and insufficient oxygenated blood will be available to nourish and supply fuel to the muscles. As lactic acid accumulates in the tissue, the onset of muscular fatigue will be more rapid. For example, if under similar conditions a static muscular effort is compared with a dynamic effort, the following will occur:

A higher rate of energy will be consumed.
Increased heart rate will be experienced.
Longer rest periods are needed to recover.

b. Repetition

Repetitive motion is the repeated utilization of the same muscle groups. Mammography technologists are often exposed to repetitive motions in their daily work tasks. Repetitive motions can result in an increase in fatigue and muscle-tendon strain (Berg Rice, 1998). Repetitive motion in itself is usually

 The good news is that musculoskeletal discomfort and injury can be prevented.

*Repetitive motion in itself is usually not a problem,
but it becomes a concern when it is combined with
high force and awkward body postures.*

not a problem, but it becomes a concern when it is combined with high force and awkward body postures. When an individual is exposed to high force and awkward postures and the activity is highly repetitive in nature, there will often not be sufficient time for the tissues to recover adequately. In other words, combined with the other accompanying stressful factors, it is beyond the body's capacity to withstand the repetitive motion without damage. An activity is considered repetitive when the cycle time is less than 30 seconds or when one fundamental cycle constitutes more than 50% of the total cycle (OSHA, 1995). It is important to note that the level of risk associated with repetition varies by body part.

c. Posture

Awkward postures are a risk factor that most mammography technologists experience on a regular basis; they result in increased muscle force, which contributes to muscle fatigue, tendon fatigue, and joint soreness, and they can increase pressure on the spine. The degree of posture deviation that can create excessive stress will vary, depending on the individual body part. Postures that position a limb in severe deviation from its normal orientation are thought to contribute to the onset of musculoskeletal disorders.

d. Contact Stress / Mechanical Compression

Contact stress, or mechanical compression, is associated with a pressure or force that is exerted over a small (limited) area. For mammography technologists, mechanical compression occurs when their body comes into contact with a hard or sharp object (cassette, cassette latches, bucky, compression paddle, compression control knob, etc.), the sharp edge of the counter or surface, or when handling items with a small diameter (some manual compression controls). When mechanical compression occurs, it will interfere with blood flow and nerve function (Greenberg & Chaffin, 1989; Putz-Anderson, 1990).

e. Duration

Duration is the amount of time an individual is exposed to a particular risk factor. Prolonged exposure increases local and generalized fatigue and tissue stress. As the duration of exposure increases so will the recovery time required for the task.

f. Vibration

Although vibration is a risk factor that most mammographers will not be exposed to in their daily work tasks, it is important to be aware of this risk factor. There are two types of vibration, whole-body and localized vibration. Whole body vibration occurs when the whole body is exposed to repeated movement, such as during the operation of a vehicle. Localized vibration occurs when a part of the body comes into contact with a vibrating object such as a hand tool. Guidelines on the measurement and evaluation of vibration have been published by the American Conference of Governmental Industrial Hygenists (ACGIH, 1995).

g. Temperature

The final risk factor related to musculoskeletal disorders is low temperature. Again, although this risk factor is not commonly experienced by mammography technologists as they perform their normal work tasks, it is important to be aware of this risk factor. Low temperatures will reduce the dexterity and sensitivity of the hand, increase grip force requirements, and can exacerbate the effects of localized vibration. The ACGIH (1995) has developed recommended temperature limits for bare skin exposure, based on the type of activity performed.

E. ANATOMICAL SITES OF MUSCULOSKELETAL DISCOMFORT

1. Leg and Foot Discomfort

Leg and foot discomfort is a frequently reported form of discomfort experienced by mammographers. In industry, risk factors that can contribute to leg and foot discomfort include:

- awkward leg postures (such as hyperextension of the knee, standing on tiptoes, or crouching)
- fixed standing postures
- fixed awkward postures (such as crouching or kneeling)
- repetitive leg motions

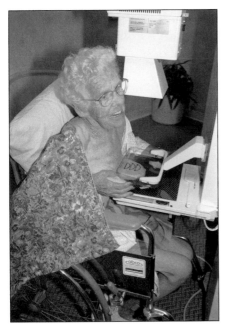

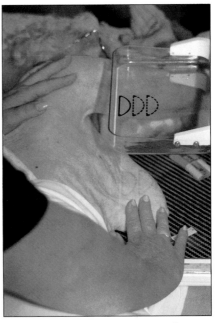

Figure 11.1 Crouching is frequently noted when technologists position patients in wheelchairs. This is difficult to avoid due to the low patient presentation and the restricted patient mobility.

Figure 11.2 Stretching over a patient on a stretcher often results in hyperextension of the knees and straining of the leg muscles.

All of the above examples are known to characterize mammography tasks.

The extent and degree of discomfort to which awkward leg postures affect mammography technologists will vary since the relationship between the mammographer's height and the patient's height often influences leg posture during the examination.

Crouching is frequently used when positioning patients in wheelchairs; this is difficult to avoid with the low patient presentation and the restricted patient mobility. Fortunately, these situations are uncommon in most facilities. Crouching and kneeling may also be noted with poor positioning techniques for the MLO projection; the technologist may bend down or kneel to observe the patient and complete positioning from beneath the C-arm. This is not recommended. Education in updated positioning techniques that avoid undue strain on the technologist's musculoskeletal system should be adopted to reduce the risk of stress and injury. Finally, crouching may be encountered when a very tall technologist is positioning a very short client.

The very nature of mammography positioning is such that maintaining a fixed stationary position or an awkward position for an extended period of time is relatively uncommon. These situations would only be encountered when working with a difficult patient (elderly, frail, kyphotic, very ill, physically impaired) and with wheelchair (Figure 11.1) and stretcher (Figure 11.2) patients.

Repetitive leg and foot motions form a major component of the mammography technologist's job profile. Careful attention to the suggestions outlined here is important in order to avoid undue stress and strain in the lower extremity area.

Prevention techniques fall into four primary categories: proper body mechanics, job design, work-area set up, and work-relief strategies. The following information reviews specific techniques you may want to incorporate into your everyday routine.

a. Body Mechanics

- When positioning the client, try to keep your legs (knees) slightly bent rather than hyperextended.
- Avoid stretching your legs into awkward positions as you work with the patient.
- Move the foot pedals close to your work area; this will minimize the need to stretch your legs excessively during patient positioning.
- Try to remain standing flat on your feet to maintain balance and good support.

b. Job Design

- Try to alternate tasks that will allow for both sitting and standing positions.
- Sit on a chair while completing and discussing the history form with the patient as you begin the examination.
- Look for opportunities that will allow you to sit down, even for a short period of time. Some examples may be these: while completing any

The very nature of mammography positioning is such that maintaining a fixed stationary position or an awkward position for an extended period of time is relatively uncommon.

paperwork related to the case, entering patient information into a computer, calling other facilities for previous examinations, or simply if you have a few moments while waiting to view your images or while waiting for access to the x-ray room. Even brief periods of change and rest are beneficial.

c. Work Area Set-Up

- Ensure the immediate area is free of obstructions so you can properly place your feet into position when working with the client and when operating the equipment. When the patient must step out of footwear for the examination, ensure that it remains well away from your working *foot* area.

- A tall chair or stool will allow the technologist to perform many of her *standing* duties in a *semi-sitting* position, without significantly changing the work height of the task. The individual should avoid using a high chair if they are unable to easily get on and off the chair; when the position or height is uncomfortable, the operator may slip or fall, creating the potential for injury.

- When viewing images on wall mounted viewboxes (usually near the film processor), stand with one foot raised on a footstool, footrest, a low shelf, or even the rung of a nearby chair. Alternate this foot position regularly throughout the day.

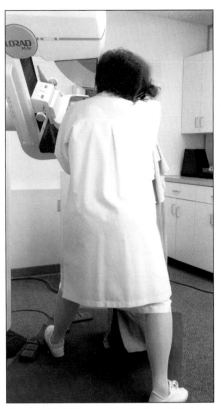

Figure 11.3 The technologist will have to stretch and hyperextend her knee to reach the foot control when the mammography equipment has only one stationary foot control.
NOTE: This foot control was placed in a stationary position only for demonstration purposes. This equipment does have multiple, movable foot pedals.

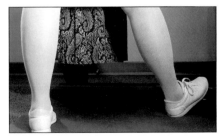

Figure 11.4 The controls on the superior surface of the foot pedals should not have a high profile; the operator will have to hyperextend her foot each time she activates the controls.

The foot pedal should always be positioned before you begin working with the patient.

- Variations in the design of the mammography equipment can have a significant influence on the leg and foot stress that the technologist will experience. The design and location of the foot pedals are a major factor affecting leg and foot discomfort. Equipment that has one stationary foot control will require that the technologist stretch and hyperextend her knee to reach the control when she is standing in various locations as she performs her work (Figure 11.3). A single, free foot control (pedal) that can be easily moved from side to side to accommodate multiple operating positions is an improved option. This pedal should be relatively lightweight; if not, it must be easily mobilized to avoid excess strain, since the technologist will have to adjust its position a number of times during each mammography examination. Two sets of foot pedals are far superior; they should still be somewhat mobile to allow each technologist to make slight positional adjustments according to their individual body habitus. The controls on the superior surface of the pedal should not have a high profile; this would require the operator to hyperextend her foot excessively to activate the controls (Figure 11.4). Finally, the controls should be activated with moderate pressure; heavy pressure would result in unnecessary strain to the foot and calf during the course of a normal workday.
- The foot pedal should always be positioned before you begin working with the patient. Additionally, because the x-ray rooms are shared by many mammographers, each technologist should always take a few moments to adjust the position of the foot pedal according to her specific needs. Balancing on one leg and *searching* for the foot pedal with the other while you are holding the patient in position would be both awkward and uncomfortable.
- Position foot pedals close to your body to allow for comfortable foot operation (Figure 11.5). Ideally, you should be able to operate the pedal while maintaining your feet no more than shoulder width apart (Figure 11.5). It is important that the foot pedal be easily repositioned; a semi slip-resistant surface should be fixed to the base of the foot pedal since it is often pushed back with the foot when the foot pedal is released. When moving the foot pedal try to maintain proper body mechanics, avoiding excessive stretching of the leg or bending at the waist. Crouch down and move a foot pedal that is not easily relocated with the foot.

- Ensure foot pedals are well maintained so they require minimal force to activate the foot pedal functions.
- Some manufacturers have incorporated a number of additional options into their foot pedals, allowing the technologist to adjust the height of the C-arm and to turn on the collimator light without having to reach for the hand controls. This attractive feature eliminates the technologist's need to repeatedly reach for these controls as she positions her patient.
- If a patient is very short in stature compared to the technologist, the patient could be asked to stand on a low stool or platform for the examination. Safety would become a very important focus here; the platform would need to be large enough that the patient would not inadvertently step off the edge and fall. Also, the platform must be able to be moved into position without undue strain on the part of the technologist.

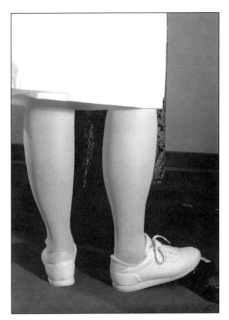

Figure 11.5 The technologist's feet should remain shoulder width apart when she operates the foot controls.

- If the floor area is a hard surface, investigate the feasibility of using high-density bevel-edged, anti-fatigue matting around the mammography machine. This will reduce leg and foot fatigue. These mats are also available with anti-static properties for areas where dryness is prevalent.
- If the patient is very tall, thereby requiring the technologist to stand on the balls of her feet, investigate the feasibility of the technologist using a light-weight platform large enough to accommodate both feet and the foot pedal; be careful not to step off the platform incorrectly. Alternately, in extreme cases, you

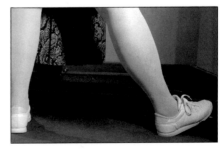

Figure 11.6 This foot pedal is incorrectly positioned too far from the technologist's work area; she must extend her leg to reach the control as she positions her patient.

might consider asking the patient to kneel in front of the machine on a pillow. She will still be fairly mobile and able to adjust her position slightly by *walking* on her knees. Although this suggestion could also create alternate positioning difficulties, you might also consider offering the patient a chair with locking castors that will allow you some mobility yet provide the security of locking the chair once the correct patient position has been achieved. These suggestions refer to extreme situations; they are relatively uncommon.

d. Work-Relief Strategies

- Avoid standing in one position for extended periods of time. Try to move your feet regularly.
- Utilize proper footwear and shoe insoles. Note: insoles should be purchased at the same time as new shoes are purchased since the insoles will tighten the fit of a shoe.
- Sit down periodically to give the legs a break from standing; even brief periods are beneficial.
- Use stretching techniques. Remember to check with your healthcare provider to ensure that these stretches are safe for you. Discontinue any stretch if it causes pain or severe discomfort.

i. Foot Rotation

- While sitting, slowly rotate foot from the ankle three times in one direction.
- Then, slowly rotate that foot three times in the other direction.
- Repeat for the opposite foot.
- Repeat the rotation for each foot three times.

ii. Toe Points

- When sitting, point toes downward as far as possible.
- Hold for three seconds. Relax.
- Repeat three times.

iii. Knee Bends

- While standing straight, slowly do small knee bends.
- Repeat five times.

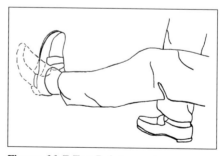

Figure 11.7 *Toe Point* exercise

iv. Leg Lifts

- While standing or sitting, lift each leg up in front.
- Repeat five times.

v. Thigh Stretch

- Stand facing a chair.
- Place your right hand on the chair.
- With your left hand, grasp your left ankle.
- Ensure the knee of your standing leg is slightly bent.
- Tighten your stomach muscles and slowly bring your left ankle towards your buttocks.
- Keep knees close together and point bent knee downwards.
- Hold for a count of 10, relaxing and breathing deeply.
- Repeat for the opposite leg.

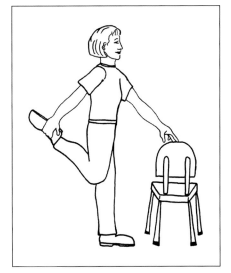

Figure 11.8 *Thigh Stretch* exercise

vi. Hamstring Stretch

- Stand on one leg with your knee bent slightly.
- Hold the opposite leg with both hands under the knee.
- Bring your knee slowly up towards your chest.
- Stretch your foot out slowly in front of you.
- Hold for a count of 10, relaxing and breathing deeply.
- Repeat for the opposite leg.

2. Lower Back Discomfort

Lower back pain has a complex etiology. Approximately 70 percent of the population will experience an episode of lower back pain at one time or another during their lifetime. Mammography technologists often report lower

Approximately 70 percent of the population will experience an episode of lower back pain at one time or another during their lifetime.

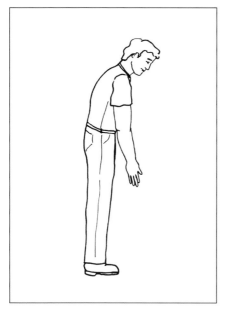

Figure 11.9 *Forward Bending*

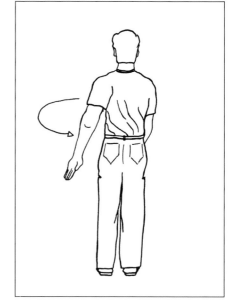

Figure 11.10 *Twisting*

back discomfort. Other back disorders that may result from physically heavy work include muscle strains and sprains and disc herniation. Risk factors that can contribute to lower back discomfort and disorders fall into two primary categories: workplace and personal.

Workplace risk factors (in industry) include:

- heavy activity (pushing, pulling, lifting, holding, and carrying)
- awkward postures of the back (Figures 11.9 through 11.11) (forward bending, twisting, and loading)
- repetitive motions
- static, fixed postures of the back
- extended task duration
- whole-body vibration

Mammography technologists experience all of the above risk factors except for whole body-vibration. The extent to which each of these risk factors occurs is dependent on the design of equipment used, the individual work habits of the technologist, the length of workday, and the type of patient that is encountered.

For example, heavy activity can occur when moving and working with patients in wheelchairs and on stretchers. Occasionally, this phenomenon may also

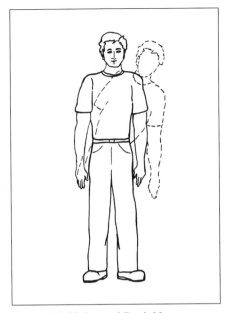

Figure 11.11 *Lateral Back Movement*

occur during the process of positioning or holding a client when the technologist is forced to bear the weight of a patient who is uncooperative during positioning or who may lean against the technologist for support during the examination. Moving heavy boxes of supplies (chemicals and film) would also fall into this category. Awkward postures of the back can occur when there is a significant difference in height between the mammographer and the patient or when the mammographer must bend sideways to reach / operate the overhead controls on the mammography equipment. Repetitive motions and static, awkward back postures can occur when moving or positioning the patient; these can be particularly awkward and stressful when working with the difficult patient (eld-

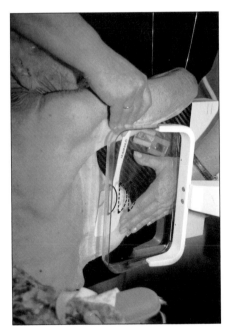

Figure 11.12 Heavy activity can occur when moving and working with patients in wheelchairs.

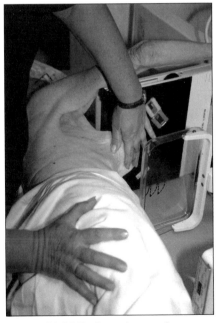

Figure 11.13 Back strain can also occur when positioning patients on stretchers.

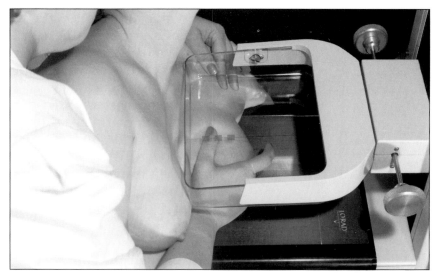

Figure 11.14 Stand as close as possible to the patient; keep your arms close to your body when positioning her.

erly, frail, kyphotic, very ill, physically impaired) or with a patient in a wheel-chair or on a stretcher.

Another less obvious example of this type of activity accurs when a mammographer performs multiple bending and twisting movements as part of their regular work tasks. For example, mammography darkrooms are typically very small and compact. The technologist can often remain in one position (or very close to one position) to unload her cassettes, turn (twisting her back) to feed the film into the processor, then turn again and bend over to remove a film from the film bin (located beneath the counter – film is usually *low* in the bin) then straighten up and turn to reload the cassette with the new film. A normal work pattern will repeat these motions two to four times for every examination.

Also, when unloading supplies in a small, confined area, avoid performing a twist and turn (to reach the item) and then another twist and turn to place the

 One of the more critical personal risk factors is an individual's own personal experience and knowledge regarding proper body mechanics and work techniques and how that knowledge is applied at work and at home.

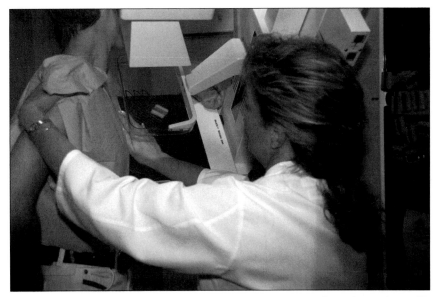

Figure 11.15 Working with outstretched arms at a distance from the patient will result in much more stress for the back and the upper extremity.

item on a nearby shelf. Instead, keep your head, back, and pelvis straight and aligned; turn your whole body to pick up the item, then, using your feet, again turn your body as one unit to place the item on a shelf or counter.

Personal risk factors for individuals include the following characteristics:

- weight of the technologist
- height of the technologist
- age of the technologist
- past medical history
- fitness level of the technologist
- the individual's work knowledge

Obesity has been associated with an increase in an individual experiencing or reporting lower back pain. One of the more critical personal risk factors is an individual's own personal experience and knowledge regarding proper body mechanics and work techniques and how that knowledge is applied at work and at home. Taking the time to set up the work environment, incorporating proper body mechanics, and using work-relief methods can reduce the risk of lower back injury. Similar precautions and strategies should be utilized in the home since both environments have a significant and cumulative impact on the overall health and general physical condition of the mammographer.

Prevention techniques fall into four primary categories: body mechanics, job design, work-area set up, and work-relief strategies.

a. Body Mechanics

- Always practice the principles of good posture.
- Encourage the client to assist you when you are moving and positioning her at the mammography equipment.
- Stand as close as possible to the client and keep your arms as close as possible to your body as you position the patient for her mammogram (Figure 11.14).
- In the darkroom, avoid using a stationary foot position combined with bend and turn movements that *twist* your entire body. Instead, keep your trunk and pelvis aligned and change your foot position to move your body as a single unit for each motion.
- Obtain assistance when working with a patient in a wheelchair or on a stretcher.

Use the following techniques when you are lifting:

- Take the time to lift properly.
- Avoid rushing. Take the time to do the job right without injury.
- Use smooth, fluid motions when lifting.
- Move in as close to the load as possible before lifting.
- Crouch rather than bend the back, keep the trunk upright on a stabilized pelvis, and lift with the legs, when possible.
- Use your legs rather than your back to turn.
- Maintain a balanced stance, with feet wide apart and arms (and elbows) remaining adjacent to your sides. Shoulders should remain in a neutral position (not stretching up) and your arms and shoulders should be stabilized – shoulders should not move; do not reach forward or sideways with arms; and do not twist and bend your back. Movement will occur by shifting your weight from one leg to the other, moving your body as one unit.

Stand as close as possible to the client and keep your arms as close as possible to your body as you position the patient for her mammogram.

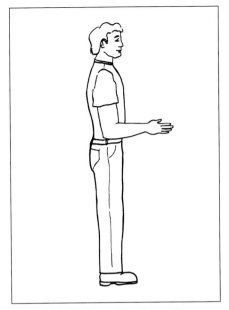

Figure 11.16 *Neutral* back position

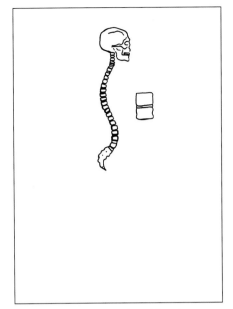

Figure 11.17 *Cervical and Lumbar* curvature of the spine

- Push or pull with a straight back (the neutral position), as illustrated in Figure 11.16, maintaining the natural curves of the back as illustrated in Figure 11.17.
- Push rather than pull whenever possible.
- Minimize the strain and pressure on the muscles and the discs by:
  - evenly distributing the load
  - sharing an oversized load with another person
  - using a lifting aid when available
  - alternating tasks when possible
  - obtaining assistance when you have a heavy load
- Obtain assistance when moving or positioning a patient in a wheelchair or on a stretcher.
- Use a footstool when lifting heavy racks out of the film processor for cleaning.
- As you work to position the client for her mammogram, be sure that you are not attempting to support her weight. The patient should always feel stable as you position her for her mammogram. Encourage the patient to remove high heels or any other footwear that may cause her to be unsteady when she assumes various body positions for her examination. Also, position her feet shoulder width apart; this will provide a broad base of balance and minimize the probability that the

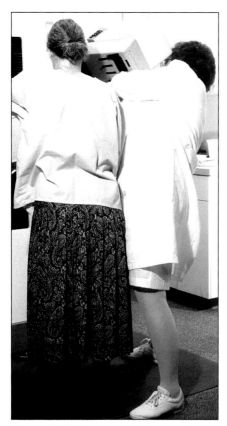

Figure 11.18 Poor positioning techniques will result in unnecessary back strain and muscle fatigue.

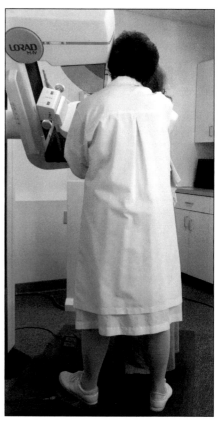

Figure 11.19 Always practice good posture habits as you position your patients.

client may lean toward or sway into your body as you position her for the examination. Take advantage of her proximity to the x-ray equipment; encourage her to *lean into* the unit and utilize the handlebars for security whenever possible.

b. Job Design

- Alternate work that will allow for a change of posture, such as sitting or standing.
- Alternate tasks that involve heavy lifting (carrying boxes of film and chemicals) or frequent bending.
- Ensure that you take regular breaks throughout the workday.

c. Work-Area Set Up

- Raise your work area whenever possible to minimize bending motions. Even small measures will be helpful over time. For example, if you frequently bend over to dispose of paper, labels, etc., during your work day, consider raising the garbage can on a stand to minimize the need to bend over.
- Ensure that frequently handled items such as cassettes, compression paddles, and alternate sizes of image receptors are conveniently located between knee and shoulder height.
- Use a step stool to reach for items above shoulder level.
- Avoid placing cassettes on the floor, leaning against the wall after each exposure. The numerous stooping motions performed are very difficult and tiring for the back. Place exposed cassettes on a counter or shelf; alternately, some facilities mount a narrow *box* to the wall at elbow level to provide a convenient receptacle for cassettes.
- The processor feed tray in the darkroom should be located at elbow level to minimize the number of stooping motions the technologist performs each day.
- Countertops in the darkroom, where film loading and unloading tasks are performed regularly throughout the day, should also be located at elbow height. This will be difficult to achieve when you have multiple technologists using the same work area, so it is advised that ergonomic design principles are used when selecting a proper counter height.
- Unexposed film storage can be located in light-tight counter-top storage units; such units are commercially available. This option would eliminate the motion (which is performed 4 times for each examination) of bending over and reaching down into the standard under-counter film bin during film loading and unloading tasks.
- Raise the position of the film boxes in the under-counter film bin so that you will not have to bend over as far to reach the film.
- When purchasing a film processor, note the height of the collection area where film will be deposited as it leaves the processor. Some manufacturers have designed their processors to deposit processed films in a tray on the top surface of the unit at the end of the processing cycle. This is a great improvement over those that deposit films in a bin

 When positioning the patient, stand as close to her as possible in order to avoid excessive reaching and bending.

Raise your work area whenever possible to minimize bending motions.

near the floor; this latter design requires the technologist to bend over each time she retrieves a film from the processor. Many mammography processors are small and compact; they are frequently mounted on a stand or base structure. This presentation will alleviate the problem of excessive bending on the part of the technologists as they retrieve their processed images.

- The countertop beneath viewbox areas should be narrow from front to back to eliminate excessive forward trunk flexion, shoulder elevation, and stretching of the legs and knees when closely examining films with a magnifying glass for detail and for artifacts.
- Shelving that houses the files with the day's previous mammography examinations should be easily accessible and located between waist and shoulder height to minimize back strain as the technologist searches to locate these documents for each examination. Clearly marked charts with large lettering and perhaps color-coding will facilitate quick access to individual charts without the need for an intense, focused search each time.

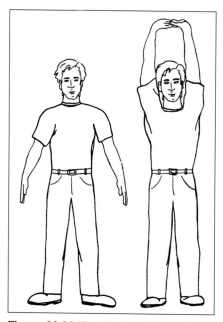

Figure 11.20 The *Overhead Stretch* exercise

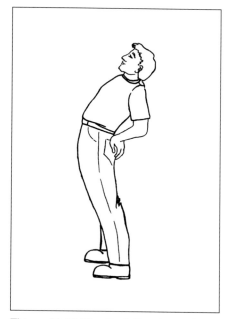

Figure 11.21 The *Back Bend* exercise

d. Work Relief Strategies

- Stretches. Remember to check with your healthcare provider to ensure that these stretches are safe for you. Discontinue any stretch if it causes pain or severe discomfort.

i. Abdominal Tucks

- Sit or stand upright.
- Slowly pull in your abdominal muscles.
- Hold for a count of three, then push outward.
- Repeat three times.

ii. Overhead Stretch

- Stand in a relaxed position.
- Bring hands together and interlock the fingers.
- Gradually raise your hands upward as if a cable were pulling your hands up.
- Hold for a count of three, then relax.
- Repeat three times.

iii. Back Bend

- Ensure this stretch is performed slowly and easily.
- Stand with feet shoulder width apart and knees slightly bent.
- Place hands on back just below the waist with fingers pointing downwards.
- Take a breath and while breathing out, with your hands slowly push your lower body forward at the hips and lean backwards with your upper body.
- Keep your head upright.
- Ensure you only stretch in comfort and do not cause pain.
- Hold position for a few seconds before returning to upright position.

3. Shoulder and Neck Discomfort

Individuals performing mammography examinations frequently report shoulder and neck pain. In some cases, job tasks can contribute to the onset of shoulder tendonitis, chronic shoulder pain, and tension neck syndrome. In industry, factors that can contribute to the onset of pain and discomfort, and over the long term, shoulder and neck disorders include:

- stressful positions or movements
- static (fixed) work
- heavy or forceful work
- high frequency of performed tasks
- insufficient recovery or rest pauses

In mammography, the primary risk factors include stressful positions, static work, high frequency, and insufficient recovery times. Stressful positions may occur when the technologist is positioning the patient and operating the mammography equipment. Both of these tasks are frequently performed with outstretched arms at elevated levels; holding these positions for prolonged times will result in a great deal of upper extremity stress (Figures 11.15 and 11.22).

Figures 11.23 through 11.29 illustrate a neutral position of the shoulder as well as non-neutral or stressful shoulder and elbow positions. It is important to note that each non-neutral position, in isolation, is not a concern. However, when it is frequently repeated or if it is held in position for extended periods of time, undue stress and strain can be placed on the musculoskeletal system. Static work and frequent positions occur when holding and positioning the patient, when performing routine darkroom and film processing duties, and when conducting clerical and general office functions. Insufficient recovery often occurs when the work pace is high with limited physical task variety such as might be experienced when working on site with a mobile mammography unit. These conditions are frequently combined with extended work hours to maximize the utility of this equipment in remote areas. As well, the mobile environment is frequently accompanied with less-than-ideal conditions for the work area set-up. Together, these factors have a greater potential to stress the musculoskeletal system; technologists must be particularly cognizant of correct body mechanics in these situations. Whenever similar working conditions (high volume, limited relief activity, and extended hours) exist in any situation, the same increased potential for stress and injury are present and should be acknowledged. Technologist education and awareness are critical to address.

Prevention strategies can be incorporated into your everyday routine. These strategies fall into four primary categories: body mechanics, job design, work-area set up, and work-relief strategies.

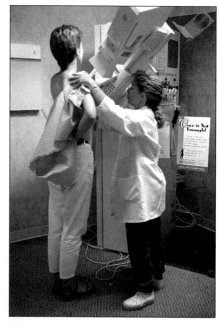

Figure 11.22 Positioning the patient with outstretched arms at elevated levels is very stressful for the upper extremities.

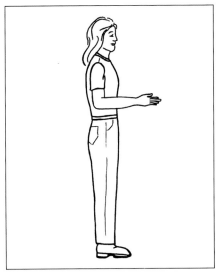
Figure 11.23 *Neutral* shoulder position

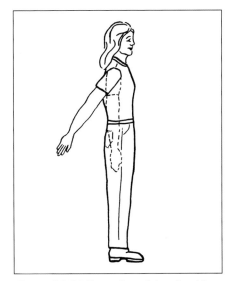
Figure 11.24 *Extension* of the shoulder

a. Body Mechanics

- When positioning the patient, stand as close to her as possible in order to avoid excessive reaching and bending (Figure 11.14).
- When adjusting the position of the equipment, try not to reach across your body to activate the C-arm controls (Figure 11.30); instead, reach with the arm that is on the same side as the C-arm control keypad.

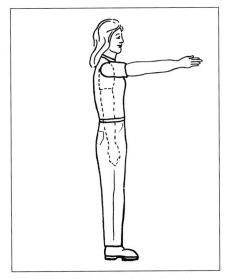
Figure 11.25 *Flexion* of the shoulder

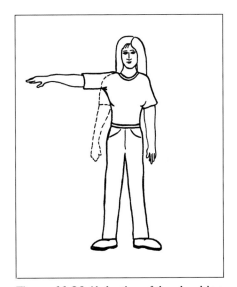
Figure 11.26 *Abduction* of the shoulder

- Encourage the patient to assist with positioning her body properly in front of the equipment whenever possible. Also encourage her to lean against the equipment for support and to use the handlebars whenever possible to help her feel secure and steady.
- Avoid postures that position your head in front of your body with your chin extending forward (poking your head forward and looking down to check your patient's position as you perform the mammogram), particularly for an extended period of time.

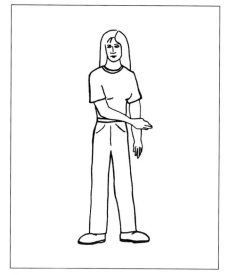

Figure 11.27 *Adduction* of the shoulder

Maintain the correct alignment of the head with the body (ears should line up with shoulders) to minimize excessive neck tension (Figure 11.32).
- Carry heavy equipment and cassettes as close to your body as possible.
- Avoid tight, restrictive clothing that will inhibit arm and shoulder movement.

b. Job Design

- Incorporate task rotation into your job: alternate tasks such as positioning patients and taking mammograms with processing films, darkroom duties, and clerical functions.
- Monitor the degree of overtime associated with your job.
- Be sure to take regular breaks; maximize these times to relieve tense muscles.
- Investigate the feasibility of alternating the work environment between the mobile unit and another office site on a regular basis.

c. Work-Area Set Up

- Position films and supplies between knee and shoulder height. If items need to be positioned above shoulder height, use a platform or step stool to reduce excessive reaching.
- Try to position items frequently used within a comfortable reach (16 to 18 inches from the body) to avoid excessive forward reaching.
- The selection of *user-friendly* equipment at the time of purchase will have a major impact on the physical parameters that the technologist

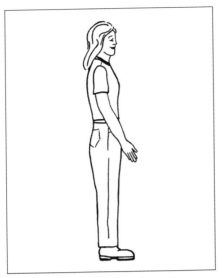

Figure 11.28 *Extension* of the elbow

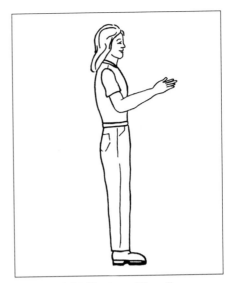

Figure 11.29 *Flexion* of the elbow

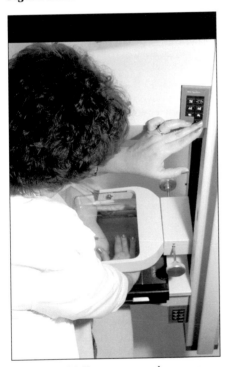

Figure 11.30 Try not to reach across your body, between yourself and the patient, using your opposite hand to activate the equipment controls; instead use the hand closest to the controls or use the foot pedal functions to prevent back strain.

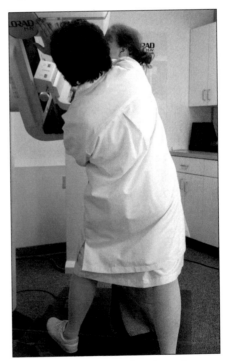

Figure 11.31 Clinical situation where *twisting* and *lateral back movement* is illustrated. Refer to Figures 11.10 and 11.11 as well.

will experience. Most modern mammography equipment has now incorporated multiple motorized movements of the C-arm. This has dramatically reduced the force and energy required to manipulate the equipment into a variety of positions during the examination; previously the technologist's upper extremities, in particular the shoulders, bore the burden of this physically demanding task. Also, the control keypads that house the C-arm drive controls are frequently located in multiple locations, all within arm's reach of the *average* technologist (Figure 4.188). This too has reduced the strain of reaching for controls that may be located in awkward or distant locations. Many of these control keypads provide tactile *codes* to allow the operator to select a variety of functions without having to stretch or strain for visual confirmation of the correct key selection.

- A large magnifying glass mounted on a flexible arm and attached to the viewboxes used to examine images as they emerge from the film processor is a helpful tool. This presentation can provide alternate relief for the technologist's arms compared to the similar raised position that they must maintain during patient positioning.

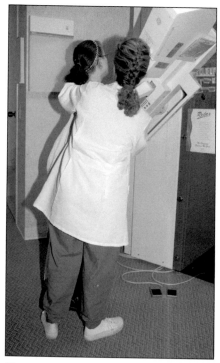

Figure 11.32 Maintain correct alignment of your head, trunk, and pelvis as much as possible while you perform your job tasks.

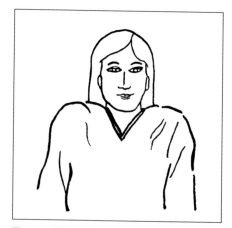

Figure 11.33 The *Shoulder Shrug* exercise

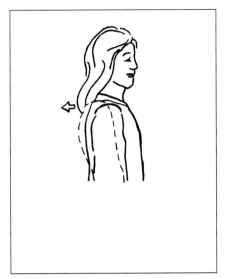

Figure 11.34 The *Shoulder Squeeze* exercise

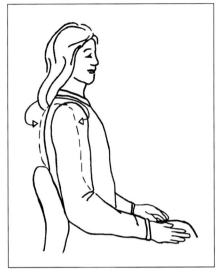

Figure 11.35 *The Shoulder Rotation* exercise

d. Work-Relief Strategies

- Incorporate a variety of stretches before work and during the workday. Remember to check with your healthcare provider to ensure that these stretches are safe for you. Discontinue any stretch if it causes pain or severe discomfort.

i. Shoulder Shrug

- Sitting up straight, slowly bring your shoulders up.
- Hold, then bring your shoulders down and hold.
- Repeat three times.

ii. Shoulder Squeeze

- Gently push your shoulders back.
- Hold for a count of three.
- Relax.
- Repeat three times.

iii. Shoulder Rotation

- Slowly rotate both shoulders backward for a count of ten.
- Then slowly rotate both shoulders forward for a count of ten.
- Repeat three times.

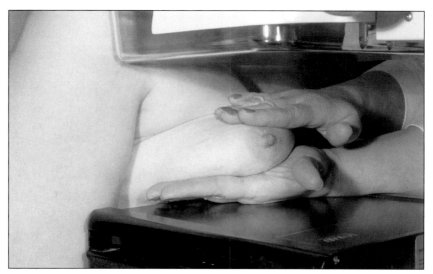

Figure 11.36 The mammographer's hands are her most valuable and most frequently used positioning *tools*; they are invaluable in performing her job tasks.

4. Hand and Wrist Discomfort

Finally, mammographers often report hand and wrist pain. The mammographer's hands are some of the most important and frequently used *tools* that are required for patient positioning (Figures 11.36, 11.37, and 11.38). They

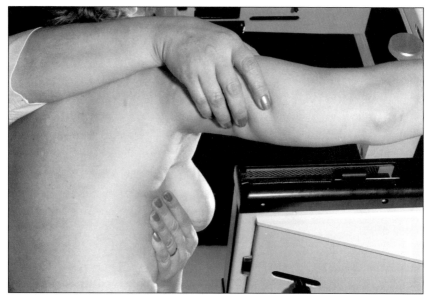

Figure 11.37 Awkward hand and wrist positions are frequently encountered during the process of patient positioning.

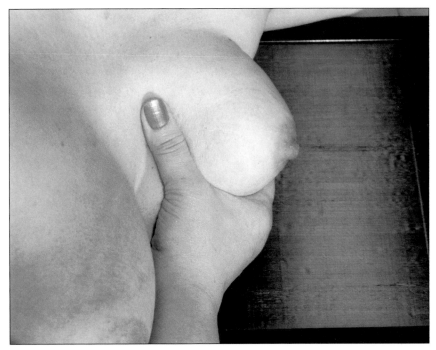

Figure 11.38 High force may also be experienced by he hand and wrist during patient positioning.

perform a critical function by continually lifting, holding, supporting, pulling, and stretching; the pressure and weight they support can be substantial with large, heavy breasts. Cumulative exposure to mammography tasks can contribute to the onset of tendonitis, tendosynovitis, carpal tunnel syndrome, and ganglionic cysts. Industry work related risk factors include:

- awkward wrist positions
- high frequency
- long duration
- high force
- vibration
- cold temperature
- exposure to hard edges

The primary risk factors that mammographers are exposed to include position, force, frequency, and duration. It is the combination of the aforementioned factors that can contribute to the onset of a cumulative trauma disorder and/or hand/wrist discomfort. High force can occur when carrying heavy items like a bucky. Concerns about force could also apply when handling cassettes, includ-

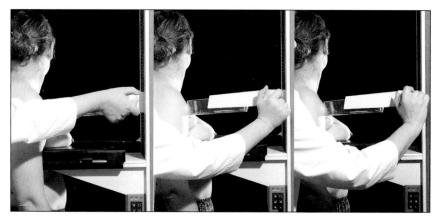

Figure 11.39 This exaggerated demonstration of operating the manual compression control illustrates the wide range of position that the wrist may encounter.

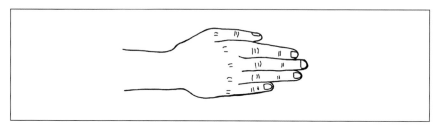

Figure 11.40 *Neutral* wrist position

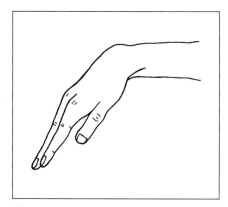

Figure 11.41 *Flexion* of wrist

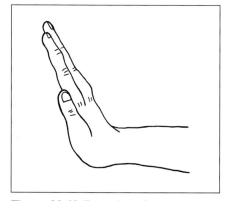

Figure 11.42 *Extension* of wrist

 When handling the breast, try to use the entire hand rather than just using the fingers or the fingertips.

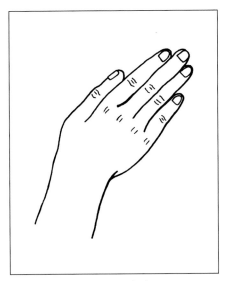

Figure 11.43 *Ulnar* deviation

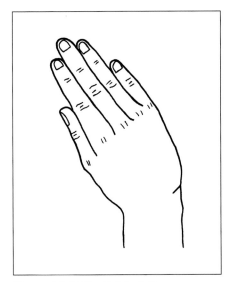

Figure 11.44 *Radial* deviation

 The mammographer's hands (and wrists) are some of the most important __tools__ that are used for patient positioning.

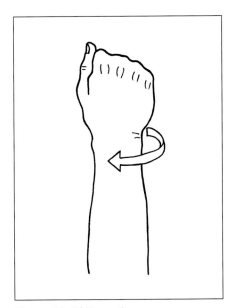

Figure 11.45 *Pronation*

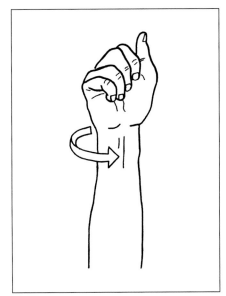

Figure 11.46 *Supination*

ing opening cassettes and pulling or pushing cassettes in and out of the mammography equipment and automatic film identification units.

Additionally, high grip forces can be associated with positioning the breast. High frequency and long duration can be associated with a heavy work pace and poor job design. Awkward hand and wrist positions may be associated with positioning the patient and the breast, operating the manual compression control (Figure 11.39), and with manipulating cassettes and equipment accessories. Figures 11.40 through 11.46 illustrate neutral and non-neutral wrist positions.

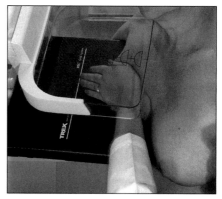

Figure 11.47 Ulnar deviation of the wrist during patient positioning

To reduce the risk associated with the hands and wrists and to prevent fatigue, discomfort, and injury, examine the following preventive strategies. The strategies fall into four categories: body mechanics, job design, work-area set up, and work-relief strategies.

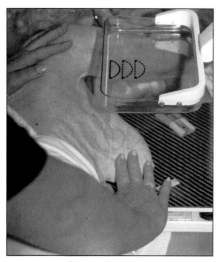

Figure 11.48 Radial deviation of the wrist during patient positioning

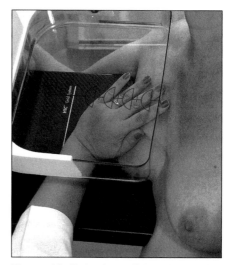

Figure 11.49 Again, radial deviation of the wrist is frequently noted during patient positioning.

Try to maintain neutral wrist positions as much as possible when performing work related tasks.

a. Body Mechanics

- Ensure the equipment is adjusted to the correct height for the patient so that the individual is comfortable. If the machine is not positioned to the proper height, the patient may compensate by standing on her tiptoes or stooping: both postures are difficult to maintain and may contribute to the patient's unsteadiness and tendency to lean against the technologist. Instruct the patient to expect the feeling that the platform where her breast is resting may appear somewhat high. Describe the fact that we deliberately elevate the breast and, although this may feel unnatural to her, this technique is important in obtaining high quality images. Emphasize that her feet should remain flat on the floor and slightly separated at all times during her mammogram. When the patient feels uncomfortable, she will compensate for the awkward posture by continually repositioning the body, thereby moving the breast out of position, and causing the mammographer to repeatedly adjust the breast. Clearly communicated instructions and proper posi-

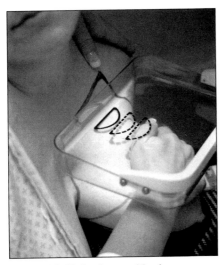

Figure 11.50 During positioning, use your entire hand rather than just your fingers to position, hold and move the breast.

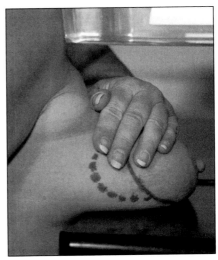

Figure 11.51 Again, the entire hand is used to position the breast; note the radial deviation of the wrist during this positioning maneuver.

tioning of the patient should mini-mize the need for multiple adjust-ments and the accompanying unnecessary, repetitive wrist and hand movements by the tech-nologist.

- When handling the breast, try to use the entire hand (Figures 11.38, 11.50, and 11.51) rather than just using the fingers or the fingertips. Using only the finger-tips can increase hand and wrist discomfort due to the high forces associated with the *grasp* that will be required to control and manipulate a heavy breast.
- When opening cassettes, try to alternate using your fingers and your thumbs. Also, using more than one finger to open the cas-sette will distribute the forces to more than one structure.

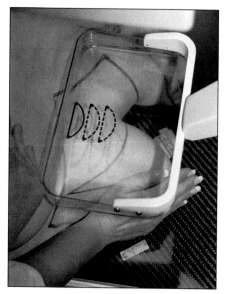

Figure 11.52 Try to maintain a neutral wrist position as much as possible when performing work related tasks.

- Vary the position of your hands and the film cassettes when opening these devices in the darkroom. Sometimes position the latches facing you and occasionally turn them away from you. For variety, you can leave the cassette standing on end while you release the latches, then lie it down on the counter top to unload the film. Using a variety of methods to open the cassettes will prevent repetitive stress on the same muscles and tendons in your hands and wrists.
- Always handle cassettes and equipment accessories with two hands rather than one.
- Try to maintain neutral wrist positions as much as possible when performing work related tasks (Figure 11.52). Avoid using wrist splints at work since splints will reduce movement and increase the risk of incorporating compensatory awkward movements of the shoulder and elbow.

b. Job Design

- Incorporate task rotation into your job.
- Try to control the work pace to prevent extended periods of muscle fatigue.
- Avoid extended hours on a regular basis.

- Take regular breaks during your workday.
- Incorporate work-relief exercises into your daily routine.

c. Work-Area Set Up

- Ensure that counter tops are at the optimum working height for cassette loading and unloading in the darkroom.
- Ensure that equipment accessories fit adequately without being overly tight; installing and removing them will then require the use of excessive force.
- When the technologists choose to wear protective gloves for mammography positioning, ensure that they fit properly. Oversized or undersized gloves can increase the grip forces required to manipulate the equipment.

d. Work-Relief Strategies

- Incorporate stretches into the work routine. Remember to check with your healthcare provider to ensure that these stretches are safe for you. Discontinue any stretch if it causes pain or severe discomfort.

i. Finger Stretch

- Stretch fingers of both hands wide.
- Slowly close them as you bring fingers together into a relaxed fist.
- Stretch fingers again.
- Hold for a count of three.
- Repeat three times.

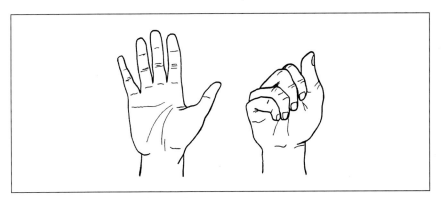

Figure 11.53 *Finger Stretch* exercise

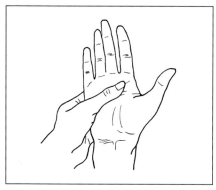

Figure 11.54 *Hand Massage* exercise

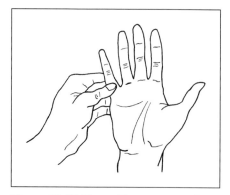

Figure 11.55 *Finger Massage* exercise

ii. Handshake
- Put you hands to your sides with your fingers pointing down.
- Shake them gently.

iii. Hand Massage
- Massage both sides of the hand by using your thumb and your fingers.
- Use gentle pressure.

iv. Finger Massage
- Massage fingers of each hand.
- Starting at the palm, move slowly toward top of the finger.
- Also massage the area between fingers.
- Use gentle pressure.

 It ultimately remains the responsibility of the individual to seriously consider the consequences of poor work habits and to take steps to adopt and use the principles of good body mechanics.

F. CONCLUSION

We all should strive to get through our workday with more comfort and more energy. We all would like to be able to leave our workplace with enough vitality and enthusiasm to enjoy our families and our leisure time. The value and the need for every mammographer to pay attention to her own personal health and fitness is an important factor in both her personal life as well as her career. The level of fitness and vitality that you bring to the workplace has an impact on your ability to cope with the physical, psychological, and emotional demands of your job. Routine mammography tasks can often place the body at risk of developing fatigue and discomfort and may possibly lead to the development of musculoskeletal disorders over an extended period of time.

The physical challenges that the mammographer encounters in her profession have been outlined in this material. The psychological component is equally demanding. Dealing with breast cancer, with women in the midst of its diagnosis, and with women who live in fear of developing it, is an extremely demanding and emotionally draining position to assume on an ongoing basis. Fortunately, mammographers report an extremely satisfying and rewarding sense of fulfillment in helping women work through these crises. Nevertheless, the need for daily renewal of physical energy and spirit is apparent. As well, attention to the work related factors that have the potential to create distress and to practices that can minimize their impact on the body are extremely important. Neglecting these factors may shorten the mammographer's career at a time when the benefit of her years of experience have the potential to be highly advantageous and profitable to her field of specialty. The good news is that musculoskeletal stress and disorders are preventable. However, it ultimately remains the responsibility of the individual to seriously consider the consequences of poor work habits and to take steps to adopt and use the principles of good body mechanics.

It's Your Body
It's Your Job
It's Your Responsibility

 Always handle cassettes and other equipment accessories with two hands rather than one.

The strategies in the preceding material are designed to help you use your body properly, to help you work smarter, and to protect yourself from pain and injury. They can be incorporated into your daily routine with minimal change to your daily work duties and with a minimal investment in time. If these strategies do not reduce fatigue or discomfort, report symptoms to your supervisor and visit a physician for examination and treatment. Additionally, you may want to consider seeking the professional expertise of an ergonomist to evaluate your work tasks and environment to help determine appropriate workplace and work-task modifications that may be applicable to your individual situation.

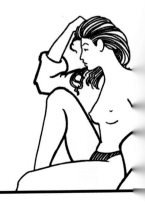

PREFACE TO CHAPTER 12

This chapter was written in hope that the mammography technologist will be able to use the material to create a more positive
experience for the patient and for herself as well. Much of the
information presented here represents the collaborative experience of Louise C. Miller, RTRM, and Shirley M. Long, RTR, CBI.
These authors have a combined practical experience of over
forty years working with mammography patients; they both
continue to work as mammographers to this date in an effort to
practice the principles of their teachings.

In order to include a level of validity and credibility to the
psychological issues that are an integral part of this material, the
advice and participation of a registered, practicing therapist
with extensive experience in these areas was sought. Sandra
Landstedt Thoma, MA, MST, has contributed invaluable information to this chapter with her keen insight and extensive
experience in communications and relationship issues. Her
professional expertise has enabled the authors to present a
more complete, well-rounded and professionally competent
document.

Thank you, Sandy, for your advice and guidance in presenting
these principles to the mammography community.

CHAPTER 12:
PATIENT RELATIONS

CHAPTER 12:
PATIENT RELATIONS

A. INTRODUCTION

Years ago when patients would come for their first, baseline mammogram, many times they had already developed a negative perception of what the examination entailed. Often their impressions were that the technologist was cruel and insensitive and that the examination was painful. Many times patients believed that mammograms were unnecessary in that they often *miss* cancers and that they may, in fact, actually *cause* breast cancer. The patient was often armed with misleading or incorrect information provided by well-meaning friends and relatives. Jokes and poems (i.e. *The Ode to a Mammogram*) and other *humorous* items (i.e. *Instructions for Preparing for a Mammogram)* are widely circulated among patients and proudly *presented* to every mammography technologist. These are understandable attempts to make light of an anxiety-laden situation, but they also can perpetuate the perception that having a mammogram is a negative experience and this consequently tends to erode the mammography technologist's sense of pride and professional respect. As a result, this may also set up a kind of *emotional standoff*. Fortunately, many of these untruths are ignored or have faded as women's familiarity and confidence in mammography has improved. However, problems still exist. Misconceptions, falsehoods, and understandable fears continue to haunt some patients. The media still publishes biased perspectives and misinterpreted data. Patients still ask about the *new procedure* that does not require compression ... or the one where they stand up to a board ... or lie down on a table. It is difficult for the layperson to understand that a new technology must undergo rigorous testing on thousands of women for an extended period of time — years, in fact — in order that we can be certain it will not miss small cancers. Also, many patients do not understand the theory behind breast cancer screening programs; they do not realize that the benefit of early detection is the single most important factor that will influence their chance of surviving this disease. Many women may have had a bad experience with mammography in the past. They may have been hurt or treated in an impersonal, less-than-compassionate fashion. Unfortunately, many negative impressions are still associated with this lifesaving examination; only in exceptional circumstances does the technologist receive compliments or accolades for her efforts. However, this is the work, the responsibility, the privilege, and, often, the frustration of the mammography technologist.

While most technologists are well prepared for the technical challenges of mammography, few have been readied, much less qualified, to deal with the psychological challenges that many patients and situations present. Most patients demonstrate some level of anxiety about mammography. This anxiety can be manifested in a number of ways, some of which, unfortunately, leave the technologist feeling frustrated and even angry. In order to understand the patient, and therefore her behavior, the source of the patient's concern must first be addressed.

B. UNDERSTANDING PATIENT ANXIETY

1. Patient's Relationship With Breasts

Without knowing it, when a mammography technologist first greets a patient that presents at the hospital or office for a mammogram, she is entering into more that just a professional relationship with this woman. She is also entering into whatever personal relationship this woman has with her breasts. Although this may sound unusual, culturally and experientially a woman relates to her breasts as two of her more significant body parts for a myriad of reasons. It is important that the technologist understand this aspect of the patient's feelings as she performs the mammogram; the patient's concerns and feelings can then be acknowledged and treated with respect. This will help to ensure that the patient's current examination will be perceived as important and meaningful. It will also have an impact on the likelihood that the woman will return for future mammography examinations and that she will also willingly participate in her own breast health care. American women, Hispanic women, Asian women, Middle Eastern women, Slavic women, and African women have each been raised with a different understanding of what their breasts mean to them; most often, their cultural teachings have helped to define these concepts. It is this engrained belief system that will influence their feelings about exposing their breasts to strangers as well as having their breasts examined and evaluated with the potential risk of losing one breast, or both, as a result.

2. Breast Symbolism

Women of all cultures generally identify their gender and many times understand themselves *by way of* their breasts. Breasts imply notions of *who we are*. One woman may relate to her breasts as sexual, another as a means to nurture, while yet another sees them as symbols that identify her with motherhood. Most often a combination of interpretations are involved. One woman may be proud of her breasts while another feels shame or embarrassment regarding hers. Identifying factors such as these exist for all women, even if only on a subconscious level.

A woman who is proud of her breasts (and who may rely on them for her identity as a woman) may experience tremendous fear that surpasses concerns with physical disfigurement if she anticipates that her breasts may change in any way. The notion that she might lose them, or that they may change after being treated for *disease* will affect her at the very root of her identity. She firmly believes that changes to her breasts will affect her perceived *identity* as a complete person. This woman may have little difficulty with the mammogram itself; her intense reaction is directed to information or an outcome that does not enhance and support her positive identification with her breasts.

Women who feel embarrassment or shame regarding their breasts may be much more uncomfortable during the mammography examination itself. The focus of their anxiety, however, relates primarily to the prospect of being *seen* and potentially compared with other women. Disease and the possibility of loss only compound the well-established frustration and troubled feelings that they already associate with their breasts. Positive experience and association of any nature regarding their breasts is completely foreign to these women.

Educated, informed women relate to their breasts very differently than do women who have had little exposure to information or who have had limited experience with analytical thinking and problem solving. Educated women are better equipped to deal with factual information regarding their breasts. They are also less likely to assign the responsibility of their personal identity to their breasts; they have no difficulty separating their breasts from the concept of their being as an individual. They are capable of examining information and processing it factually and logically, from an impartial standpoint. They also acknowledge that their questions are valid and that answers to them can and should be pursued. Women with little education or training or those who lack basic information about breast health may not be able to isolate the *condition of their breasts* from the concept of their person as a whole. This would also apply to women who have blindly *bought into* erroneous information or

---

misinformation. They may be unable to logically formulate questions about care, testing, treatment, and outcome; they may be completely paralyzed by the prospect of breast disease.

3. Type of Examination

First time examinees have very different concerns than do women who are repeating the examination in accordance with routine screening guidelines. It is also a completely different experience for the patient who presents with a clinical finding. Each and every patient has her own concerns, her own special needs. If the mammogram is a new experience, the technologist fulfills the role of the teacher who will alleviate stress and familiarize the patient with the procedure to set the stage for future positive experiences. The success of this initial experience is critical. However, when the woman has a history of breast cancer, or is currently being evaluated for this disease, the mammographer will be dealing with fear, anxiety, and anger, all at the same time. The patient's reaction to these emotions can range from denial to apparent disinterest to anger and irritation. The patient may also be imagining what it would be like to lose her breast(s) and to ultimately face impending death. She frequently wants to share these emotions at the time of the mammogram; the anticipation may be that the technologist, who has a wealth of information and experience in these matters, will help to alleviate her feelings and fears.

4. Cultural Considerations

Special consideration should be given to women from different cultures. Those who have maintained a strong identity with that culture and its beliefs even after becoming more *westernized* require special attention. Anecdotal accounts show that most older women who have emigrated from other *less open* cultures (regarding open display of the female body as wrong or unacceptable) are much more uncomfortable about mammography and potentially more embarrassed about exposing their breasts to a stranger. Most of these women do understand the need for mammography, but they still come to the examination reluctantly. This is often the case for older women of the North American culture, where modesty was the norm in their day.

Some cultures prohibit the uncovering of a woman's body for any purpose — extreme sensitivity and patience must be exercised with these patients who are literally entering a new world. The technologist should remain highly sensitive to this patient's needs during the mammogram, and only expose one breast at a time, as required, during the course of the examination.

---

a. Language Barrier

Many times patients speak little, if any, English. This instantly sets up a huge barrier between the technologist and the patient. If at all possible, make sure that a friend or relative who can translate your questions and instructions accompanies the patient into the room. If this is not possible, you may want to try to demonstrate what is about to happen, showing them especially how the compression paddle works: go slowly!

Special attention should be devoted to facial expressions and other visible signs of anxiety. Every attempt should be made to use eye contract and express compassion with demonstrations of caring and concern; a sincere smile goes a long way, particularly when verbal communication is difficult.

b. Cultural Influence

Technologists must also be sensitive to cultural differences regarding mammography, radiation, and breast cancer in general. These differences may influence the patient's individual experience. Ignoring these factors could cause the patient unnecessary concern and embarrassment.

i. Anecdotal Accounts

In order to better understand the effect of cultural influences, an informal survey was done by the authors. The survey was given to mammographers and health care workers who have professional or personal information relating to this topic. The following anecdotes are interesting and revealing; they may be helpful in understanding and caring for these special populations. Please note, however, that these observations may not be typical of all women from the individual cultures represented here. They are only used as examples of varying cultural concerns that relate to mammography; many of them reflect the universal concerns of women from all countries and cultures.

> One time an Indian woman (North American, nation unknown) who lives in our town was diagnosed with breast cancer. Other Indian women would see her on the street and cross to the other side to avoid having to be close to, or possibly touching her ... they were afraid of catching breast cancer.

> My mother emigrated from China ... she is very shy and embarrassed about her breasts ... but she goes to have a mammogram ... only because I drag her there.

I did a patient one time who was from the Middle East ... I didn't know what country ... but it was really difficult to do her mammogram because she was all wrapped up in these robe-type garments. She would not put on a gown. She would not let the radiologist (who is a male) examine her ... even though she had a lump.

I had a patient who was in her mid seventies ... just like my grandmother. When I told her we were going to start her mammogram she kind of looked at me nervously and asked: "Don't I have to take my gown off?" I told her No, not completely...we will just take one arm out at a time when I do the side views. She looked shocked and said "This is the first time anyone has let me keep it on ... every other time I had to stand in front of some stranger half naked ... feeling terribly embarrassed. Thank you SO much!" Then she hugged me. She was obviously very relieved. All I could think of was my grandmother being in the same situation and no one thinking about her feelings.

While working in Japan I learned that it is generally considered rude to look a Japanese person directly in the eye. So, when working with these women or asking for information from them, I now focus on the history sheet or the mammography equipment and I tend to demonstrate how things are done. I try to avoid looking directly at her as much as possible; that way she may be more comfortable with me and with the procedure.

We do a lot of Russian and Polish women. Even though they appear to be stoic I can almost see the fear in their eyes. In their home countries many times the diagnosis of breast cancer means certain death. I think this belief is still well engrained in their minds.

Lots of women from the Navajo community will not come for mammography because the local medicine man told them that radiation was bad for them ... so now they are even more afraid of mammography.

I was in a Latin American country working as a volunteer. The women would come to the mobile van for screening. There were no dressing rooms, no hangers, and no gowns to change into.

About six of them just took off their blouses and sat together in the waiting area in the van and they would go in to have their mammograms one at a time. While they waited I noticed them clutching their blouses to their chests, attempting to cover themselves. They seemed embarrassed. When they had their mammogram, the technologist tucked the patient's shirt into the waistband of her pants or skirt.

During this same visit we were sharing information with their health care professionals about mammography. They wanted to do a TV interview about our work and the new mammography units that were donated to their country. It was decided that it would be helpful if the women of this country could actually see a mammogram being done. Out of possibly twenty of the women working with us from this country, none would volunteer to be the "model". They expressed real concern that someone (especially one of their husbands) may recognize them, even though we promised not to show the model's face. (One of the volunteer group finally agreed to model for us.)

I organize positioning workshops for mammographers throughout the U.S.; we always need models and we pay well for this service. When I ask for volunteers from our attendees, perhaps one in twenty will offer. Everyone has her personal reason for not wanting to do this ... and of course I respect that. However, I am always surprised by how many techs say "I'm way too embarrassed" or "My boobs are too small (or too big)!" or "You wouldn't want me!" Yet I think to myself ... why do they not see themselves as representatives of real patients? and then I think again ... they are! Not only physically ... but even more so in their attitudes about their own breasts.

On a personal level, every technologist can relate to every one of these concerns. However great the anxiety may be with the *average* patient, these feelings will be even more pronounced when dealing with women who exhibit strong cultural influences. In these circumstances the best approach is to be hypersensitive and acutely aware of the issues that have *piqued* the patient's sensitivity in each individual situation and respond accordingly each time.

5. Body Image

Women of all cultures frequently exhibit conflicting thoughts about their personal body image ... and how others may perceive it ... especially the mammographer, who is often, virtually, a complete stranger. An interesting phenomenon we see in North American culture is the *glorification* of *perfect* breasts. Average, *normal* women may frequently compare themselves, their bodies and in particular, their breasts with those of models, actresses, and others whose representation in the media exemplifies this unrealistic form of perfection. Many times women may feel that they do not *measure up*. This perception and the associated negativity will further complicate their feelings about having a mammogram. Often modest, self-conscious, or unsure about her breasts (*Are they normal?*), the patient may internalize this conflict. This represents a major source of patient anxiety.

a. Normal vs. Abnormal

Occasionally women's feelings of inadequacy may go so far as to affect their desire to have a mammogram. They realize that the examination may indicate that their breasts *have a problem*; some women may even lose their breast(s) as a result of the mammogram. These *outcomes* fit very conveniently into their well-established negative mindset. Because they believe their breasts are not *perfect*, they may secretly suspect that they are probably *damaged*. An insecure patient may believe that diseases are indeed *warranted* or even *expected*; this follows the pattern of disappointment and inferiority that they have always associated with their breasts.

A woman may be extremely reluctant to have a mammogram if insecurity or negativity relating to her breasts has left her feeling *defeated* and *crushed*. If the patient is already convinced that she is inadequate, she may resist putting herself in a situation where this information may be blatantly confirmed, and in fact, *made public* (reports to doctor, etc.). Furthermore, this whole process will focus a lot of attention on a part of her anatomy that she would prefer to ignore. Doctors may have to examine her; she may incur additional appointments and more examinations. She will have to talk about her breasts; a lot of people will have to *look* at them — they will be the focus of far too much attention. To complicate matters further, she may then proceed to gather more information (i.e. a *bad* diagnosis) that supports these feelings of inadequacy. For any patient who is struggling with uncomfortable feelings such as these, it is an act of courage to make and follow through with their initial mammography examination.

Patients whose breasts have been scrutinized or made fun of (i.e. too flat, too big, etc. compared to someone else's, etc.), even if this has been done in their closest circles, may already be dealing with some level of shame about their body. They may have reacted to this treatment in either a defensive manner or simply with defeat. The technologist may experience this anger, depression, and/or fear when the patient comes for the mammogram. Often these underlying feelings are difficult to interpret and the technologist may simply experience undue negativity from the patient.

The mammography patient population includes women who represent a wide variety of experiences, thoughts, and impressions; their behavior will often serve as a signal for understanding their underlying emotional state. It is essential for the mammographer to acknowledge the gamut of emotions that the patient may be experiencing and consider how these perceptions may have an impact on the examination at hand. No matter how unrealistic or unfounded these feelings may be, to the patient they are very real; never dismiss or trivialize the patient's emotions.

C. MANIFESTATIONS OF ANXIETY: HOW IT AFFECTS PATIENT BEHAVIOR

Chinese Proverb:

A little anxiety helps to focus the mind ...
but too much paralyzes it.

It is important that the mammography technologist has some understanding of the anxiety phenomenon that often accompanies examinations of all types.

1. Anxiety Defined

Anxiety is an apprehension, tension, or uneasiness that comes from the anticipation of danger, the source of which is unknown or unrecognized. It also results from the threat of losing something we believe to be essential to our well being, such as an important relationship or physical wholeness. Both of these definitions apply to the mindset of the woman coming for a mammogram. The patient anticipates an unfamiliar examination process, discomfort, and uneasiness during the examination itself, and the anticipation of an unknown result with the very real potential for the loss of well-being. This very accurately describes many aspects of the mammography examination from the patient's perspective: Will it hurt? Will the technologist think my breasts are ugly? Will I have to wait a long time for the results? What will the results be? It is important that they realize that all of these *unanswered* questions, initially at least, represent the perspective of a typical mammography patient; they also contribute to and serve as a basis for anxiety.

2. Indications of Anxiety

Patients experience anxiety in a variety of ways and with varying intensities. There are many characteristic signs of anxiety that the mammography technologist should be aware of and watch for with her patients.

a. Physical Signs

- Sweating.
- Shortness of breath.
- Increased pulse and respiration.
- Dizziness.
- Fidgeting (with clothing, tissues, jewellery, etc.).

b. Behavioral Signs

- Seeming unable to hear clearly and needs you to repeat instructions.
  How to change: the classic example is telling the patient to take everything off from the waist up only to return and find she may still be confused as to what to do.

- Childlike responses.
  Giggling, making jokes, need to be led and shown what to do.

- Hypersensitivity — both physically and emotionally.
  Excessive or inappropriate laughing or crying.

- Over-personalizing any comment you may make pertaining to her.
  What do you mean I am too dense?

- Being unable to follow instructions (literally).

- Amplifying certain trigger words and taking them out of context (i.e. tumor, mass, cancer, abnormality, dense).
  Technologist: *We have to do two more (films).*
  Patient: *I have a tumor?*

- Blanking out.
  Emotional discomfort is so high that she may be dizzy or unre-sponsive.

- Lack of affect: numbness or blocking.
  Patient may not speak at all because anxiety is so high that she is unable to formulate her thoughts into words. By the same token, she may react to stress by blocking her feelings. Her feelings may not register at all; this patient appears to be numb.

- Fear of going crazy or dying, in extreme cases.

c. Hiding Anxiety

Some patients may handle their anxiety by attempting to mask it. They may do this by:

- Excessive Talking.

- Attempting to control the examination by directing or instructing the technologist.
  You're not doing it the same way I had it done last time ... what you are doing is not right.

- Insisting on speaking with the Radiologist or other authority.
  I will not leave until the doctor tells me the results!

- Being embarrassed and making derisive comments about themselves
  I'll bet you have never done breasts this small before ... there's not much to work with.

- Making derisive comments to and about the technologist.
  How can you stand to do this all day? What a terrible job.

- Becoming angry.
  I will not let you take any more films ... NO ... you are done ... that's it!

- Over intellectualizing: talking only about terminology and research to stay above or to distract from her emotional feelings.
  I read a study that says that compression can actually spread cancer cells throughout the breast. Why don't you have the new equipment that doesn't require compression, such as MRI?

3. Technologist Interaction

The most important factor for technologists to recognize is that patient anxiety and the accompanying behavior the patient manifests are not personal in nature. They represent coping mechanisms that the patient is using in order to personally manage the experience of the examination at hand. It is important to recognize what is happening and especially to avoid reacting to the inappropriate behavior(s). Reaction to these types of behaviors will intensify the emotional component of the interaction and the situation will deteriorate rapidly. A professional technologist will not enter the patient's emotional state; instead she will continue to guide and reassure the woman through the examination.

4. Anxiety and Fear

It is also important to distinguish between anxiety and fear. Anxiety is the uneasiness associated with the unknown, while fear is the anticipation of what is known, or thought to be known. The mammography technologist will deal with both of these emotions in her patient interactions. The patient may be anxious about the unfamiliarity of both the examination and the outcome, or actually fearful of the examination itself or the potential results (i.e. tumor, abnormality, *I may lose my breast, I may die*). The technologist must respond to all of these feelings in a professional manner.

With the information presented in this chapter, the technologist will better understand patient anxiety and the resulting behavior. However, it is not the job of the technologist to sort out the motivation of fear or anxiety for each patient. It is much better to handle these symptoms very objectively and to answer the patient's questions directly, without the need to fully analyze their meaning and origin. It is better to simply reassure the patient about the wisdom of baseline and screening examinations and the improved statistics for everyone who perseveres through their anxiety to have them done. Furthermore, the patient may not expect answers to all of her personal questions. Instead she may simply need to be reassured by the technologist's ability to relay basic, general information and she may want to analyze the technologist's comfort level in addressing her inquiries. Subtle, telltale signs of insecurity may disclose that the technologist is hesitant to discuss a subject — the anxious patient may immediately interpret the reluctance to indicate that a very serious problem exists (breast cancer, which the technologist is attempting to mask or hide).

In your interaction with your patient, rather than personalizing and using the word *You* (when explaining to or reassuring the patient) it is best to be objective and speak in the *third person* concerning technical information. This is helpful in explaining the more *impersonal aspects of the examination.* Examples of this third person type of information would be:

Most women tend to be concerned about the compression.

Studies (or research) show that mammography is very safe and does not harm the breast with compression or radiation.

Statistically many women are nervous about having a mammogram ... but they find, after their first examination, that many of their concerns have been alleviated.

Note: Please see the Communication section of this chapter for additional examples.

Also, it is important for the technologist to demonstrate warmth and caring about the non-technical components of the examination. Examples include greeting the patient, telling the patient how to change, and other such issues that are more *personal*.

Another important consideration when addressing patient anxiety is to remember that:

Anxiety Clouds Intake

In a highly anxious state, a patient will only hear a limited amount of your explanations, instructions, and reassurances. Repetition may be necessary for the technologist and the patient in order to overcome this barrier.

The patient's behaviour will often serve as a signal to indicate her underlying emotional state. It is essential for the mammographer to acknowledge the gamut of emotions that the patient may be experiencing and consider how these perceptions may have an impact on the examination at hand. No matter how unrealistic or unfounded these feelings may be, to the patient they are very real; never dismiss or trivialize the patient's emotions.

5. Detecting Anxiety: Quick Survey

Mammography technologists deal with emotionally charged situations on a regular and rather constant basis. It is important to become skilled in the process of quickly surveying *who* it is you are dealing with; then try to anticipate what her potential concerns are likely to be. Later in this chapter we will continue to explore ways to address patient anxiety within the bounds of the mammographers' professional role.

a. What to look for . . .

Avoidance of eye contact
Arms crossed across chest
Fidgeting with purse, tissues, or clothing
Perspiring noticeably
Shortness or holding of breath

b. What to listen for . . .

Talking excessively
Not talking at all
Blocking behavior ... seems not to take in any information
Nervous laughter
Repeating questions
Asking for reassurance that they are doing right
Comments about their personal (or other patients') breast size
A *Let's get this over with* message

The information that has been presented here will serve as a basis for understanding the mammography patient. With this information, the technologist is able to be more empathetic. The ability to recognize and detect the behaviors that indicate anxiety will help the technologist to address the emotional condition of the patient. Rather than reacting to inappropriate comments or behavior in a negative manner or becoming needlessly defensive, the technologist can work toward easing the patient's stress by addressing her questions and comforting her in a professional manner. Perhaps more importantly, the technologist will be able to guide the patient through the examination with competence and confidence. This will set the stage for creating a more positive experience for both the patient and the technologist for this and future examinations.

D. CREATING THE POSITIVE MAMMOGRAPHY EXPERIENCE

There are several factors involved in creating a positive experience for the mammography patient. In additional to understanding her concerns and behavior, there are specific skills and traits that are both important and necessary in order to ensure success. There are four components that will help address the issues that are important for a successful interaction with the patient.

Key Components for a Positive Mammography Experience

- ***Competence***
- ***Communication***
- ***Comfort***
- ***Caring***

Although each of these components will be discussed separately, it is important to remember that each individual component interacts with the others in order to create a complete and successful interaction with and for the patient.

1. Competence — Purpose and effectiveness

Competence equates to *Confidence*. The more competent that the technologist is, the more confident she will appear to the patient. The patient senses when the technologist knows what she's doing. The patient also senses when this is not the case; uncertainty and hesitancy on the part of the technologist may be evident, and these perceptions could result in additional patient anxiety.

The patient is often acutely aware and alert to every small detail that she senses during the mammography examination: her hyper-anxious state will be very attuned to the most subtle hints from the technologist's behavior, body language, etc.

In the current environment of ongoing controversy regarding the efficacy of mammography, some patients may question the validity of the examination as well as the qualifications of the technologist. When the technologist does not demonstrate confidence or appears hesitant or uncertain, the patient may interpret this behavior as a lack of competence. As a result, the patient may feel that she has received an inadequate examination.

Conveying confidence to the patient may pose significant problems for technologists whose basic personality may be unusually shy and reserved, and for those who are exceptionally soft spoken, or have a very youthful appearance (see section on Role-playing for suggestions). While these are certainly not adverse qualities, the patient's heightened state of anxiety may misinterpret these characteristics as a lack of competence or, at the very least, as evidence of inexperience.

In order to instill a sense of competence and confidence in mammography patients, the technologist must, in fact, possess and emanate these two qualities. Specialized training and experience are not difficult to acquire given the numerous educational opportunities that are required and available for licensed mammography technologists.

a. Instilling Confidence and Competence

- Display licenses, continuing education and seminar certificates, and evidence of other *achievements.* Matte and frame and display them in a prominent area where the patients can easily see them.

- Dress your best ... a professional appearance says a lot.

- Wear your society pins or badges; they are reminders of your accomplishments.

- Exhibit professionalism: makeup, nails, perfume, hairstyle, personal hygiene, etc.

- Maintain an awareness of the patients' feelings and of the sensitive nature of the examination.

- Use appropriate communications skills (see section on Communication).

It is generally not difficult to emulate the qualities that we would each look for when seeking out the services of a health care professional.

The patient is often acutely aware and alert to every small detail that she senses during the mammography examination: her hyper-anxious state will be very attuned to the most subtle hints from the technologist's behavior, body language, etc.

2. Communication — Purpose and Effectiveness

Communication skills are essential in creating a positive experience for your patients. These skills can be extremely effective in alleviating patient anxiety and projecting a professional, yet caring atmosphere.

a. Guidelines ... to Improve Patient Communications

i. Skills

A. Avoid Personalizing ... Use Broad Terminology

Example:
Addressing obvious patient anxiety
INEFFECTIVE RESPONSE:
You look like you are scared.
EFFECTIVE RESPONSE:
Most patients are somewhat anxious about having a mammogram; is there anything I can do to make you more comfortable today?

B. Acknowledge Feelings and Concerns ... Even if You Don't Think They are Valid

Example:
Addressing a previous bad experience reported by the patient
INEFFECTIVE RESPONSE:
I'm sure it couldn't have been that bad.
EFFECTIVE RESPONSE:
I am sorry that you had a bad experience with your last mammogram, but let me tell you how this will be different.

C. Use Understandable Terminology ... be Understandable, Without Being Condescending

Example:
Describing what you are doing when performing the mammogram
INEFFECTIVE RESPONSE:
Now I am going to do the MLOs.
EFFECTIVE RESPONSE:
Now we are going to do some side views of your breasts.

D. **Non-Verbal Signals ... to Help Guide You**
Use the *Quick Test* that was described earlier for detecting anxiety.

E. **Invite Questions ... Before, During, and After the Examination**

F. **Scripts**
Develop samples that are concise, correct and caring
Know each script well enough so you can personalize them
(examples to follow).

G. ***Ease* the Unknown**
Provide explanations whenever possible before each step of the
procedure.

There are many additional situations, other than those described here, in which
these principles can be applied. These suggestions will help prepare you to
deal with each situation in an appropriate manner.

b. Communication Guidelines ...
Effective Use in Mammography Setting

i. Scripts ... samples:

A. Greeting / Introduction:

Introduce yourself. Tell her who you are and what you do ... ask her how she
would like to be addressed.

> *Hi, my name is Joy. I am the technologist who will be working
> with you today. Should I call you Mrs. Smith, or is Kathy OK?*

B. Obtaining History:

Go over pertinent history prior to greeting your patient. Read the intake form
so you understand her history ... and to reassure her that you are familiar with
her individually.

> *I see that you have been here every year for the past three years
> ... and all your mammograms were normal. I also see that you
> had a biopsy on your right breast a few years ago and the results
> were negative.*

c. Examination Preparation:

Ask the patient if she has any questions or concerns ... or if there is anything she would like you to know before you get started.

Do you have any questions or concerns before we get started?

d. Changing ... and Waiting:

In addition to the verbal information that the patient will receive, it is advantageous to have these instructions in written form, printed or posted for the patient's easy access (i.e. on changing room wall). Waiting can be a difficult time for the patient. Give her an approximate time that she will be waiting ... and explain what she is waiting for. It can be helpful to give her some suggestions of things to do while waiting.

I'm going to put on a tape on Breast Self Examination that you can watch while I get the room ready for you. I'll be back in about three minutes.

Here are some brochures on Breast Self Examination that you can read while I'm developing your films. I will be gone about five minutes.

e. Examination Explanation:

It is best not to tell the patient *how many* films you are taking. You may want to develop a script that goes something like this:

We are going to start by taking some pictures of each breast. Some will be from the side, some from the top to bottom. After taking these I will develop them and check to make sure that we have seen all of your breast tissue ... and that we can see through it clearly. If not, I'll be back to take some more pictures to complete the examination. You also probably remember the compression part. It is really important that I position and image your breast properly to get the best pictures possible. Compression is an important part of this process.

This also opens the door to additional films and will help reduce any potential or projected anxiety should this, in fact, be necessary. This explanation also addresses:

a) What will happen

b) In what order

c) The possible variations in routine (additional views)

d) The importance and necessity of your role as a mammography technologist in positioning and compressing the breast. Otherwise the patient may experience *touching* as arbitrary, and not part of the procedure.

F. Apologizing ... When Appropriate

If the patient has had to wait for an unreasonable amount of time, acknowledge this. Not only is this important for the sake of common courtesy, but it also will help to diffuse anxious anger, which we may still have to bear despite our apologies.

> *Mrs. Smith, I am so sorry you have had to wait. I know how frustrating it must be, but I should be with you within five minutes.*

G. Acknowledging Feelings:

Do not discount or minimize her concerns by making light of the situation. Saying things such as *I'm sure everything will be fine* may alleviate immediate anxiety but it may also be untrue and/or very misleading.

> *Most patients are anxious when we have to do additional views ... but I can tell you honestly that it is quite common. They really are just a completion of the examination ... the first four views are just the beginning; from there we continue and add what is needed to give the radiologist (doctor) all the information he/she needs. I will see what I can do to make sure you get the results as soon as possible.*

H. Empathizing:

If the mammogram is especially uncomfortable for her, let her know how much more ... and/or how much longer it will be until you are done. Remind the patient that it is important to do a good and thorough examination.

> *I wish we could do this differently as I can see you are uncomfortable, but we're almost done. We only have the side views left to do. I will try to go quickly, but at the same time make sure we get really good films.*

I. Informing the Patient:

When you leave the room, tell the patient why and when to expect you back.

> *I'm going to develop your films ... that will take about five to ten minutes ... then I'll be back to tell you what else we need to do to finish up your examination.*

This again opens the possibility for additional views and reminds them that possibility exists — in case they did not hear this earlier in your conversation.

J. BSE and CBE ... Providing Information:

Ask you patient whether she has had a physical examination by her doctor (or nurse or NP); encourage her to do so if she has not. You and your patient are partners in her breast health care.

> *Have you had an examination done by your doctor recently and did he/she or you notice any changes? It is such an important part of your breast health care ... as is Breast Self Examination. I have some brochures I can give you ... or perhaps I can answer some questions about it. Please let me know.*

K. Inviting Feedback ... Ask For This

Patients may not offer information readily, especially if they believe the mammogram should hurt (or it won't be good). They may also be *tuning you out*.

> *How are you doing? Is it getting too tight? Compression is not supposed to be painful ... but may be uncomfortable ... please tell me if it gets to be too much, I don't want to hurt you.*

L. Patient Questions ... Prepare For Awkward Questions

It is important to do a visual breast examination to provide information to the radiologist concerning asymmetry, scars, raised skin lesions, nipple characteristics, etc. It may be difficult to ascertain what is *normal* for the patient, and what is not. An example would be when addressing obvious breast asymmetry, or an inverted nipple.

> *Have you noticed any recent change in the size or shape of your breasts (or nipples) when comparing one to the other?*

Be prepared to answer any questions appropriately and with sensitivity. This may be the only time that the patient feels comfortable in asking, and you may

---

be her only resource for information. Answer honestly and with compassion, when appropriate. If the question extends beyond your expertise (i.e. surgical and or treatment options), recommend that she discuss this issue with her doctor. If you don't know the answer to the questions, again, refer her to her physician.

Many of the questions and situations above could be avoided or at the least eased by the development of a *information card* handed to the patient upon her arrival that will explain the mammography procedure in detail: what to expect, when and why. The patient could keep it with her before, during, and after the examination. It will serve as a reference and source of correct information for each patient. This in itself can be a very effective measure in *easing the unknowns.*

Patients may find it helpful to have a bulletin board mounted in an accessible area that is posted with a wide variety of information on breast heath and other women's health issues, such as osteoporosis and hormone replacement therapy. Free brochures are available from many sources for this purpose. A binder may also be kept with the latest news and information about breast cancer detection and/or letters of thanks and appreciation from previous patients.

C. Barriers to Effective Communication

In anxiety-laden situations, there are barriers that may inhibit effective communication despite the skill and desire of the technologist. Each of these barriers must be dealt with appropriately.

i. Anxiety Clouds Intake

Despite your repeated directions or reassurances, a patient may *tune out* what you are saying. This is where repeated instructions or reassurances, whether written, or verbal, may be helpful.

ii. Judgmental Language ... Avoid This With Your Patient

Avoid the use of *should* or *ought to*.

INEFFECTIVE RESPONSE:

> *You really should come and have a mammogram every year between the ages of forty and fifty.*

EFFECTIVE RESPONSE:

> *It is really in a woman's best interest to have a mammogram every year especially between the ages of forty and fifty.*

iii. Overcoming Inexperience

Many of us have never been taught good communication skills; we simply learn as we go. Great strides can be made in this area by merely asking your *non-mammography* technologist friends or simply close friends or family members what made them feel comfortable or uncomfortable about the experience they had during a mammogram. During this discussion, pay attention to detail, like warming your cold hands and staying focused on the patient and not how many people are in the waiting room.

iv. Non-English Speaking Patients

If possible, have brochures available in many languages for your non-English speaking patients. Audio tapes explaining the mammography procedure have been developed for this purpose. Should these resources not be available at your mammography facility, a family member or companion who speaks the language should accompany the patient into the mammography room. The same information and instructions should be given to the patient through the *interpreter*, as described in the section on cultural differences on page 452. This is where eye contact and smiles can go a long way to bridge the gap. Go a little slower and be a little more patient in these situations.

3. Comfort

a. Physical Comfort

Physical comfort plays an extremely important part in creating a positive experience for your patient. Providing comfort involves attention to details. This in turn, will make your patient feel cared for.

i. Décor

- The waiting area can make a strong impression. Décor is important; if possible it should be pleasing and comfortable. Make available current magazines and information about breast health. Offer the patient a printed explanation of the mammography procedure and what she should expect.

ii. Temperature

- Temperature must be monitored so that the patients are comfortable when waiting, especially after changing and during and after the mammogram. Have shawls for thin, elderly patients.

iii. Patient Gowns

- Storage: Patient gowns can be stacked on the top of the processor (if convenient). When grabbing a gown for the next patient, take one from the bottom of the pile, closest to the processor. The gown will be nice and warm, and the patient pleasantly surprised.

- Sizes: A variety of gown sizes should be available so that they will cover each patient appropriately. This is especially important for the large woman. She should never be given two gowns to piece around her.

iv. Information Cards

- Patient information cards and instructional videos should be available for the patients after changing and while they are waiting.

v. Warming the Bucky

- Put a heating pad on the bucky and be sure to keep the heat setting on low. It can be wrapped on top of and under the bucky in a small pillowcase. A strip of Velcro can be placed on the underside of the bucky and a corresponding piece placed on the heating pad cover. This is important so that the cold undersurface of the bucky can also be warmed; this is the part that comes in contact with the patient's abdomen, and most often what they complain about. The top of the heating pad can be held in place with the compression paddle in the down position; the bottom of it will also be heated. Be sure to check with your manufacturer to make sure that the use of the heating bad will not damage the grid. An alternate suggestion is to use a microwave-able pad to warm the bucky. Gel- and bean-filled pads are available for this purpose; they need to be reheated every few hours in the micro-wave oven.

vi. Music

- Have music and/or head phones for patients undergoing longer proce-dures, i.e. core biopsy. Invite the patient to bring her own tapes or CDs or provide an assortment of relaxing music. This has a soothing effect on all involved, and may distract the patient from the anxiety she is feeling. Soft background music can also create a relaxed, soothing environment in the main reception area and in the mammography rooms.

vii. Aromatherapy
- Aromatherapy can be very effective. Many studies have been done that validate the soothing effect of certain scents.

viii. Amenities
- Amenities should be available for your patients: deodorant, baby wipes, lotion, and hairspray are welcome sights for a patient; this demonstrates your attention to detail and your regard for her comfort.

- Clothing Storage: Designate a place to put clothes and have hangers available so clothes don't get wrinkled. Many times a patient is coming from or going to work, or just going about her day. The simple act of pulling a blouse or sweater over her head, and leaving it crumpled on a chair would be unappealing.

b. Emotional Comfort

In most cases, technologists and their patients are meeting for the first time and they are usually complete strangers. Within a very short period of time the technologist is asking the patient for very personal information that even a best friend may not know about, and she then proceeds to be *in the patient's face* (literally, almost face-to-face) for the examination. This very close and personal interaction can make even the most confident patient uncomfortable.

Therefore, one of the more important aspects of the technologist's job is to provide emotional comfort. Understanding and utilizing the concepts that have been presented in this chapter can help to accomplish this. However, the technologist must be cognizant of other issues affecting patient comfort.

i. Patient Modesty

As the examination proceeds, the technologist will need to perform a brief visual examination of the patient's breasts; she will also need to touch the woman's breasts as she is positioned for the mammogram. These functions should be done in a professional manner with a great deal of sensitivity. Do not *linger* when performing the visual examination; be thorough but also be as professional and as brief as possible. Convey the positioning process (using good communication skills), through the interpreter if necessary. Examples have been provided for your reference. A very important consideration is to be sure that the patient is adequately covered during the examination. It is not necessary to remove the gown completely for the examination. In fact, the gown can remain on for both CC views; one arm at a time can be removed from the gown as the MLO for each side is positioned. A patient should never be asked to completely disrobe from the waist up; as well, the side that is not being imaged should always be covered. Also consider the guidelines that have been outlined in the section dealing with *personal space* issues.

ii. Compression

Compression during mammography is an issue that is appropriate to address with respect to both physical and emotional comfort. Perhaps, more than actual physical pain, compression is an issue of control. Studies have shown that given the option to apply compression to their own breasts, patients tended to compress themselves more than the technologist did. In circumstances where the patient can tolerate little, or perhaps inadequate compression, the following techniques can be used in order to achieve the proper goals of positioning and imaging excellence in mammography.

- Use manual compression rather than the foot pedals. This will allow the compression to be applied more slowly and with more precise control.

- Offer to let the patient compress herself. Show her how to use the foot pedals and then have her practice on her fist. Position the breast as she applies compression.

- If the patient states she has very tender breasts and just cannot tolerate any compression, offer to let her reschedule her mammogram until just after her menstrual period begins.

- If she still cannot tolerate compression explain to her that to continue with the examination under these circumstances would result in a mammogram that would be unacceptable and therefore unable to be evaluated by the radiologist. Tell her that you will notify the radiologist and her doctor that she simply could not tolerate the examination. Do not chastise her for this, or attempt to place blame or guilt. Simply state the facts.

iii. Personal Space

More important than a generalized number of inches (i.e. 18-24" as most people believe) the technologist is better served to understand that each person and each culture have different perceptions of *personal space*. It is significantly different in various cultures and even for various ethnic backgrounds. You might be safely outside of this space (and thus within the patient's comfort zone) of an American woman, but with this same proximity you may have the invaded the comfort zone of a Middle Eastern or Asian woman. What is most important for the technologist to acknowledge is that the process of observing and touching another woman's breasts universally crosses this line, no matter how liberal and accepting an individual may be.

The technologist can prepare the patient and hopefully minimize her perception of inappropriate *invasion* by:

a) first getting permission from the patient, and

b) explaining the exact boundaries and limitations of what you will be doing while you are within the patient's *personal space* and about how long you will be there.

> *While we (remember, you have already established a partnership between you and the patient) are doing your examination today, I will be asking you various questions in order to ensure your comfort as I position your breasts for the mammogram. I will need to position them in a very specific manner, so the x-ray machine will take the views that are necessary for a complete examination. It should only take a few minutes. Do you have any questions about what I will be doing before we get started?*

4. Caring

Most technologists enter into the healthcare profession because they like people and they want to work with them, and hope to make a positive contribution by doing so. While years of doing the same thing over and over can, at times, be tedious, the technologist must stay focused on the good she is doing. Perhaps the last ten patients have been very challenging and the frustration level of the technologist is at its peak: she must remember that the next patient is different. She may be the thirtieth patient that has been seen on that day, but the technologist who is doing her mammogram may be the only contact this woman has for breast health care for an entire year. How she perceives her experience at this time may well influence her decision to ever return for a mammogram again.

a. Professional boundaries ... Maintain these Boundaries

While most technologists want to express their caring attitude for their patients, the empathizing must remain within professional boundaries. Here we can also suggest guidelines for trying to make this the best experience for both the patient and the technologist.

i. Appropriate Demonstration of Caring

- Greet the patient with a two-handed handshake. This exudes warmth and caring.

- Don't personalize the situation or your patient's behavior. If she appears angry or anxious and expresses it in a rude or condescending way, she is most likely anxious and upset about the situation. Do not interpret this as directed at you, personally. It is often hard to ignore this type of treatment by a patient, but try to remain focused on the probable reasons for her behavior, rather than the behavior itself.

- Remember there is appropriate and inappropriate sharing with your patient. It is best not to share your own personal breast history. For example, *I had a mastectomy ten years ago because my breast cancer was found on a mammogram, and it saved my life.* To do so would set up a comparison situation which may result in over-personalization for the patient; she may compare her individual situation and her treatment protocol (should this be necessary) with yours. This can increase confusion and ambivalence. You can, however, share a part of your experience by telling her that you have had a mammogram and you honestly do understand how she is feeling. If you are under screening age have a technologist position and compress your breasts so that you are able to understand and empathize with the patient appropriately.

- Do not be overly personal when addressing your patient. Call your patient by her first and last name when greeting her in the waiting room, then ask her how she would like you to address her: i.e., *Should I call you Alice or Ms. Smith?* (see Communications section.) Give her the options. Do not assume.

- Do not use overly familiar terms of endearment; terms such as *Sweetie* and *Honey* are inappropriate and unprofessional.

- Assure the patient that the questions you present are directly related to clinical information the radiologist needs to know when he examines and interprets her films. Her answers are an important part of the complete examination; this information is very important and will remain confidential. As you proceed, relate all questions to the reason for asking them and they won't be regarded as personal.

- Never minimize her feelings or the situation by saying or implying that the mammogram is *no big deal.* Finding breast cancer early is, in itself, a very big deal.

- Focus on easing the unknown (examples in Communication section).

- Encourage patients to become breast educated and co-practitioners in their breast health care.

    I am examining your breasts with x-ray today, as we do your mammogram, to see any changes that cannot be felt. You are examining your breasts for any changes you may see or feel when you are doing your breast self examination at home.

Intermingle the education process so you are also teaching, not just examining. This alternating focus (instruction and examination) may diffuse some of your patient's anxiety, or at the very least, distract her from it regularly as she focuses on learning something new. The patient may also feel that her anxiety is not as obvious, or the focus of your attention; a more relaxed exchange can occur under these circumstances. This instructional opportunity also expands the technologist's role and her feelings of contribution to *the cause.*

- Invite your patient into a partnership with you by simply stating

    You and I are going to do this together.

This simple phrase can speak volumes in caring, and at the same time provides the patient with a level of control in the examination process that she so often feels she has lost.

E. ROLE-PLAYING:
COMMON QUESTIONS AND RESPONSES

In the course of the day many technologists will hear similar comments and questions from patients repeated over and over again. It is often difficult to think of appropriate responses on the spur of the moment.

There are both *ineffective* and *more effective* answers to the questions and comments that patients frequently present. Examples of each are listed below. The *ineffective responses* are generally curt and tend to dismiss the patient and her remarks. The *effective responses* provide a more helpful alternative. Of course, each technologist must develop her own answers that reflect her own personality and style.

In some situations it may be difficult to answer or address your patient's questions and comments. The professional technologist will remain focused on her work; she will not buy into her patient's anxiety or negativity.

Patient:

I bet this machine was made by a man!

Technologist: (INEFFECTIVE)

All the patients say the same thing.

Technologist: (EFFECTIVE)

Actually a female physician designed the compression device, because she realized that in order to see through the breast tissue properly it must be compressed to the same thickness. No one has yet found another way that is as effective.

Patient:

If I didn't have cancer before, I probably will get it now from this squeezing

Technologist: (INEFFECTIVE)

There is no way the government would let us do such a thing.

Technologist: (EFFECTIVE)

Actually many studies have shown that compression and mammography is very safe and effective.

Technologist:

We need to do some additional pictures.

Patient:

Why — what's wrong? Do you see something?

Technologist: (INEFFECTIVE)

You moved, so the film didn't come out right.

Technologist: (INEFFECTIVE)

The doctor just wants some more.

Technologist: (EFFECTIVE)

Actually, we do additional views for several reasons. The most common is because breast tissue piles up on top of each other and we can't see through it clearly. This (these) view(s) is (are) needed to complete the examination so the doctor can have the information he/she needs.

Patient:
>*Are you sure there is nothing wrong?*

Technologist: (INEFFECTIVE)
>*I don't know, I can't read the films.*

Technologist: (INEFFECTIVE)
>*I'm sure everything will be fine.*

Technologist: (EFFECTIVE)
>*You know, most patients are anxious when we have to do extra pictures, but I can assure you it is quite normal to take extra films. Because breasts are all different sizes, shapes, and textures it's often very difficult to get all the information we need on the first set of films.*

Patient:
>*You look much too young to do this. I'm sure you can't even imagine what it's like.*

Technologist: (INEFFECTIVE)
>*I am too young to have a mammogram, but I'm certainly old enough to do this.*

Technologist: (EFFECTIVE)
>*Thanks for the compliment. I can assure you that you are in good hands; I have had a lot of experience (or training) doing mammograms. Even though I am not in the screening age yet, I have been positioned and compressed by another technologist so I would know what my patients are experiencing.*

Patient:
>*I have never let my husband touch me like this!*

Technologist: (INEFFECTIVE)
>*Well, this is what we have to do to get the pictures.*

Technologist: (EFFECTIVE)
>*Most women find this awkward, but it is necessary in order for me to position your breast properly to get the best pictures possible.*

It is very important for the mammography technologist to maintain an emotional balance that will enable her to objectively meet the challenges of her interactions with the patient on an ongoing basis.

Patient:

My doctor recommended a biopsy. What to you think I should do?

Technologist: (INEFFECTIVE)

Well, I would probably wait six months and have another mammogram. The calcifications look benign to me.

Technologist: (EFFECTIVE)

I understand that sometimes these are difficult decisions so be sure to talk with your doctor about all your questions and concerns; that way you both can make the best decision for you.

Probably the most commonly asked question is:

Patient:

Is this all you do all day long?

Technologist: (INEFFECTIVE)

Actually, after I am finished doing you I am going to go down the hall to clean out the toilets.

Technologist: (INEFFECTIVE)

I do mammograms because my mother (best friend, sister, etc.) died of breast cancer

Technologist: (INEFFECTIVE)

Yes. And what do YOU do?

These examples are inappropriate in that they are sarcastic, defensive, and will only serve to create additional tension between the technologist and the patient. In some situations it may be difficult to answer or address your patient's questions and comments. The patient may exacerbate the situation by speaking in a rude or condescending manner; she may be curt and mean-spirited. But the professional technologist must remained focused on her work and not buy into the patient's negativity. The technologist's work is important and essentially life saving; she must focus on her professional pride rather than the reactions that anxiety laden patients may be projecting. To do so requires skill, patience, understanding, and empathy. Perhaps the most important consideration of all is that the technologist maintains an emotional balance that will enable her to objectively meet these challenges on a regular basis.

F. MAMMOGRAPHER STRESS AND BURNOUT

No input — no output.

Professionals in caring vocations need to be aware that burnout, both emotional and physical, is a phenomenon to watch for. For the mammography technologist who is dealing with patient anxiety and stress on a daily basis, this is a very real concern. Unfortunately, the personal characteristics that mammography technologists commonly share can predispose them to developing and experiencing work related stress and burnout.

1. Common Characteristics of Mammography Technologists

Mammography technologists share many common traits. First and foremost is a keen interest in helping people. Many seem to have found a special place that gives them a great sense of personal and professional satisfaction. Other common characteristics include the following positive traits:

- A desire to make things better — to make a contribution.
- Compassionate feelings towards people in general.
- Pride in their profession and the contribution they make.
- Generally optimistic.
- Intellectually curious.
- Motivated to master new skills and technology.
- Meticulous nature, often perfectionistic.
- Display autonomy — can make decisions independently and enjoy doing so.

Unfortunately, many of the traits that are characteristic of the best mammographers can also work against them, if they are not kept in check with reality. For example, a compassionate nature is extremely important to relate to the patient. However, an overly caring mammography technologist will go too far; she may tend to absorb her patient's anxiety. Little by little, this will amount to a great deal of internal pressure; stress and burnout will follow. Also, the desire to *make things better* or to *make a difference* can, at times, seem like an overwhelming task when cancer is diagnosed in younger women and in women who are *doing all the right things*. After years of exposure to these realities, the dedicated mammographer may begin to feel that the task is too big to tackle and she may lose her drive and motivation.

a. Effects of Stress:

After she has spent many years working at the same job, stressors can tend to erode her positive traits and the technologist may begin to experience the following feelings:

- Lack of appreciation — due to infrequent positive feedback.
- Lack of respect from patients, co-workers, the public and others — resulting from the frequent *negative* association with their job (compression, pain, cruel nature, and examination).
- Recognition of inappropriate balance of responsibility and power.
- Not treated as true colleague by other health care professionals (MDs, RNs, Administrators, etc.); often seen as glorified *button-pushers — anyone can take a photograph!*
- Powerless in decision-making processes.
- Inadequate compensation relative to overwhelming responsibilities.
- Ineffective — work does not really make a difference (late stage burnout).
- Less trusting of co-workers abilities and of management

Thus the technologist may exhibit the emotional effects of stress and these feelings, which contribute to burnout:

- Frustration.
- Defensiveness.
- Apathy.
- Anger.
- Loss of self-respect (pride slipping rapidly).
- Embarrassment or shame about her job (buy into patient's negative comments).

Stress can also manifest itself physically. Many times the technologist may exhibit the following symptoms:

- Mood swings
- Loss of /or increase in appetite
- Headaches
- Chronic fatigue
- Interruption of sleeping patterns
- Loss of productivity at work and at home

2. Identification With Patients

Mammographers soon become aware that their personal attachment to patients and their outcomes has a definite (and sometimes profound) personal effect on them. The constant exposure to an intensely emotional environment that is focused on discovering abnormalities and serious breast disease may eventually begin to erode the technologist's professional distance; technologists frequently will begin to over-personalize their work. This is not unusual. As each technologist grows in her own career she will see an ever-increasing number of patients her own age who are diagnosed with breast cancer. Identification with these patients may be internalized and contribute markedly to the technologist's own stress and anxiety. Her personal fears and concerns may be intensified; this will only be further compounded when co-workers and other mammographers are diagnosed with breast cancer. There is a feeling of heightened vulnerability resulting in increased anxiety and stress. The technologist must work to resolve these feelings and recognize her own needs and respond to them appropriately.

a. Empathy: Appropriate Use of Empathy

Should the technologist note a tendency to internalize the patient's fears and concerns and then transfer them to her own fears of breast cancer and well-being, an attempt should be made to redirect these feelings to a more useful purpose. Rather than allowing these feelings to cause the technologist increased anxiety and stress, she can use this as an opportunity to be empathetic. The technologist may truly understand many of her patient's feelings and resulting behaviors as she may be experiencing these same feelings herself. This common bond often enables the technologist to remain compassionate and more accepting of her patient's anxiety. Empathy can be used as a powerful, positive tool to increase understanding and decrease stress for both the patient and the technologist.

3. Basic Principles of Self-Care for Stress Reduction

While meeting the needs of her patients, the technologist needs to be continually aware of her own need structure as well. A basic rule for healthy practice in a helping profession is that the individual must be taking into themselves enough nurturing and personal enhancement to offset the amount that they give out on a regular basis. Basic areas such as physical exercise, satisfying relationships, and mental stimulation in areas other than her vocation are essential. Spiritual and inspirational resources are also important to provide balance in one's life and to rejuvenate one's spirit; this will facilitate ongoing professional competence in conjunction with a healthy personal lifestyle.

a. Stress Reduction

Strategies for stress control and reduction can be divided into four areas. Examples of each are listed.

i. Physiological

Research has shown that a change in behavioral habits related to self-care can be very beneficial in reducing stress and its related physical symptoms. Suggestions such as those listed below are believed to contribute to lower blood pressure, improved cardiovascular performance, decreased cancer risk, and an overall improvement in one's general health. As well, the benefits of pursuing good general health habits extend far beyond the primary focus of reducing stress and burnout.

- Eat a controlled and balanced diet.
- Exercise regularly.
- Practice relaxation techniques.
- Reduce noise.
- Dress comfortably — supportive, comfortable shoes are mandatory for mammographers; avoid tight, restrictive clothing — comfort is very important.
- Get rest; sleep well.

ii. Emotional

Emotional factors have a significant influence on the level of stress that an individual experiences. A positive and healthy emotional environment is important for an overall sense of well-being; it can also dramatically affect one's perception of her work and her life in general.

- Express cheerfulness and joy.
- Plan ahead to decrease worries and last minute panic.
- Develop self-respect.
- Express gratitude.
- Develop positive attitudes and thinking habits.
- Be realistic and thereby eliminate unnecessary fear.

iii. Psychosocial

Successful interactions with patients and colleagues can directly affect the technologist's job performance as well as her sense of well-being and personal power. Unfortunately, health professionals are seldom taught these important psychosocial skills. The proactive technologist will search out reference and resource material and work toward building these interpersonal skills. Hopefully the material in this chapter will begin this process.

- Develop and practice good interpersonal skills
- Develop and practice good communication skills
- Remember kindness
- Help others.
- Forgive and forget.
- Simplify your lifestyle.
- Look for good in others.
- Learn to say no; don't take on more than you can handle.

iv. Spiritual

As referenced earlier, meditation and relaxation techniques are known to be very effective in reducing stress. Many individuals also consider these practices to be a form of *spiritual* connection. The specific activity or method that one adopts is relatively unimportant; different individuals may find that one technique works better for them than another. In fact, pursuing a variety of techniques can be even more stimulating and beneficial. It is also important to:

- Learn self-control.
- Give of your time and means to worthy causes.
- Clarify your values and motives.
- Confess your wrongs.
- Accept forgiveness.
- Learn to pray and meditate effectively.
- Read material that inspires you.

b. Specific Antidotes for Stress

Randi Gunther, Ph.D., a Psychotherapist from the U.S. addressed many aspects of a mammographer's work in an article entitled *Hearkening to the Mammography Technologist*. In this article, Dr. Gunther suggested the following antidotes to help mammographers reduce stress:

1. *Learning personal empowerment.*
   This comes from the realization that mammographers have something important to offer and they are going to do their job right unless someone can show them a better way to do it.

2. *Learning to be comfortable with assertiveness and confrontation.*
   There are clear, effective ways to state what they believe is right. Certain

---

communication skills and rules must be mastered, such as the knowl-edge that effective communication must be in the language of their superiors.

3. *Leaving their unresolved conflicts behind them.*
This is done by re-evaluating goals and values and by being unwilling to compromise honor or ethics.

4. *Making certain they have tribal support.*
This means developing a support network of people who both chal-lenge and support them.

5. *Learning quality interpersonal communication skills with peers, supe-riors, staff and patients.*

6. *Learning how to assess situations and take appropriate risks.*

7. *Making certain that their life has recreation, exercise, meditation and relaxation to balance out the tension in their work.*

8. *Learning to have concern and detachment at the same time so that they do not over-identify with their patients.*

9. *Feeding their bodies with quality food, not fast foods and sweets to compensate for helplessness and depression.*

10. *Planning healthy escapes.*

11. *Sleeping well.*

12. *Understanding crisis and stress.*

Knowing when to fight, when to accept, when to leave and when to transcend are important skills in understanding and combating stress.

Source: Gunther, R.: Hearkening to the Mammographic Technologist, Admin-istrative Radiology; 5/91:39.

It is most important to remember *You can't take care of your patients if you are not taking care of yourself.*

You, as a mammographer, are a key link in the breast imaging chain. Not the best machine, or the most highly skilled radiologist, or the most expensive and impressive decor can do what you do. You make the patient feel comfortable and cared for. This in itself can determine whether the patient will ever have a mammogram again. This in itself, saves lives.

So when a patient asks you, *Is this all you do all day long?* or *How can you stand to do this all day long?* You say to her, honestly:

> *Actually, as a mammography specialist there are lots of things I do during the day, but one of may favorite things is working with patients, because I know I can make a difference in their lives.*

This is, again, the work, the responsibility, and the privilege of the mammography technologist.

G. CONCLUSION

The following new *Ode to a Mammogram*, although written by a technologist, hopefully represents our patient's real perception of our effort as mammographers. It is dedicated to all mammography technologists who endeavor to make a difference.

Ode to a Mammogram (Revisited)

My doctor had ordered an x-ray of breasts
Although I was frightened, I knew it was best.

The tech was most gentle and equally kind;
She answered the questions that cluttered my mind.

She told me to practice my breast self-exam;
An exam by my doctor; they're part of the plan.

Tho' it's not the most fun, I know it's done right;
If it finds cancer early, she's just saved my live.

So I'll tell all my friends, with our fears we can cope.
This tech, this experience, have given me hope.

Copyright Louise C. Miller, 1995

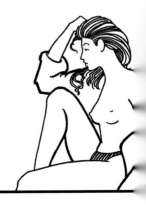

APPENDIX A: ABBREVIATIONS

ACR _____ American College of Radiology
AEC _____ Automatic Exposure Control
AG _____ Average Gradient
AGD _____ Average Glandular Dose
ALARA _____ As Low As Reasonably Achievable
AT _____ Axillary Tail
B+F (BF) _____ Base plus Fog
BSE _____ Breast Self Examination
Bx _____ Biopsy
C/kg_____ Coulomb per Kilogram
CAR_____ Canadian Association of Radiologists
CBE _____ Clinical Breast Examination
CC _____ Craniocaudal
CTD _____ Cumulative Trauma Disorder
CV _____ Cleavage
DD _____ Density Difference
ESE _____ Entrance Skin Exposure
FB _____ From Below (Caudocranial)
FBCV_____ From Below Cleavage
FBXCCL _____ From Below Exaggerated Craniocaudal
Gy _____ Gray
HVL_____ Half Value Layer
Hz _____ Hertz
ID _____ Implant Displaced
IMF _____ Inframammary Fold

KeV	Kiloelectron volts
kVp	Kilovolt peak
L	Left
LCNB	Large Core Needle Biopsy
LET	Linear Energy Transfer
LIQ	Lower Inner Quadrant
LM	Lateromedial
LMO	Lateromedial Oblique
LOQ	Lower Outer Quadrant
lp/mm	Line Pairs Per Millimeter
Lux	Lumen Per Square Meter; Unit of Luminance
M	Magnification
MAP	Mammography Accreditation Program
MAP	Mammography Aid for Positioning
mAs	Milliampere Second
MD	Mid Density
MGD	Mean Glandular Dose
ML	Mediolateral
MLO	Mediolateral Oblique
MPD	Maximum Permissible Dose
MQSA	Mammography Quality Standards Act
MSD	Musculoskeletal Disorder
MSDS	Musculoskeletal Disorder Syndrome
MTF	Modulation Transfer Function
NCRP	National Council on Radiation Protection
Nit	Candela Per Square Meter; Unit of Illuminance
OD	Optical Density
pH	Acid / Base Balance
PNL	Posterior Nipple Line
QA	Quality Assurance
QC	Quality Control
R	Right
R	Roentgen
Rad	Radiation Absorbed Dose
RBE	Relative Biological Effectiveness
Rem	Radiation Equivalent Man
RMI	Radiation Measurements Inc.

RI _____ Rolled Inferior
RL _____ Rolled Lateral
RM _____ Rolled Medial
RS _____ Rolled Superior
RSI _____ Repetitive Stress Injury
SI _____ Standard International
SID _____ Source-to-Image-Receptor-Distance
SIO _____ Superolateral to Inferomedial Oblique
SSD _____ Source-To-Skin-Distance
Sv _____ Sievert
TAN _____ Tangential
UIQ _____ Upper Inner Quadrant
UOQ _____ Upper Outer Quadrant
WMSD _____ Workplace Musculoskeletal Distress
XCCL _____ Exaggerated Craniocaudal

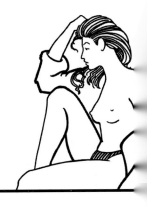

APPENDIX B: GLOSSARY

MEDICAL DEFINITIONS

ABSCESS

A localized area of infection, usually very painful; common in lactating breasts.

ACCURACY

The percentage of cases correctly diagnosed by a study.

ACINUS (alveolus)

In the breast, one of the tiny sacs lined with gland cells which extract ingredients from nearby blood vessels and recombine them to produce milk (plural: acini).

ADENOLIPOMA

A benign tumor containing glandular and fatty tissue.

ADENOCARCINOMA

A malignant adenoma arising from a glandular organ.

ADENOMA

A benign tumor composed of glandular tissue, usually well circum-scribed.

ADENOSIS

A benign breast change marked by an increase in the proportion of glandular (adeno-) tissue to the other kinds of tissue in the breast. This change is not associated with an increased risk of breast cancer.

ADIPOSE

Fatty tissue.

ADJUNCTIVE

A helping, assisting auxiliary (although subordinate) process.

ADJUVANT THERAPY

A type of treatment of breast cancer; utilized when metastases are anticipated, usually due to lymph node involvement; commonly chemotherapy or hormone therapy.

AESTHETIC

A pleasing appearance or effect.

AMASTIA

The absence of breast development; often also associated with the absence of pectoral muscle.

AMBIENT

The surrounding atmosphere (environment).

AMPULLA

A local dilation of the excretory duct; functions as a milk reservoir.

ANASTOMOSES

Connections between structures.

ANXIETY

Apprehension, tension, or uneasiness that comes from the anticipation of danger, the source of which is unknown or unrecognized. It also results from the threat of losing something we believe to be essential to our well being, such as an important relationship or physical wholeness.

ARCHITECTURE (BREAST)

The arrangement of structures within the breast.

AREOLA

The dark pigmented skin around the nipple.

ARTIFACT

An unwanted irregularity or defect on an image.

ASPIRATION

Drawing of fluid or cells by means of a needle.

ATHELIA
The absence of nipples; often associated with amastia.

ATROPHY
A wasting; a decrease in size of an organ or tissue.

ATYPISM
Deviation from the normal.

AUTOMATIC EXPOSURE CONTROL (AEC)
Systems, often referred to as phototimers, designed to automatically select the exposure and to produce a pre-determined density by sampling the x-ray intensity after passage through the patient and image receptor.

AVERAGE GLANDULAR DOSE (AGD)
The energy deposited per unit mass of glandular tissue (the most radiosensitive tissue in the breast) averaged over all the glandular tissue in the breast; calculated from values of entrance exposure in air, x-ray beam quality (half-value layer), and compressed breast thickness.

AVERAGE GRADIENT
An indication of contrast that is calculated with the useful density levels found in medical radiography (2.0 and 0.25 plus B+F).

AXILLA
The armpit or underarm area.

BASE DENSITY
Optical density due to the supporting base of the film.

BASE OF BREAST
Referring to the chest wall; the portion of breast adjacent the chest wall.

BASE PLUS FOG DENSITY
Optical density of film due to its base density plus any unintentional exposure the film may have received.

BATCH PROCESSING
Mass development of images at one time.

BENIGN
Not cancerous or malignant.

BIOPSY

Surgical removal of a piece of tissue to be examined microscopically to diagnose disease.

BLIND AREAS

Areas of breast tissue with the potential for exclusion on mammography images due to the natural curvature of the rib cage.

BREAST SELF EXAMINATION (BSE)

Inspection and palpation of breasts by a woman herself.

BROMINE DRAG

A depression of optical density due to the accumulation of bromine ions from an adjacent high optical density area.

CANCER

Disease characterized by abnormal and uncontrolled growth of cells; the resulting mass can invade and destroy surrounding normal tissue; cells can travel to other areas of the body and start new cancers.

CARCINOMA

Cancer or malignancy.

CASSETTE

Light-tight case, usually made of thin, low x-ray absorption plastic, for holding x-ray film in close contact with an intensifying screen.

CELLULAR

Pertaining to the cells or composed of cells.

CHARACTERISTIC CURVE

A graphic representation of the relationship between the exposure given to a photographic material and the resulting optical density (see sensitometric curve).

CHEMOTHERAPY

Anti-cancer drugs used when cancer has spread to the lymph nodes, indicating possible spread to other parts of the body.

COLLAGEN

The main supportive protein of skin, tendons, and connective tissue.

COLLAGENOUS

Pertaining to collagen.

COLOSTRUM
A watery milk secreted for a few days after parturition which has a high protein and antibody content.

COMEDO-CARCINOMA
A malignant disease of duct-like acini in which they become filled with hardened secretions.

COMPRESSION DEVICE
Plastic paddle used to help hold the breast stationary for the x-ray exposure.

COMPTON SCATTERING
The absorption process that occurs when only part of the incoming photon's energy is used to eject an electron from an atom; the remaining energy is scattered in the tissue.

CONES
Photoreceptors in the eye that function in bright light conditions and are responsible for color vision.

CONTRAST
A difference in optical density between an object and surrounding structures (background).

CONTROL LIMIT
Upper and lower control limits are those values that when reached or exceeded indicate that the process being monitored is "out of control" and requires that some action be taken immediately.

CONTROL CHART
Graphic means of displaying data pertinent to the processing environment.

CONTROL FILM
A box of film of the same type used clinically, reserved in the film bin for quality control purposes.

CONTRAST FILM
A film that demonstrates high contrast: black and white film with few shades of gray.

COOPER'S LIGAMENTS
Curvilinear connective tissue septa connecting the posterior and anterior fascial planes of the breast.

CORRECTIVE MAINTENANCE

Action taken to correct a problem that has occurred frequently and results in interruption of the work flow.

COSMIC RADIATION

A source of background radiation resulting from extraterrestrial phenomena.

COSTOCHONDRITIS

Arthritis affecting the junction of the ribs medially along the sternum.

CYCLE TIME

a) Time it takes for the leading edge of the film to enter and exit the processor; b) time it takes the leading edge of the film to enter and the trailing edge to exit the processor (most commonly used).

CYST

Any sac or capsule containing a liquid or a semi-solid substance.

CYSTOSARCOMA

Sarcoma with cysts; malignant.

CYTOLOGY

Study of cells.

DENSITOMETER

A device that provides an indication of optical density by measuring transmitted light.

DESMOPLASIA

The formation and development of fibrous tissue, often forming adhesions.

DEVELOPER

The chemical solution that changes the film latent image to a visible image composed of black metallic silver.

DIAGNOSTIC MAMMOGRAPHY

Mammography performed on women who, by virtue of symptoms or physical findings, are considered to have substantial likelihood of breast disease.

DOSE

The amount of energy deposited in tissue due to x-ray exposure.

DUCT ECTASIA

A benign breast change in which large or small ducts in the breast become dilated and retain secretions, often leading to nipple discharge, and sometimes a lump in the nipple/areola area and/or nipple retraction. This change is not associated with an increased risk of breast cancer.

DYNAMIC EFFORT

Repetitive motion, characterized by a lengthening and shortening, tension and relaxation of the muscles.

DYSPLASTIC

Abnormality of development; alteration in size, shape or arrangement of cells; poorly structured tissue in a breast.

ECTOPIA

Displacement or malposition.

EDEMA

Accumulation of fluids in the tissue.

EFFLUENT

Waste material discharged into the environment.

EPITHELIAL

Cellular substance of skin and mucous membrane.

ERGONOMICS

The science that examines human performance and safety as it relates to an individual's work environment, equipment, and tools, and the design of the job.

ESTROGEN

A female hormone which, every month before menopause, readies the breast for possible milk production and transport by multiplying and enlarging breast cells.

EXPOSURE

The amount of x-irradiation.

EXTRANEOUS

Existing or coming from other sources.

FALSE NEGATIVE (FN)
Cancer is present in a breast that has been incorrectly diagnosed as normal.

FAT NECROSIS (Traumatic fat necrosis)
A benign breast change in which the breast responds to trauma (including surgical biopsy sometimes) with a firm, irregular mass, often years after the event. This breast change is not associated with an increased risk of breast cancer.

FEAR
An unpleasant, strong emotion caused by the anticipation of what is known or thought to be known; an awareness of danger.

FIBROADENOMA
Adenoma containing fibrous tissue; usually mobile and of rubbery texture; these often calcify.

FIBROCYSTIC
Overgrowth of fibrous tissue and development of cystic spaces.

FIBROSIS
The formation of fibrous tissue.

FINE NEEDLE ASPIRATION BIOPSY (FNAB)
Cells from a lump are removed with a small-calibre needle; they are smeared on glass slides for pathological study.

FIXER
The chemical solution that removes the undeveloped silver halide crystals from film.

FIXER RETENTION
The inadequate removal of fixer from the film by the water in the wash tank of the processor. This results in poor archival quality.

FLOODED REPLENISHMENT
A process of using a timed cycle to automatically add a pre-determined amount of chemical replenisher to the processing tanks; this maintains chemical activity in a low volume setting.

FOCAL SPOT SIZE

The focal spot is the area of the target or anode that is bombarded by electrons from the cathode of the x-ray tube to produce x-rays. The smaller the focal spot the better the resolution of the x-ray system, especially in magnification mammography.

FOG

An unwanted density added to a radiograph: due to light, radiation, or heat exposure during storage, handling, and processing problems.

FOVEA

The 6 mm central area of the retina that contains the highest density of cone receptors and is responsible for the optimum level of visual acuity.

FROZEN SECTION

Tissue section is quick-frozen and sliced for immediate pathology; used during a surgical procedure.

FUSION

The act or process of liquefying.

GALACTOCELE

A cystic enlargement of the mammary gland, containing milk.

GALACTOGRAPHY

Injection of a duct with contrast media.

GRAVIDA

A pregnant woman, regardless of the duration of pregnancy.

GRIDS

A set of thin, closely spaced lead strips interspaced by fiber or aluminum for mammographic grids. The grid is placed between the breast and the film-screen image receptor to absorbe scattered radiation and reduce the amount reaching the film.

GYNECOMASTIA

Excessive development of the male mammary glands, sometimes even to the functional state.

HALF-VALUE LAYER (HVL)

The thickness of a specified substance that, when introduced into the path of a given beam of radiation, reduces the exposure rate by half. HVL is a measure of beam quality and usually is specified in mm of aluminum for diagnostic units. The higher the HVL, the more penetrating the x-ray beam.

HOMOGENEOUS

Having a similarity of structure.

HORMONE THERAPY

Manipulation of hormones to slow the growth of breast cancer.

HYPERPLASIA

Abnormal, but benign, increase in number of normal cells.

HYPERTROPHY

Overgrowth or enlargement of an organ or part due to increase in size of the constituent cells.

IONIZATION

The process whereby an electron is ejected from an atom.

ILLUMINANCE

The amount of light falling on a surface (units = lux).

ILLUMINATOR

See viewbox.

IMAGE CONTRAST

The optical density difference between adjacent areas resulting from a difference in attenuation.

IMAGE QUALITY

The overall clarity and detail of a radiographic image. Limiting spatial resolution (or resolving power), image sharpness, radiographic noise, and image contrast are common parameters of image quality.

IMAGE SHARPNESS

The overall impression of detail and clarity in a radiographic image.

IMMERSION TIME
a) The time period from when the leading edge of a film enters the developer to when it exits the developer; b) the time period from when the leading edge of a film enters the developer to when it enters the fixer (current).

INFLAMMATION
Condition in which tissues enter as a reaction to injury resulting in pain, heat, redness, and swelling.

IN SITU
Confined to the site of origin; not having invaded adjoining tissues or metastasized to other parts of the body.

INSPISSATED
Being thickened, dried, or rendered less fluid through evaporation; hardened secretions that form intraductal calcifications.

INVASIVE BREAST CANCER
Disease in which breast cancer cells have penetrated (invaded) surrounding breast tissue.

KILOVOLTAGE PEAK (kVp)
The maximum potential difference setting between anode and cathode in an x-ray tube.

LACTATION
Secretion of milk.

LACTIFEROUS
Producing or conveying milk.

LATENT
Not visible or apparent but capable of becoming so.

LATITUDE FILM
A film that demonstrates latitude; many shades of gray with small density differences between them.

LESION
Any change in tissue structure or function due to any process, including injury.

LINEA ALBA

An anatomical line of connective tissue extending down the middle of the abdomen from the sternum to the pubis; provides a pathway for metastases.

LIPID

Any one of a group of organic substances which are insoluble in water, but soluble in alcohol, ether, and other fat solvents.

LIPOFIBROMA

A fibroma containing fatty elements.

LIPOMA

A fatty tumor.

LOBULE

Functional unit of the breast; termination of branching ducts.

LUMINANCE

The amount of light emitted or scattered by a surface (units =nit).

LUMPECTOMY

The simplest type of surgical procedure; only the tumor and surrounding tissue are removed through a small incision.

LYMPH NODES

Small bean-shaped glands scattered along lymphatic vessels; act as filters to infection and cancer.

LYMPHOMA

A primary tumor of the lymph tissue.

MACROCYST

A cyst large enough to be palpated.

MALIGNANT

Cancer or carcinoma.

MAMMOPLASTY

Plastic reduction of the mammary glands.

MASKING

The process of blocking out extraneous light (glare) from around an image on an illuminator or viewbox.

MASTECTOMY
Removal of the breast.

MASTITIS
Inflammation of the mammary glands.

MEAN GLANDULAR DOSE (MGD)
See average glandular dose.

MEDULLARY CARCINOMA
Carcinoma arising from the central part of the breast; frequently large and defined; often misdiagnosed as cystic disease; soft on palpation.

MELANOMA
A tumor made up of melanin (dark) pigmented cells; usually skin lesion.

METASTASIS
The spread of cancer from the initial tumor to other body parts.

MICROCALCIFICATIONS (Calcifications)
Tiny white specks of calcium salts which can sometimes be seen on mammograms. In clusters, they can be the only sign of duct carcinoma in situ or early invasive cancer, or they can be associated with benign breast changes.

MICROCYST
A cyst too small to be palpated.

MILLIAMPERE (mA) SETTING
The electron current passing from cathode to anode in an x-ray tube.

MILLIAMPERE SECONDS (mAs)
The product of electron current (mA) and exposure time (in seconds).

MODIFIED RADICAL MASTECTOMY
This involves removal of the breast, underarm lymph nodes, the lining over the chest muscles and sometimes the smaller of the two chest muscles.

MODULATION TRANSFER FUNCTION (MTF)
The ability of an imaging system to reproduce the available image information. A higher number indicates more information represented. This is a concept that was formulated to provide an objective measurement of the combined effects of sharpness and resolution.

MONTGOMERY GLANDS

Small nodular prominences on the areola that secrete lipid material to lubricate the nipple during nursing.

MOTTLE

Random, undesirable variations in optical density on a radiograph that has received a uniform x-ray exposure.

MULTICENTRICITY

Occuring in more than one place.

MULTIPARA

A woman who has had two or more pregnancies to the stage of viability.

MYOBLASTOMA

A tumor of striated muscle made up of groups of cells which resemble primitive myoblasts; a benign circumcised lesion.

MYXOID

Resembling mucous.

NEEDLE ASPIRATION

Removal of fluid or cells with a needle.

NEEDLE LOCALIZATION

Procedure where radiologist marks a suspicious, non-palpable area with a needle, hookwire, or dye; assists surgeon to locate exact area for surgical biopsy.

NEGATIVE PREDICTIVE VALUE (NPV)

Percentage of women called negative by a study who truly do not have breast cancer.

NEOPLASIA

Formation of a neoplasm.

NEOPLASM

New or abnormal growth; tumor.

NEOPLASTIC

Pertaining to neoplasm.

NEVUS

A circumscribed growth of skin; congenital origin; a mole.

NIPPLE
> A conical projection in the centre of the areola which acts as the outlet for milk.

NIPPLE DISCHARGE
> Secretion of fluid from nipple; spontaneous or elicited with pressure.

NODULARITY
> "Lumpiness" of normal tissue.

NOISE
> Unwanted fluctuations in optical density.

ONCOLOGIST
> A doctor who treats cancer (tumors).

OPERATING LEVEL
> The average value about which we expect day-to-day measurements to fluctuate.

OPTICAL DENSITY (OD)
> The exposure level or the degree of darkness (blackness) of an image.

OPTIMIZE
> To make as perfect, effective, or functional as possible.

ORTHOGONAL
> Perpendicular to; 90 degrees to.

OXIDATION
> The action of losing electrons.

PAGET'S DISEASE
> An inflammatory cancerous affection of the areola and nipple; usually associated with underlying ductal carcinoma.

PALPATION
> To feel; examine by touch.

PAPILLOMA
> A branching of lobulated benign tumor derived from the epithelium; usually inside mammary duct near nipple; produces clear or bloody discharge.

PAPILLOMATOSIS
The development of multiple papillomas, often in UOQ.

PARA
refers to past pregnancies that have produced an infant of viable age, whether or not an infant is dead or alive at birth.

PARA I
A primipara.

PARA II
A woman who has had two children of viable age (and so on up numerically: para III, para IV, and so forth).

PARENCHYMA
Essential elements of an organ; functional portions.

PARTIAL MASTECTOMY
The segment of the breast containing the tumor is removed, together with some skin and the lining of the chest muscle below the tumor.

PARTURITION
The process of giving birth.

PATHOLOGIST
A doctor who studies tissue under a microscope to make a diagnosis.

PECTORALIS MAJOR MUSCLE
A large triangular muscle on the anterior upper portion of the chest.

PECTUS CARINATUM
Abnormal prominence of sternum; pigeon chest.

PECTUS EXCAVATUM
Abnormal depression of sternum.

PENUMBRA
The blurred margin that is imaged at the edge of an object.

PERMANENT SECTION
Producing definitive (detailed, clear) slides of biopsied tissue for pathology; takes 24 hours.

PHANTOM (Breast)

A test object that simulates the average composition of and various structures within the breast.

PHOTOELECTRIC ABSORPTION

The absorption process that occurs when all of the incoming photon's energy is used to eject an electron from an atom. This type of absorption is primarily responsible for image contrast.

PHOTOMETRY

The science of light measurement.

PHOTOPTIC VISION

A component of vision that functions in bright light conditions and is responsible for color vision.

PHYLLODE

A term applied to tumors which on section show a lobulated, leaf-like appearance.

POLYTHELIA

Presence of extra nipples.

POLYMASTIA

Presence of excess number of breasts.

POSITIVE PREDICTIVE VALUE (PPV)

Percentage of women who are suspected of cancer by a study, who prove to have cancer.

POSTERIOR NIPPLE LINE (PNL)

A landmark that represents the alignment of the nipple to the chest wall.

PREVENTATIVE MAINTENANCE

Action taken on a regular basis to prevent deterioration of image quality and breakdown of the components in the imaging chain.

PRIMIGRAVIDA

A woman pregnant for the first time.

PRIMIPARA

A woman who has given birth once to a fetus that has reached the age of viability.

PROGNOSIS
Prediction of survival or recurrence.

PROLIFERATE
Fast growing tissue.

PROCESSING TIME
The time from when the leading edge of a film enters the processor until the trailing edge of the film exits the processor.

PROCESSOR
An automated device that transports film at a constant speed by a system of rollers through developing, fixing, washing, and drying cycles.

QUALITY ASSURANCE
The overall management program that has been designed to ensure that high quality imaging will be consistently produced.

QUALITY CONTROL
The segment of a quality assurance program that is responsible for measurement and monitoring of the image quality and the integrity of the imaging equipment.

QUALITY CONTROL TECHNOLOGIST
A technologist assigned the task of testing and maintaining records of radiographic imaging systems.

QUANTUM MOTTLE
Random variations in optical density on a radiograph that are due to the random distribution of x-ray quanta in the x-ray beam.

RADICAL (Halsted) MASTECTOMY
The skin, breast, chest muscles, and all underarm lymph nodes are removed; popular in past years but not frequently used today.

RADIOGRAPHIC NOISE
Unwanted fluctuations in optical density on the mammographic image.

RADIOGRAPHIC SHARPNESS
The distinctness of perceptibility of the boundary or edge of a structure on a mammogram.

RADIOLOGIST
A doctor who reads x-rays and ultrasound examinations.

RADIOTHERAPY
High energy x-rays that are used as a primary treatment to destroy early tumors or after surgery to prevent recurrence of cancer.

RECIPROCITY FAILURE
The phenomenon that occurs with extended times (1-2 seconds) in screen-film imaging where an increase in radiation intensity does not proportionally produce a corresponding increase in optical density.

RECONSTRUCTIVE SURGERY
Surgery to restore the normal shape to the chest wall after a mastectomy.

REPEAT ANALYSIS
A systematic approach to determine the causes for radiographs being repeated.

REPLENISHMENT RATE
The amount of chemicals added per sheet of film to maintain the proper chemical activity.

RESOLUTION
The ability to detect closely spaced objects as being separate.

RODS
Photoreceptors in the eye that function in low levels of illumination and are responsible for colorless, gray tones; they are instrumental for night vision.

SAFELIGHT
A lighting fixture with appropriate filters that produces light that will not fog radiographic film within a specified time period.

SANGUINEOUS
Abounding in blood.

SARCOMA
A tumor made up of closely packed cells.

SENSITIVITY
The percentage of malignancies correctly identified by a study.

SENSITOMETER
A device that produces controlled light exposure of a series of graduated steps; used to indicate photographic chemical performance.

SENSITOMETRIC CURVE

See characteristic curve.

SENSITOMETRY

A method of quantitatively estimating the relationship between exposure and density.

SCIRRHOUS

Pertaining to, or of a scirrhus nature; hard, indurated.

SCIRRHUS

A hard cancer with a marked predominance of connective tissue.

SCLEROSING ADENOSIS

A common form of adenosis which occurs in two phases: 1)solid benign breast lump develops; 2)sclerosis (hardening) replaces the cells of the breast lump. If the areas of sclerosis calcify, they may lead to misleading findings on a mammogram.

SCOPTIC VISION

Is stimulated by low levels of illumination and provides colorless gray tones.

SCREEN

Microscopic phosphor crystals coated on a plastic support that emits visible light when exposed to x-irradiation, thereby creating a latent image on x-ray film.

SCREEN-FILM MAMMOGRAPHY

Mammography performed with a high detail intensifying screen in close contact with a film in a cassette.

SCREEN-FILM COMBINATION

A particular intensifying screen used with a particular type of film. It is important to match the light output spectrum of the screen with the light sensitivity of the film.

SCREENING MAMMOGRAPHY

The x-ray breast examination of asymptomatic women in an attempt to detect cancer when it is small, nonpalpable, and confined to the breast.

SENSITOMETRIC STRIP

A sheet of film exposed by a sensitometer that demonstrates a representative range of densities, from minimum to maximum.

SIMPLE MASTECTOMY
> The entire breast is removed but not the underarm lymph nodes.

SOLARIZATION REGION
> The region beyond D-max in which increased exposure results in decreased film density.

SPECIFICITY
> The percentage of normal cases correctly identified by a study.

SPICULATED
> A star-shaped lesion, characterized by radiating "arms" of connective tissue (see STELLATE).

SPOT COMPRESSION VIEW
> An image obtained with localized, focal compression using a small compression paddle: for clarifying tissue detail by minimizing superimposition.

STAGING
> Using all the information about the cancer to find out how much of the body may be involved; indicates the extent of the disease.

STARTER SOLUTION
> A chemical solution which is added to fresh developer solution; it is designed to retard the overly active nature of fresh chemicals. With flooded replenishment, starter solution is added to the replenishment tank.

STASIS
> Stoppage of the flow or other body fluid in any part.

STATIC EFFORT
> A stationary state in which the muscle does not change length, but remains in a state of heightened tension; force is exerted over the entire duration of time.

STELLATE
> Star-shaped (see SPICULATED).

STROMA
> Supporting framework of breasts.

SUBAREOLAR
> Beneath the areola.

SUBCUTANEOUS
Situated or occurring beneath the skin.

SUSPENSORY LIGAMENT
A ligament which serves to hold up a part; Cooper's ligaments in the breasts.

SYMMETRY
Having balanced proportions; correspondence in size, shape, and position of parts.

TAUT COMPRESSION
The degree of compression achieved when a gentle tapping of the breast with one finger does not indent the tissue; this degree of compression is rarely painful.

TERRESTRIAL RADIATION
A source of background radiation resulting from radioisotope deposits in the earth.

TRIANGULATION
A process in determining in which area of the breast a lesion will be located based on its known position on two other images.

TRUE NEGATIVE (TN)
A breast without a cancer that has been interpreted as a normal examination.

TRUE POSITIVE (TP)
Breast cancer that is correctly diagnosed.

TUMOR
A mass of fast growing tissue (as compared to normal tissue) which may either be benign or malignant.

TYLECTOMY
A lumpectomy.

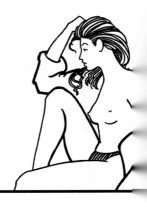

APPENDIX C:
BIBLIOGRAPHY

1. American College of Radiology, American Cancer Society: Mammography Quality Control Manual, Revised Edition, 1994.

2. American College of Radiology, Committee on Quality Assurance in Mammography: Mammography Quality Control Manual, 1999.

3. Andolina, Valerie F., Lill, Shelly L., Willison, Kathleen M.: Mammographic Imaging, A Practical Guide, J.B. Lippincott, 1992.

4. Burns, Ellen F.: Radiographic Positioning, A Guide for Producing Quality Radiographs, W.B.Saunders, Philadelphia, 1992.

5. Bushong, Stewart C.: Radiation Protection, Essentials of Medical Imaging Series, McGraw-Hill, 1998.

6. Eastman Kodak Co., Health Sciences Division: Positioning Techniques in Mammography, Rochester, NY, Publication #M7L025, January 1998.

7. Eastman Kodak Company, Health Sciences Division: Quality Control Mammography 1, April 1990.

8. Eklund, G.W., Busby, R.C., Miller, S.H., Job, J.S.: Improved Imaging of the Augmented Breast, AJR 151; 469-473, September 1998.

9. Fieg, S. M.D,: Categorical Course Syllabus, AARS Breast Imaging, RSNA 1988.

10. Gould, Robert G. ed.: Syllabus: A Categorical Course in Physics, RSNA 1996.

11. Gray, Joel E.: Quality Control in Diagnostic Imaging, Aspen Publication, Rockville, MD, 1983.

12. Haus A.G., Yaffe M.J., eds.: Categorical Course in Physics-Technical Aspects of Breast Imaging 2nd Edition; RSNA Publications, December 1993.

13. Haus, A.G. ed.: Film Processing in Medical Imaging, Medical Physics Publishing, Madison, WI, 1993.

14. Haus, A.G., Yaffe, Martin J. eds.: Syllabus: A Categorical Course in Physics, RSNA 1994.

15. Haus, Arthur G. ed.: Film Processing in Imaging, Medical Physics Publishing, 1993.

16. Haus, Arthur G., Jaskulski, Susan H.: The Basics of Film Processing in Medical Imaging, Medical Physics Publishing, 1997.

17. Huda, Walter, Slone, Richard: Review of Radiologic Physics, Williams & Wilkins, 1995.

18. Kopans, Daniel B., Mendelson, Ellen B., eds.: Syllabus: A Categorical Course in Breast Imaging, RSNA 1995.

19. Kopans, Daniel B.: Breast Imaging, Lippincott-Raven, 1998.

20. Logan-Young, Wende, Hoffman, Nancy Yanes: Breast Cancer, A Practical Guide to Diagnosis, MT Hope Publishing, Rochester, NY, 1994.

21. McKenney, W.E.J.: Radiographic Processing and Quality Control, J.B. Lippincott Company, Philadelphia, PA, 1998.

22. Peters, M.E. ed.: Handbook of Breast Imaging, Churchill Livingston, NY, 1989.

23. Reference Articles, 10th Annual Breast Imaging Seminar, Pittsburgh, PA, July 1990.

24. Sickles, E.A.: Fundamentals of Mammography: The Quest for Quality, Positioning Handbook, 1990.

25. Tabár, L.: Optimum Mammography Technique, May 1989.

26. Wentz, Gini: Mammography for Radiologic Technologists, McGraw-Hill, 1997.

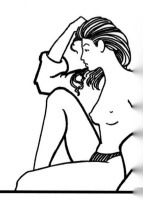

INDEX

BB marker   128, 139, 165, 183, 217, 226-228, 242-245, 263

beam quality   44

benefit versus risk   393

benefit-risk   393, 394

bent corners   339

biopsy   116, 127, 227, 279-283, 466, 472, 480

birth control pills   166

black light   323

blind areas   144

body habitus   89, 90, 95, 115, 128, 137, 189, 195, 219, 220, 257, 292, 307, 410

body image   456

body mechanics   143, 264, 402, 403, 408, 410, 416-418, 424, 425, 434, 435, 438, 439

body powder   162, 163, 166, 327

breast health care   135, 450, 469, 475, 477

breast implants   163, 250, 251, 254-256

breast mobility   139, 140, 144, 216, 217, 220, 229

breast pain   149-151

breast self examination   467, 469, 477

breast symbolism   451

breathing technique   201

brittle films   379

bromide ions   24-26

brown films   338, 339

BSE   167, 469

bucky   82, 85-90, 98, 100, 101, 106, 107, 111, 116, 117, 127, 128, 150, 152, 168, 184-198, 217, 222-227, 230, 235, 238, 240, 252, 264, 270, 271, 283, 292, 293, 296, 326, 347, 348, 351, 389, 405, 431, 472

burnout   481, 482, 484

C

calcium oxalate   281

camel's nose   102, 103

caring   152, 170, 453, 461-466, 475-477, 481

cassette identification   51

ceiling air ducts   54

change of posture   420

characteristic curve   9-16

chatter   333

chemical stability   57

chest wall lesions   144

clean up film   61

clear margins   279

clearing   25, 332

cleavage view   111, 206-210, 213, 266

clinical breast examination   165

clinical symptoms   163-165, 202

collimate   123, 155, 291

collimation   44, 156, 291

collimators   326, 349, 350

color temperature   361, 366

comfort   88, 137, 152, 162, 168, 170, 178, 179, 182, 190, 196, 211, 221-223, 240, 258, 264, 269, 271, 274, 362, 364, 402, 410, 423, 426, 435, 439, 454, 460-465, 469-475, 484, 486

communication   157, 165, 289, 302, 443, 453, 461-466, 470-473, 485, 486

competence   41, 462-464, 483

compressed air   48, 49

compression   15, 44, 45, 46, 49-53, 66, 82, 85-88, 98-103, 106-108, 111, 116, 118, 121-129, 139-141, 145-156, 161, 162, 168-170, 178-201, 204, 205, 208-243, 249-257, 261-265, 268-279, 282, 283, 289-297, 300, 307, 310-314, 326, 348-351, 372, 375, 376, 388, 405,

254, 281, 310, 312, 316, 346, 361, 363, 387, 422, 463, 464, 470-473

detecting anxiety 462, 466

development 5, 9, 12, 16, 23, 25, 28, 34, 59, 92, 273, 297, 298, 326, 348, 392, 394, 401, 439, 470

deviation 56, 89, 180, 295, 378, 405, 433-435

diagnostic examinations 392

differential absorption 310, 387

difficult patient 112, 128, 129, 218, 263, 265, 321, 408, 415

difficult to position patients 263, 265

discharge 55, 167

discomfort 88, 126, 148-153, 184, 185, 188, 195, 259, 265, 293, 365, 397-407, 410-414, 423, 429-431, 434-440, 457, 459

documentation 44-47, 52, 61-66, 74, 164, 298

dose evaluation 44

dose parameters 388

double exposure 9, 376

draping 184, 187

drying 27, 30, 31, 322, 335, 379

drying streaks 335

duration 401-406, 414, 431, 434

dye stains 339

dynamic effort 404

E

early detection 135, 138, 366, 393-396, 449

electrostatic air cleaner 55

emotional comfort 473, 474

emotional state 457, 460

empathize 476

encapsulated implants 254, 255, 258, 259

entrance roller 332

entrance roller assembly 28, 56, 332

entrance roller marks 332

entrance rollers 332

entrance skin exposure 388, 389

environmental factors 402

equipment design 402

equipment motion 49, 348, 376

equipment performance 44

equipment preparation 168

equipment related artifacts 326-328, 349

ergonomic techniques 401-403

ergonomics 401-403

estimator strip 52

exaggerated CC view 109, 203

exaggerated CC view lateral 109

examination identification 158

exhaust 27

exhausted chemicals 322, 336, 338, 378, 379

experience 17, 45, 81, 82, 144, 148-153, 161, 167, 169, 184, 185, 222, 250, 259, 263, 264, 298, 364, 365, 391, 401-406, 410, 413-417, 424, 428, 431, 439, 443, 449-453, 457-465, 468, 471, 475, 476, 479, 482, 484, 487

explantation 461, 466, 467, 471

exposure control 154, 182, 298, 390

exposure factors 13, 289, 296, 388, 389

exposure technique 13-16, 66, 135, 155, 163, 208, 217, 225-228, 237, 250, 251, 254-257, 283, 294, 296, 307

extended cycle processing 34, 59

eye contact 170, 178, 462, 471

F

face shield   82, 106, 107, 111, 168, 180, 182, 185, 283

family history   165

fear   151, 161, 164, 265, 439, 449-454, 457-460, 483, 484, 487

feed tray   28, 54, 57, 60, 324, 330, 340, 343, 421

feedback   43, 169, 302, 469, 482

film bin   8, 52, 54, 326, 330, 345, 348, 416, 421

film creases   345

film emulsion log   71, 72

film handling   49, 307, 316, 324, 325, 343, 374

film handling related artifacts   324, 325, 343

film identification   289, 434

film loading   29, 34, 49, 54, 57, 59, 323, 340, 343, 344, 347, 348, 421

films jammed   379

filter artifacts   351, 352

filters   30, 56, 323, 324, 343, 378

filtration   26, 326, 390

fingerprints   7, 136, 324, 344, 345

fixer retention   46, 52, 322, 323, 338

fixing   25, 26, 51, 339, 378

flaccid muscles   149

flaccid, pancake breasts   243

flame patterns   339

flooded replenishment   25, 29, 30

fluctuations   23, 61, 67, 150, 377

fluid retention   150

fluorescent lamps   361

fluorescent tubes   54

focal compression   118, 123, 155, 156, 235

fog   10, 11, 14-16, 34, 46, 55, 56, 60, 64, 324-326, 342, 343, 348, 349, 376, 378

fog related artifacts   326, 348

fog test   46, 55, 325

foot control   409-411

foot pedal   408-411, 427, 474

footwear   178, 190, 409, 412, 419

forced exhalation   201

fovea   359, 363, 364

free margins   85-89, 195

from below view   211

frozen shoulder   265

G

glandular breast tissue   85, 95, 105-109, 122, 154, 242, 293

glandular tissue   16, 59, 65, 107, 108, 112, 118, 123, 140, 141, 154, 176, 203-206, 215, 223, 225, 229, 233, 273-277, 298, 300, 311, 373, 376, 387-389, 392

gloves   167, 187, 437

gowns, patient   472

greeting the patient   163, 461, 466, 476

grid flaws   326

gross fog   16

guide shoe marks   331

guide shoes   28, 56, 331, 334

H

hand and wrist discomfort   430, 436

handling artifacts   49, 324

heat exchangers   31

heating pad   168, 472

heavy activity   414, 415

height of the image receptor   180, 191, 208, 217, 256

pectus excavatum   220, 221, 260, 262, 265

penumbra   313, 314

perceived pain   149, 151

personal risk factors   416, 417

personal space   474, 475

personalize   466, 476, 483

pH   33, 57

phantom   45, 46, 53, 55, 65-72, 325-327, 333, 340, 350, 351

phantom imaging   46, 55, 65, 66

phantom scoring protocol   68

photocell   98, 129, 182, 227, 251, 256, 257

photoelectric absorption   386, 387

photometric measurements   359, 366

photoptic vision   363

physical challenges   439

physical comfort   471

physical pain   149, 474

physiological   484

pick off   336, 337

pink coloration   339

PNL   85, 90-97, 100, 102, 105, 106, 113, 124, 140, 177-180, 195, 212, 232, 294

polarized light   281

posterior nipple line   85, 92, 140, 294

posture   143, 152, 267, 401-407, 414, 415, 418, 420, 426, 435

powders   167

pre-exposed sensitometric strips   13, 63

pre-menstrual   150

preclinical detection   136

pregnancy   166

premixed chemicals   57

pressure marks   338, 346

preventative maintenance   34, 46, 322

prevention   393, 408, 418, 424

previous examinations   163, 365, 409

previous mammogram   164

previous studies   300

processing   5, 9, 12, 13, 17, 19-35, 41, 52-68, 72, 281, 298, 307, 311, 316, 321-324, 330, 332, 339, 371, 374-377, 421, 424, 426, 451

processing environment   17, 32, 58, 61, 307, 322

processing time   29

processor Q.C.   5, 46, 52, 59, 61, 63, 64, 67, 339, 377

processor related artifacts   321, 323, 327, 329, 331, 336

professional boundaries   475

protection program   43

psychological   265, 401, 439, 443, 450

Q

Q.C. technologist   43, 44, 45, 46, 54, 65, 71, 374, 375, 377

quadrant division of breast tissue   157, 158

quality assurance   41, 42, 47, 51, 63

quality control   8, 9, 13, 32, 34, 37, 39, 41, 43, 44, 45, 46, 55, 56, 58, 60, 61, 63, 64, 65, 67, 68, 71, 72, 74, 307, 321, 325, 326, 352, 361, 365, 371, 372, 373, 374, 377, 380

quantum mottle   47, 315, 337

R

radiation dose   42, 147, 389, 390, 391

radiation measurement   66, 395

radiation output   44, 63

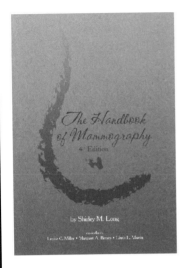

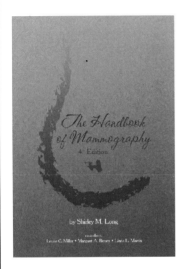